Medical-Surgical Nursing
DeMYSTiFieD

Notice

Medicine is an ever-changing science. As new research and clinical experience broaden our knowledge, changes in treatment and drug therapy are required. The authors and the publisher of this work have checked with sources believed to be reliable in their efforts to provide information that is complete and generally in accord with the standard accepted at the time of publication. However, in view of the possibility of human error or changes in medical sciences, neither the editors nor the publisher nor any other party who has been involved in the preparation or publication of this work warrants that the information contained herein is in every respect accurate or complete, and they disclaim all responsibility for any errors or omissions or for the results obtained from use of the information contained in this work. Readers are encouraged to confirm the information contained herein with other sources. For example and in particular, readers are advised to check the product information sheet included in the package of each drug they plan to administer to be certain that the information contained in this work is accurate and that changes have not been made in the recommended dose or in the contraindications for administration. This recommendation is of particular importance in connection with new or infrequently used drugs.

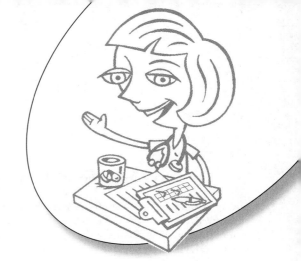

Medical-Surgical Nursing
DeMYSTiFieD

Jim Keogh, DNP, RN-BC

Third Edition

New York   Chicago   San Francisco   Athens   London   Madrid
Mexico City   Milan   New Delhi   Singapore   Sydney   Toronto

Medical-Surgical Nursing Demystified, Third Edition

1 2 3 4 5 6 7 8 9   LCR   23 22 21 20 19 18

ISBN 978-1-259-86181-9
MHID 1-259-86181-3

This book was set in Minion Pro by Cenveo® Publisher Services.
The editors were Susan Barnes and Kim J. Davis.
The production supervisor was Richard Ruzycka.
Project management was provided by Dolly Sarangthem, Cenveo Publisher Services.

Library of Congress Cataloging-in-Publication Data

Names: Keogh, James Edward, 1948- author. | Preceded by (work): DiGiulio, Mary.
Medical-surgical nursing demystified.
Title: Medical-surgical nursing demystified/Jim Keogh.
Description: Third edition. | New York: McGraw-Hill Education, [2019]|
    Includes index. | Preceded by: Medical-surgical nursing demystified/Mary
    DiGiulio, Jim Keogh. Second edition. 2014.
Identifiers: LCCN 2018018922 (print) | LCCN 2018019799 (ebook) | ISBN
    9781259861826 (ebook) | ISBN 1259861821 (ebook) | ISBN 9781259861819 (pbk.
    : alk. paper) | ISBN 1259861813 (pbk.: alk. paper)
Subjects: | MESH: Perioperative Nursing—methods | Nursing Process | Nursing
    Care—methods
Classification: LCC RD99.B78 (ebook) | LCC RD99.B78 (print) | NLM WY 161 |
    DDC 617.0231—dc23
LC record available at https://lccn.loc.gov/2018018922

McGraw-Hill Education Professional books are available at special quantity discounts to use as premiums and sales promotions, or for use in corporate training programs. To contact a representative, please visit the Contact Us pages at www.mhprofessional.com.

This book is dedicated to Anne, Sandy, Joanne, Amber-Leigh Christine, Shawn, Eric, and Amy without whose help and support this book couldn't have been written.

—Jim Keogh, DNP, RN-BC

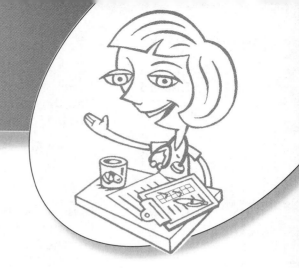

Contents

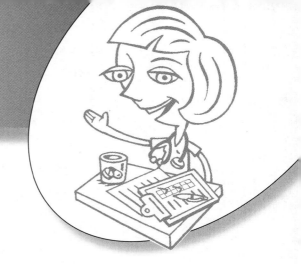

Contributors

Gerti E. Heider, PhD, ANP, GNP-BC
Associate Professor
Coordinator, Adult Gerontology Primary Care
Nurse Practitioner Program
Rutgers School of Biomedical and Health Sciences
Newark, New Jersey
16. Geriatrics

Jon Sugarmann, DNP, APRN, GNP-C, ANP-BC
Geriatric Nurse Practitioner
Emergency Department
Morristown Medical Center
Morristown, New Jersey
16. Geriatrics

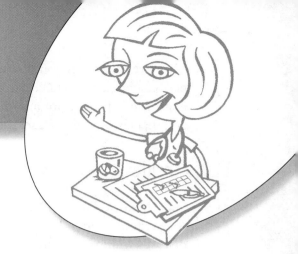

Introduction

Every patient knows to seek medical help when his or her aches and pains become too much to bear, but how does the healthcare provider determine what is wrong and what to do to restore the patient to good health? The answer depends on the patient's signs and symptoms and the results from medical tests. In this book, you will learn to identify these signs and symptoms, interpret the medical test results, and perform the nursing interventions that will assist in solving or alleviating the patient's medical problem.

Medical-Surgical Nursing Demystified contains 18 chapters, each providing a description of a major body system and the diseases and disorders which can affect that system. The discussion of each disease or disorder is divided into the following sections:

- What Went Wrong
- Prognosis
- Hallmark Signs and Symptoms
- Common Test Results
- Treatment
- Nursing Diagnoses
- Nursing Intervention
- Common Diagnostic Tests

The "What Went Wrong" section presents a brief description of how the body is affected when the particular disease or disorder occurs.

The "Prognosis" section discusses the possibilities of curing this disease and permanent damage which can occur. The remaining sections present the information as lists of symptoms, diagnoses, etc. that makes it easy for you to learn and that also serve as a useful tool for later reference.

A Look Inside

Since Medical-Surgical Nursing can be challenging for the beginner, this book was written to provide an organized, outline approach to learning about major diseases and the part the nurse can play in the treatment process. The following paragraphs provide a thumbnail description of each chapter.

Chapter 1 Cardiovascular System

The mere mention of the cardiovascular system brings all sorts of images to mind; however, these impressions are based on our experience as patients. Healthcare providers have a different view because they see it as a system that distributes nutrients and oxygen throughout the body and delivers carbon dioxide and metabolic by-products to various organs for removal from the body. Failure of the cardiovascular system has a compound effect because it interacts with the body's other systems causing a chain reaction of events. Healthcare providers need a thorough understanding of what can go wrong with the cardiovascular system; in this chapter, you will learn to recognize cardiovascular system disorders and to perform the interventions that can assist in restoring its function.

Chapter 2 Respiratory System

The respiratory system interacts with cells in the body to exchange oxygen and carbon dioxide, enabling the oxygenation of all cells in the body. In this chapter, you will learn which diseases and disorders can disrupt the respiratory system, how to recognize these conditions, and what steps you can take to assist in curing the respiratory system problems.

Chapter 3 Immune System

Remember the last time you experienced a bad cut. The site of the injury became swollen and red and you might have felt feverish. This happened because your immune system was trying to heal the wound by attacking the microorganisms that were invading your body. However, the abilities to fight off disease and to heal a wound are compromised when the immune system malfunctions. In this chapter, you will learn about immune system disorders and what actions the nurse can perform to assist in the patient's recovery.

Chapter 4 Hematologic System

The hematologic system produces and circulates blood cells throughout the body. Any disorder of this system jeopardizes the functioning of every organ in the body. This chapter explores the hematologic system and its common disorders and discusses how to care for patients who experience them.

Chapter 5 Nervous System

The nervous system is the body's command center that receives impulses and sends an appropriate response. In this chapter, you will learn about the disorders that cause the malfunctioning of the nervous system and the interventions that mitigate neurological problems.

Chapter 6 Musculoskeletal System

The musculoskeletal system is the body's superstructure that provides strength and movement. In this chapter, you will learn about disorders of the musculoskeletal system and the treatments for restoring its functions.

Chapter 7 Gastrointestinal System

The body receives nourishment and excretes waste through the gastrointestinal system. Any disorder of the GI tract might disrupt the body's ability to store carbohydrates, lipids, and protein, all of which are used to energize cells. You will learn about these disorders and what to do about them in this chapter.

Chapter 8 Endocrine System

The endocrine system is the body's messenger. It turns on and off messages that direct the action of organs. Endocrine disorders cause chaos, as messages become misdirected. Endocrine system disorders and what to do about them are presented in this chapter.

Chapter 9 Genitourinary System

Reproductive organs and the urinary system come from the same embryological origin that is why they are combined in the genitourinary system. Disruptions of the genitourinary system are caused by a variety of disorders, some associated more with one gender than the other. In this chapter, you will learn about these disorders and the treatments which can correct them.

Chapter 10 Integumentary System

Diseases and disorders of the integumentary system expose the body to invasion of viruses, bacteria, and other microorganisms because the primary defense—the skin—is disrupted. In this chapter, you will learn about these diseases and disorders and discover ways to mitigate them.

Chapter 11 Fluids and Electrolytes

Fluids and electrolytes must be in balance for the body to properly function. An imbalance causes the body to compensate in ways that can have a rippling effect throughout other systems. In this chapter, you will learn about fluids and electrolyte disorders and how to intervene to restore their balance.

Chapter 12 Mental Health

Disorders that affect the mind can interfere with daily activities and lead to self-destructive behaviors. In this chapter, you will learn about mental health disorders, how to recognize them, and steps that can be taken to minimize their influence on the patient.

Chapter 13 Perioperative Care

Surgical intervention is a radical but, at times, necessary treatment for a patient's condition. However, surgery can expose the patient to a set of disorders that would otherwise be avoided if no surgery had occurred. You will learn about these disorders and how to handle them in this chapter.

Chapter 14 Women's Health

The women's health chapter covers a multitude of conditions that affect women. Here you will learn how to recognize these conditions, the medication used to treat them, and the interventions that can mitigate their ill effects on the patient.

Chapter 15 Pain Management

Pain is associated with many disorders and must be successfully managed to reduce its disruptive effect on the patient's well-being. You will learn the techniques for managing pain in this chapter.

Chapter 16 Geriatrics

Geriatrics focuses on diseases and disorders common in the elderly. Managing a geriatric patient is challenging because the decline in the physiological reserve of the patient's organs increases the complexity of treatment. In this chapter, you will learn techniques for managing geriatric conditions.

Chapter 17 Substance Abuse Disorders

Substance abuse disorders affect all ages and demographics. You will learn the pathophysiological effects of commonly addictive substances. In addition, you will learn to recognize signs/symptoms and treatment of substance abuse disorders. You will also learn techniques for managing patients diagnosed with substance abuse disorders.

Chapter 18 Common Laboratory and Diagnostic Tests

This chapter focuses specifically on what you need to know to understand commonly performed tests, including how to educate the patient and how to provide safe, effective care before, during, and after the test.

About the Author

Jim Keogh is on the faculty of Saint Peter's College in Jersey City and New York University. He is the author of more than 100 books including Pharmacology Demystified, *Microbiology Demystified, Nurse Management Demystified, Nursing Fundamentals Demystified, Psychiatric and Mental Health Nursing Demystified, Cardiovascular Nursing Demystified, Pediatric Nursing Demystified, Nursing Laboratory & Diagnostic Test Demystified, Medical Billing and Coding Demystified,* and *Charting Demystified.*

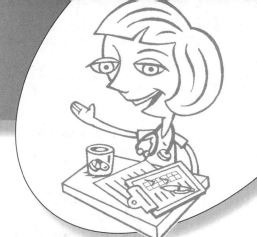

Chapter **1**

Cardiovascular System

LEARNING OBJECTIVES

At the end of this chapter, the student will be able to:

- Identify normal anatomy and physiology related to the cardiovascular system
- Discuss the disease-causing pathologic changes within the cardiovascular system
- List four signs or symptoms of specific cardiovascular disease or injury
- Recognize expected nursing and medical management of cardiovascular injury or disease

1

KEY CONCEPTS

1. Aortic aneurysm
2. Angina (angina pectoris)
3. Cardiac tamponade
4. Cardiogenic shock
5. Cardiomyopathy
6. Coronary artery disease
7. Endocarditis
8. Heart failure (congestive heart failure [CHF])
9. Hypertension
10. Hypovolemic shock
11. Myocardial infarction
12. Myocarditis
13. Pericarditis
14. Peripheral arterial disease
15. Pulmonary edema
16. Raynaud's disease
17. Rheumatic heart disease
18. Thrombophlebitis
19. Atrial fibrillation
20. Asystole
21. Ventricular fibrillation
22. Ventricular tachycardia
23. Aortic insufficiency
24. Mitral insufficiency
25. Mitral stenosis
26. Mitral valve prolapse
27. Tricuspid insufficiency

KEY TERMS

Aneurysm
Angina
Aortic valve
Atherosclerosis
Atria
Atrioventricular (AV) valves
Cholesterol
Diastolic
Embolism
Infarction
Ischemia
Mitral valve
Necrosis
Occlusion
Pericardium
Pulmonic valve
Stenosis
Systolic
Tamponade
Tricuspid valve
Ventricle

How the Cardiovascular System Works

The cardiovascular system is responsible for delivery of blood, which carries oxygen and other nutrients, to the tissues of the body. The heart pumps the blood to the body where it delivers nutrients and oxygen, picks up waste products, and then returns to the heart.

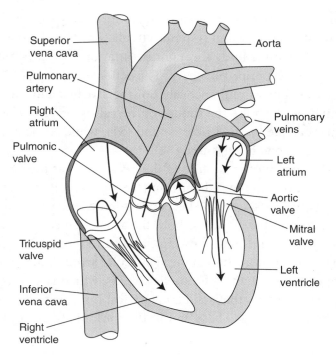

FIGURE 1–1 · Basic anatomy of the heart and pathway of blood flow.

Source: Reproduced with permission from: Mohrman DE, Heller LJ: *Cardiovascular Physiology*, 7th ed. New York, NY: McGraw-Hill; 2010, Fig. 1–4.

The heart has four chambers (see Fig. 1–1). The upper chambers are the **atria** and the lower chambers are the **ventricles**. In the middle, there is a septum, a wall that separates the right side of the heart from the left side of the heart. **Atrio-ventricular (AV) valves** control the blood flow between the upper and lower chambers of the heart. The **tricuspid valve** is on the right side, while the **mitral valve** is on the left side between the atria and the ventricles. The **pulmonic valve** controls the flow between the right ventricle and the pulmonary artery, while the **aortic valve** controls the flow between the left ventricle and the aorta.

Deoxygenated blood empties into the right atrium from the systemic circulation via the inferior vena cava and superior vena cava. During diastole, the right atrium contracts, and the tricuspid valve opens, in response to passive filling of the right ventricle. With contraction of the right ventricle, the pulmonic valve opens, allowing the unoxygenated blood to enter the pulmonary artery to go to the lungs to pick up oxygen. Once oxygenated, the blood returns to the heart through the pulmonary vein and enters the left atrium. As the left atrium contracts, the mitral valve opens, allowing the blood to flow into the left ventricle. As the left ventricle contracts, the aortic valve opens, allowing the blood to flow into the aorta and systemic circulation. The blood will return to the heart from the lower body through the inferior vena cava and from the upper body via the superior vena cava. The actions on the right side and left side of the heart happen simultaneously. So when we listen to a normal heartbeat, the sounds we hear are the sounds of the valves closing. The mitral and tricuspid valves create the first heart sound (S1), while aortic and pulmonic valves create the second heart sound (S2).

The electrical conduction system of the heart starts at the sinoatrial (SA) node, which is located in the right atrium (see Fig. 1–2). It initiates the heartbeat, ranging between 60 and 100 beats per minute, every day, for a lifetime. The electrical current travels across both the atria, then converges on the AV node, where the current slows, allowing the atria to repolarize. The AV node is located in the superior portion of the ventricular septum. In the bottom portion are located the right and left bundles of His, which is a group of special cardiac conduction fibers that send an electrical impulse to the ventricles to begin cardiac contractions. These end in the Purkinje fibers and spread out

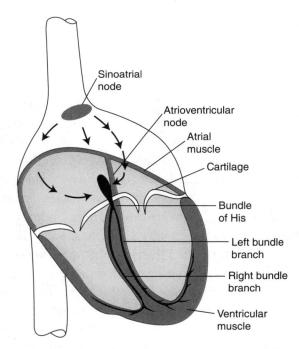

FIGURE 1–2 · Electrical conduction system of the heart.

Source: Reproduced with permission from: Mohrman DE, Heller LJ: *Cardiovascular Physiology*, 7th ed. New York, NY: McGraw-Hill; 2010, Fig. 1–6.

through the ventricles. The current passing through these fibers causes ventricular contraction, forcing the blood from the right ventricle to the lungs and from the left ventricle to the aorta, and thus the systemic circulation.

Just the Facts

1. Aortic Aneurysm

What Went Wrong

An **aortic aneurysm** is a weakening in the wall of a portion of the aorta resulting in a balloon-like bulge as blood flows through the aorta. The blood flow within this bulging area of the aorta becomes very turbulent. Over time this turbulence can cause the dilated area to increase in size, creating an aneurysm (see Fig. 1–3). The aneurysm can rupture causing a disruption in blood flow to everything below the affected area, and it may even result in death.

This is commonly due to **atherosclerosis** where fatty substances, **cholesterol**, calcium, and the clotting material fibrin, referred to as plaque, build up in the inner lining of an artery resulting in thickening and hardening of the arteries. It may also be caused by degeneration of the smooth muscle layer (middle) of the aorta, trauma, congenital defect, or infection. The aneurysm may be found incidentally on radiographic studies done for other reasons, or the patient may have developed symptoms indicating that something was

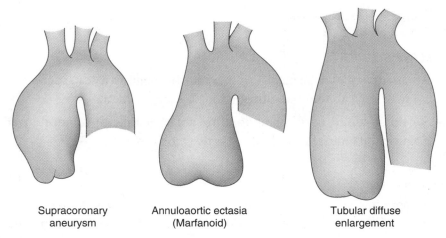

| Supracoronary aneurysm | Annuloaortic ectasia (Marfanoid) | Tubular diffuse enlargement |

FIGURE 1–3 · Three common patterns of ascending aortic aneurysm: supracoronary, annuloaortic ectasia, and tubular.

Source: Reproduced with permission from: Fuster V, Walsh RA, Harrington RA: *Hurst's The Heart*, 13th ed. New York, NY: McGraw-Hill; 2013, Fig. 106–6.

wrong, such as severe back or abdominal pain, or a pulsating mass. Severe hypotension and syncope (fainting caused by insufficient blood supply to the brain) may indicate rupture.

Prognosis

Outcome will vary depending on size and location of aneurysm. Some patients have aneurysms for months before a diagnosis is made, because they are asymptomatic. Treatment decisions will depend on the size and location of the aneurysm. Some patients with an aneurysm will have watchful waiting with periodic imaging to monitor the size of the aneurysm while other patients may need emergent surgery.

Hallmark Signs and Symptoms

- Asymptomatic
- Abdominal pain
- Back pain that may radiate to posterior legs
- Abdominal pulsation
- Diminished femoral pulses
- Anxiety
- Restlessness
- Decreased pulse pressure
- Increased thready pulse

Common Test Results

- An aneurysm may be displayed in a routine diagnostic test, such as chest x-ray (CXR), abdominal ultrasound, CT scan, or MRI.
- Swishing sound over the abdominal aorta or iliac or femoral arteries because the natural flow of blood is disturbed (bruit).

Treatment

- Surgery to resect the aortic aneurysm by removing the section containing the aneurysm and replacing it with a graft. This may be done either via an open surgical technique or endoscopically.
- Administer certain antihypertensives, reducing the force of the pressure within the aorta to decrease the likelihood of rupture.

- Administer analgesics to treat patients who may be having pain from pressure on nearby structures (nerves, etc.) or tearing of the vessel.
- Administer oxycodone and morphine sulfate as needed to decrease oxygen demand.

Nursing Diagnoses

- Ineffective peripheral tissue perfusion
- Risk for deficient fluid volume
- Acute pain
- Anxiety

NURSING INTERVENTION

- Monitor vital signs by looking for changes in blood pressure or elevated pulse and respiratory rates. During aortic dissection, the blood pressure (BP) may initially increase due to severity of pain. It may then become difficult to impossible to obtain both the BP and pulse in one or both arms because of blood flow disruption to the arm(s). The patient may go into shock quickly if the aneurysm ruptures.
- Monitor cardiovascular system by checking heart sounds, peripheral pulses (upper and lower extremities), and checking for abdominal bruits, swishing sounds heard over the blood vessel when flow is disturbed.
- Measure intake and output.
- Hypovolemia is suspected if there is a low urine output and high specific gravity of urine.
- Palpate abdomen for distention or pulsatile mass.
- Abdominal distention, which is an enlarged abdomen, may signify imminent rupture of the aneurysm.
- **Check for:**
  - Signs of severe decrease in blood or fluid (hypovolemic shock). The BP decreases as less blood circulates. Pulse rate increases as the heart tries to pump the blood faster to meet the oxygen demands of the body. Respiratory rate increases to meet oxygen needs while peripheral pulse sites are harder to find as BP lowers. The further away the pulse is from the heart, the more difficult it will be to find; it will be harder to locate the dorsalis pedis and posterior tibialis pulses earlier than the radial pulses.
  - Pale, clammy skin will be present as circulation decreases.
  - Severe back pain due to rupture or dissection.
  - Anxiety due to uncertainty of what is happening.

- Restlessness due to anxiety, discomfort, and decreased oxygenation.
- Decreased pulse pressure due to less circulating volume, increased heart rate, and less filling time between heartbeats.
- Increased thready pulse.
- Limit patient's activity to a prescribed exercise and rest regimen.
- **Explain to the patient:**
  - Decreased peripheral circulation.
  - Numbness.
  - Tingling.
  - Decrease in temperature of extremities.
  - Change in skin color in extremities.
  - Absence of peripheral pulses.
- Reduce patient anxiety.
- Maintain a quiet place.
- Have the patient express his or her feelings.

2. Angina (Angina Pectoris)

What Went Wrong

Angina is the narrowing of blood vessels to the coronary artery, secondary to arteriosclerosis, resulting in inadequate blood flow through blood vessels of the heart muscle, causing chest pain. An episode of angina is typically precipitated by physical activity, excitement, or emotional stress. There are three categories of angina.

1. **Stable angina**—pain is relieved by rest or nitrates and symptoms are consistent.

2. **Unstable angina**—pain occurs at rest; is of new onset; is of increasing intensity, force, or duration; is not relieved by rest; and is slow to subside in response to nitroglycerin.

3. **Prinzmetal's or vasospastic angina**—usually occurs at rest or with minimal formal exercise or exertion; often occurs at night.

Atherosclerotic heart disease occurs when there is a buildup of plaque within the coronary arteries. Angina is often the first symptom that heart disease exists. When the demand for oxygen by the heart muscle exceeds the available supply, chest pain occurs.

Prognosis

Patients can often be managed with lifestyle modifications and medications to control symptoms of angina. The most important factor is patient education. Patients need to understand the importance of their symptoms and when to seek medical attention. The pain must be evaluated initially and whenever a change in pattern or lack of response to treatment occurs. Additionally, a Duke treadmill score is often used to determine an individual's prognosis.

Hallmark Signs and Symptoms

- Chest pain lasting 3 to 5 minutes—not all patients get substernal pain; it may be described as pressure, heaviness, squeezing, or tightness. Use the patient's words.
- Can occur at rest or after exertion, excitement, or exposure to cold—due to increased oxygen demands or vasospasm.
- Usually relieved by rest—a chance to reestablish oxygen needs.
- Pain may radiate to other parts of the body such as the jaw, back, or arms—angina pain is not always felt in the chest. Ask if the patient has had similar pain in the past.
- Sweating (diaphoresis)—increased work of body to meet basic physiologic needs; anxiety.
- Tachycardia—heart pumping faster trying to meet oxygen needs as anxiety increases.
- Difficulty breathing, shortness of breath (dyspnea)—increased heart rate increases respiratory rate and increases oxygenation.
- Anxiety—not getting enough oxygen to heart muscle, the patient becomes nervous.

Common Test Results

- Electrocardiogram (ECG) during episode.
  - T-wave inverted with initial ischemia, which is reduced blood flow due to an obstructed vessel, usually first sign. Also, hyperacute T-waves are early signs of myocardial injury.
  - ST-segment changes occur with injury to the myocardium (heart muscle).
  - Abnormal Q-waves due to infarction of myocardium.

- Labs: troponins, creatine kinase-MB (CK-MB), which is an enzyme released by damaged cardiac tissue 2 to 6 hours following an infarction, electrolytes.
- CXR to determine signs of heart failure.
- Holter monitoring: a portable ECG which the patient wears for 24 to 48 hours, giving that many hours of continuous cardiac monitoring.
- Coronary angiography to determine plaque buildup in coronary arteries.
- Cardiac positron emission tomography (PET) to determine plaque buildup in coronary arteries.
- Stress testing to determine symptoms/electrocardiography (ECG) changes when at exercise or under pharmacologic stress.
- Echocardiogram or stress-echo to determine any abnormality of wall motion due to ischemia.
- Consult cardiologist.
- Nonemergent labs: complete blood count (CBC) used to determine the general health status of the patient, chemistry (provides information about the status of electrolytes, kidneys, acid/base balance, blood sugar, and calcium levels), prothrombin time/international normalized ratio (PT/INR), activated partial thromboplastin time (PTT) (helps to detect and diagnose bleeding disorders and the effectiveness of anticoagulants), proBNP (BNP) measures the presence and severity of heart failure.
- Cholesterol panel to evaluate risk.
- Increased risk for coronary artery disease (CAD) with increased total cholesterol, increased low-density lipoproteins (LDL), increased triglycerides, and decreased high-density lipoproteins (HDL).

Treatment

The goal of treatment is to deliver sufficient oxygen to the heart muscle to meet its need. When suspecting chest pain, always give oxygen as the first line of defense. Medications are used initially to treat symptoms and increase blood flow to the heart muscle. Medications are used for symptom control and cholesterol management in the long term. Cardiovascular interventions are used to maintain adequate blood flow through the coronary arteries.

- 2 to 4 L of oxygen.
- Administer beta-adrenergic blocking agents—this class has a cardioprotective effect, decreasing cardiac workload, and likelihood of arrhythmia.

- Drugs like propranolol, nadolol, atenolol, metoprolol, and carvedilol.
- Administer nitrates—aids in getting oxygenated blood to heart muscle.
- Nitroglycerin—sublingual tablets or spray; timed-release tablets.
- Topical nitroglycerin—paste or timed-release patch.
- Aspirin for antiplatelet effect.
- Analgesic—typically morphine can be given intravenously during acute pain. The medicine is very fast-acting when given this way and will decrease myocardial oxygen demand as well as decrease pain.

The following should be watched separately.

- Percutaneous transluminal coronary angioplasty—this is a nonsurgical procedure in which a long tube with a small balloon is passed through blood vessels into the narrowed artery. The balloon is inflated, causing the artery to expand.
- Coronary artery stent—this is a small, stainless steel mesh tube that is placed within the coronary artery to keep it open.
- Coronary artery bypass graph (CABG)—this is a surgical procedure in which a vein from a leg or an artery from an arm or the chest is removed and graphed to coronary arteries, bypassing the blockage and restoring free flow of blood to heart muscles.
- Low-cholesterol, low-sodium, and low-fat diet.

Nursing Diagnoses

- Anxiety
- Decreased cardiac output
- Acute pain

NURSING INTERVENTION

- Monitor vital signs—look for change in BP, P, R; irregular pulse; pulse deficit; when a discrepancy is found between an atrial rate and a radial rate, when measured simultaneously; pulse oximetry.
- Notify physician, nurse practitioner, or physician assistant if systolic blood pressure (SBP) is less than 90 mmHg. Nitrates dilate arteries to the heart and increase blood flow. You may have an order to hold nitrates if SBP is less than 90 mmHg to reduce risk of patient passing out from lack of blood flow to the brain.

- Notify physician, nurse practitioner, or physician assistant if heart rate is less than 60 beats per minute. Beta-adrenergic blocking agents slow conduction through the AV node and reduce heart rate and contractility. You may have an order to hold beta blockers if heart rate goes below 60 beats per minute; you should continuously monitor the patient's pulse rate.
- Assess chest pain each time the patient reports it.
- Remember PQRST (an acronym for a method of pain assessment) as follows:
- Determine the **p**lace, **q**uality (describe the pain—stabbing, squeezing, etc.), **r**adiation (does the pain travel anywhere else?), **s**everity (on a scale of 1 to 10), and **t**iming (when it started and how long it lasts and what preceded the pain).
- Monitor cardiac status using a 12-lead ECG while the patient is experiencing an angina attack. Each time the patient has pain, a new 12-lead ECG is done to assess for changes, even if one was already done that day.
- Record fluid intake and output. Assess for renal function.
- Place the patient in a semi-Fowler's position (semi-sitting with knees flexed).
- **Explain to the patient:**
  - Take rest when pain begins to decrease oxygen demands.
  - Take nitroglycerin when any pain begins—it helps dilate coronary arteries and get more oxygen to heart muscle.
  - Avoid stress and activities that bring on an angina attack.
  - Call 911 if the pain continues for more than 10 minutes or as the patient is taking the third nitroglycerine dose (1 sublingual dose every 5 minutes, if BP allows, for a maximum of 3 doses).
  - Stop smoking! Smoking is associated with heart disease.
  - Adhere to the prescribed diet and exercise plan. Lower cholesterol and fat intake to decrease further plaque buildup, and decrease excess salt intake to help BP control. Slowly increase exercise to build up activity tolerance. Possibly exercise with cardiac rehabilitation.
  - How to recognize the symptoms of a myocardial infarction (MI)? Pay attention to chest pains as well as changes in patterns of pain and response to treatment. Be aware of changes in respiratory patterns, increase in shortness of breath, swelling, and general feelings of malaise.

3. Cardiac Tamponade

What Went Wrong

Cardiac **tamponade** occurs when a large amount of liquid accumulates in the sack around the heart (**pericardium**), creating pressure on the heart that reduces the filling of ventricles with blood. This results in a low volume of blood being pumped with each contraction. The accumulating pressure within the pericardium may be due to fluid, pus, or blood. The end result is decreased stroke volume and cardiac output.

The cause of tamponade may be trauma, postoperative, post-MI, uremia, or cancer. The fluid may develop rapidly or over time, depending on cause. Tamponade is a life-threatening condition. The seriousness is related to the amount of pressure within the heart and the resulting decrease in ventricular filling.

Prognosis

Cardiac tamponade is a medical emergency requiring immediate intervention, such as drainage of the fluids. Stabilization occurs quickly once the fluid is removed and pressure is alleviated. If fluid recurs, surgery may be necessary. The prognosis depends on the etiology of the tamponade.

Hallmark Signs and Symptoms

- Neck vein distention—accumulation of fluid within the pericardium causes pressure on the heart, which prevents the venous return from the jugular veins. This causes distention, more pronounced on inspiration.
- Restlessness due to decreased oxygen to the brain.
- Muffled (dull) heart sounds on auscultation because it is harder to hear through fluid.
- Pulsus paradoxus—decrease of 10 mmHg or more in SBP during inspiration—change in pressure within the chest during inspiration, resulting in decreased ventricular filling, decreased output, fall in SBP.
- Sweating (diaphoresis).
- Difficulty breathing (dyspnea).
- Tachycardia.
- Hypotension.
- Fatigue.

Common Test Results

- Echocardiogram: ultrasound image of the heart to assess the heart's position, structure, and motion. Ventricle and atria are compressed. Fluid found within pericardial sac.
- Cardiac catheterization.
- CXR shows an enlarged heart if large effusion present.
- Electrocardiogram used to rule out other cardiac problems.

Treatment

Treatment is directed at reducing the pressure on the heart from the accumulating fluids in the pericardial sac. The following may be necessary to support and stabilize the patient:

- Pericardiocentesis—a needle is inserted into the pericardium, and fluid is aspirated or drained.
- Pericardial window.
- Administer adrenergic agent—increases heart rate and blood pressure.

Nursing Diagnoses

- Anxiety
- Ineffective tissue perfusion
- Decreased cardiac output

NURSING INTERVENTION

- Monitor vital signs.
- Ensure adequate oxygenation.

4. Cardiogenic Shock

What Went Wrong

A drop in blood pressure and blood flow caused by the heart's inability to pump blood as a result of a cardiac emergency, such as cardiac tamponade, myocardial ischemia, myocarditis, or cardiomyopathy (a disease of the heart that deteriorates the heart muscle). Blood pools in the left ventricle, which causes a backup of blood into the lungs, resulting in pulmonary edema. Contractions increase to compensate for the decreased cardiac output, causing an increase in demand for oxygen by the heart. However, the lungs are not oxygenating the blood sufficiently due to decreased blood flow; and therefore, heart muscles are starved for oxygen.

Prognosis

Treatment needs to find a balance between improving cardiac output and reducing oxygen needs and cardiac workload of the myocardium. This balance must be achieved while maintaining perfusion of the heart muscle. Prognosis depends on finding and treating the underlying cause. Cardiogenic shock requires immediate treatment, often before the cause is known.

Hallmark Signs and Symptoms

- Hypotension, because blood flow decreases below normal.
- Tachycardia, because the heart is trying to pump faster to maintain adequate blood flow to the body, or occasionally bradycardia, where the heart rate is less than 60 beats per minute due to myocardial damage.
- Arrhythmias—when the heart muscle does not have enough oxygen, it becomes irritable, making arrhythmias more likely.
- Clammy skin, because oxygenation to tissues is reduced.
- Drop in skin temperature because of reduced circulation as a result of hypotension.
- Urine output less than 30 mL/h (oliguria) because the kidneys are not being perfused.
- Crackles heard in the lungs secondary to pulmonary edema, meaning fluid is building up in lungs.
- Confusion due to poor perfusion.
- Distended jugular veins—sign of fluid overload, inability of heart to manage fluid flowing into heart.
- Narrow pulse pressure.
- Cyanosis of lips, peripheral extremities due to poor perfusion.

Common Test Results

- Chemistry—check electrolytes, kidney function to ascertain kidney perfusion; calcium level is increased or decreased secondary to muscle contractility.
- Echocardiogram—to look for ventricular rupture, pericarditis, or valve dysfunction.
- Electrocardiogram.
  - Q-wave enlarged due to heart failure.
  - Elevation of ST-waves is a sign of ischemia.

Treatment

Treatment is based on medical support for the heart until etiology (cause) can be determined. In cardiogenic stroke, the stroke volume and the heart rate must be increased to keep the organs perfused. The effects of the following medications should accomplish this:

- Administer vasodilator—dilates blood vessels (arterial and venous) to decrease the venous return to the heart and reduces the peripheral arterial resistance (what the heart has to pump against).
- Administer adrenergic agent—to increase the heart rate and blood pressure.
  - epinephrine
- Administer inotropes—strengthens the heartbeat, improves contractions, produces peripheral vasoconstriction.
  - dopamine
  - dobutamine
  - inamrinone
  - milrinone
- Administer vasopressor—decreases blood flow to all organs except the heart and brain.
  - norepinephrine
- Provide supplemental oxygen—may need to be through intubation.

Nursing Diagnoses

- Ineffective tissue perfusion
- Decreased cardiac output

NURSING INTERVENTION

- Monitor vital signs—look for changes in BP, P, R.
- Monitor heart sounds.
- Monitor Swan-Ganz catheter—is a catheter placed into the pulmonary artery to check for pressures in the heart, vessels, and lungs.
- Test capillary refill.
- Monitor arterial blood gas (ABG) to learn pH, acidosis or alkalosis, bicarb level.
- Monitor respiratory status—due to poor perfusion, these patients are in respiratory distress; mechanical ventilation may be needed.

- Place the patient on bed rest.
- Monitor intake and output of fluids—look for adequate renal perfusion. Without sufficient cardiac function, the patient will not have enough blood flow to the kidneys to get adequate filtration.
- **Explain to the patient:**
  - Be aware of particular symptoms and call the doctor.
  - Take rest periods.
  - Call the physician, nurse practitioner, or physician assistant if there are signs of fluid overload—weight increase, shortness of breath, fatigue, dependent edema.
  - Record weight each day and call the physician, nurse practitioner, or physician assistant if there is an increase of 3 lb (1.4 kg).
  - Change to a low-sodium, low-fat diet.

5. Cardiomyopathy

What Went Wrong

The middle layer of the heart wall that contains cardiac muscle (myocardium) weakens and stretches, causing the heart to lose its pumping strength and become enlarged. The heart remains functional; however, contractions are weak, resulting in decreased cardiac output. Most are idiopathic and not related to the major causes of heart disease. The three types of cardiomyopathy are

1. Dilated cardiomyopathy (common): The heart muscle thins and enlarges, which leads to congestive heart failure (CHF). Progressive hypertrophy and dilatation result in problems with pumping action of ventricles.

2. Hypertrophic cardiomyopathy (HCM): The ventricular heart muscle thickens, resulting in outflow obstruction or restriction. There is some blood flow present.

3. Restrictive cardiomyopathy (rare): The heart muscle becomes stiff and restricts blood from filling ventricles, usually as a result of amyloidosis, radiation, or myocardial fibrosis after open-heart surgery.

Prognosis

Prognosis is variable. Sudden cardiac death is a possible outcome in dilated or HCM; arrhythmia is often a precursor to sudden death.

Hallmark Signs and Symptoms

- Asymptomatic—Many clients with HCM are asymptomatic. The first sign is often cardiac arrest. Those with signs do not present until their mid-twenties.
- Dyspnea—The most frequent symptom is shortness of breath due to increase pressure in the lungs. The heart may not sufficiently relax resulting in higher pressure and a backup of blood into the lungs.
- Angina—Clients experience chest pain due to decrease in oxygen demand of the extra heart muscle and due to thick, narrowing coronary blood vessels within the heart's wall.
- Syncope—Fainting is caused by heart arrhythmias related to the inability of the cardiac muscle to conduct electrical impulses.
- Sudden death—Young adults are at risk of sudden death during physical exercise resulting from ventricular fibrillation, which is a cardiac arrhythmia.
- Abnormal heart sounds.
- Murmur is the sound of turbulence resulting from abnormal blood flow.
- S3 is a third heart sound commonly heard in heart failure. S3 is a soft sound made by the vibration of the ventricular wall when the ventricle fills too rapidly. S3 is heard after the S2 heart sound and is best found over the apex of the left ventricle, which is the fourth intercostal space along the mid-clavicular line.
- S4 that is the heart sound heard before the S1 heart sound is the result of the heart being too stiff. This is vibration of the valves and the ventricular walls when the atria contract and the ventricles fill.

Common Test Results

- CXR shows enlarged heart, pulmonary congestion.
- Echocardiography shows left ventricular hypertrophy (LVH) and dysfunction in dilated and HCM; small ventricular size and function in restrictive cardiomyopathy.
- ECG: ST changes, conduction abnormalities, LVH.
- LVH shows as a broad QRS wave, usually in leads 4, 5, and 6 because of high voltage.

- Cardiac catheterization—to measure chamber pressures, cardiac output, ventricular function, but is often unable to add to information that has already been received from echocardiogram.
- Exercise testing may show poor cardiac function not evident in a resting state.

Treatment

Treatment is based on the specific cause. Avoiding the offending drug/treatment is imperative. Manage the underlying disease and provide cardiac support; however, few therapies can halt the process of cardiomyopathy.

- Change to a low-sodium diet.
- Beta-adrenergic blocking agents—cause the heart to beat slowly, allowing more time for ventricular filling and improve contractile function.
  - propranolol, atenolol, metoprolol (for hypertropic cardiomyopathy)
- Angiotensin-converting enzyme (ACE) inhibitors—to decrease left ventricular filling pressures.
- Calcium channel blockers—reduced cardiac workload by increasing contractile ability.
  - verapamil or diltiazem (for HCM)
- Diuretics reduce fluid retention.
  - furosemide, bumetanide, metolazone (for dilated cardiomyopathy)
  - spironolactone (aldosterone antagonist)
- Administer inotropic agent to enable the heart to have greater contractile force.
  - dobutamine
  - milrinone
  - digoxin (for dilated cardiomyopathy)
- Administer oral anticoagulant to reduce the coagulation of blood.
  - warfarin, dabigatran, rivaroxaban, or apixaban (for dilated and HCM)
  - Implantable cardioverter-defibrillator for high risk.
  - Myectomy—incision into septum and removal of tissue.
  - Septal ablation—Injection of alcohol into the affected area to destroy muscle tissue.

Nursing Diagnoses

- Activity intolerance
- Impaired gas exchange
- Decreased cardiac output

NURSING INTERVENTION

- Place patient in a semi-Fowler's position for comfort, which eases respiratory effort.
- Record intake and output of fluids.
- Monitor vital signs to assess for increased respiratory rate, arrhythmias.
- Monitor electrocardiogram to look for changes from previous tracing.
- **Explain to the patient:**
  - Fluids restriction may be necessary as heart failure is a concurrent disease with dilated cardiomyopathy.
  - Record daily weight and call physician, nurse practitioner, or physician assistant if weight increases 3 lb (1.4 kg).
  - No smoking or drinking alcohol.
  - No straining during bowel movements.
  - Increase exercise.

---

6. Coronary Artery Disease

What Went Wrong

Cholesterol, calcium, and other elements carried by the blood are deposited on the wall of the coronary artery resulting in the narrowing of the artery and the reduction of blood flow through the vessel. This impedes blood supply to the heart muscle. These deposits start out as fatty streaks and eventually develop into plaque that inhibits blood flow through the artery. Elevated cholesterol levels and fat intake can contribute to this plaque buildup, as can hypertension (HTN), diabetes, and smoking. When the plaque builds up within the artery, the heart muscle is deprived of oxygen and nutrients ultimately damaging the heart muscle (see Fig. 1–4).

Prognosis

Lifestyle changes and medications can significantly impact the risks of the individual. Dietary modification, activity, and medications can help to alter the

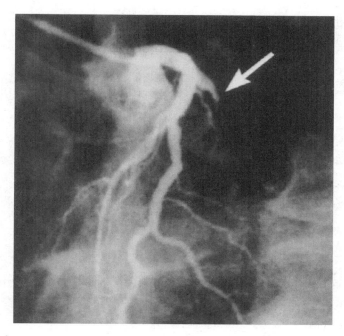

FIGURE 1–4 · Coronary arteriogram demonstrating severe stenosis (white arrow) in the right coronary artery, a common sign of coronary artery disease.

Source: Reproduced with permission from: Usatine RP, Smith MA, Mayeaux EJ Jr, Chumley H, Tysinger J: *The Color Atlas of Family Medicine.* New York, NY: McGraw-Hill; 2008, Fig. 45–1.

disease process. Patients who continue with prior bad habits will continue with disease progression. Risk factors include age, male gender, and family history.

Hallmark Signs and Symptoms

- Asymptomatic.
- Chest pain (angina) because of decreased blood flow to heart muscle and/or increase in myocardial oxygen demand resulting from stress.
- Pain may radiate to the arms, back, and jaw.
- Chest pain occurs after exertion, excitement, or when the patient is exposed to cold temperatures because there is an increase in blood flow throughout the body, raising the heart rate.
- Chest pain lasts between 3 and 5 minutes.
- Chest pain can occur when the patient is resting.

Common Test Results

- Blood chemistry.
  - Increased total cholesterol.
  - Decreased HDL—helps with reverse transport of cholesterol.
  - Increased LDL.
- Electrocardiogram during chest pain.
  - T-wave inversion—sign of ischemia.
  - ST-segment depressed—sign of injury to muscle.
  - The waves are depressed because of tissue injury.
- Stress testing.

Treatment

Treatment consists of risk factor modification, lifestyle changes, medications, and revascularization.

- Weight loss.
- Diet change: lower sodium, lower cholesterol and fat, decreased calorie intake, increased dietary fiber.
- Administer low doses of aspirin.
- Administer beta-adrenergic blocking agents to reduce workload of heart.
  - metoprolol, propranolol, carvedilol, atenolol.
- Administer calcium channel blockers to reduce heart rate, blood pressure, and muscle contractility; helps with coronary vasodilation; slows AV node conduction.
- Administer nitrate if the patient has symptomatic chest pains to reduce discomfort and enhance blood flow to myocardium.
- Platelet inhibitors.
  - dipyridamole
  - clopidogrel
  - ticlopidine
  - prasugrel
- Administer HMG CoA reductase inhibitors (statins)—lowers cholesterol.
  - lovastatin

- simvastatin
- atorvastatin
- fluvastatin
- pravastatin
- rosuvastatin
- Fibric acid derivatives reduce synthesis and increase breakdown of VLDL particles.
  - gemfibrozil
- Bile acid binding resins binds bile acid in the intestine.
  - colestipol
- Nicotinic acid reduces production of VLDL.
  - niacin

Nursing Diagnoses

- Acute pain
- Activity intolerance
- Impaired gas exchange

NURSING INTERVENTION

- Monitor vital signs—signs of hypertension, irregular heart rate.
- Monitor electrocardiogram—look for end-organ damage, signs of heart disease.
- Monitor labs—periodic lipid panel, liver function for patients on statins.
- Monitor for myalgias (muscle aches).
- **Explain to the patient:**
  - Stop smoking.
  - Reduce alcohol consumption.
  - Change to a lower-fat, lower-cholesterol diet, as well as increased dietary fiber intake.
  - Increase daily activity.
  - Weight reduction.
  - Stress management.
  - Hospital-based cardiac rehabilitation programs.

7. Endocarditis

What Went Wrong
Microorganisms, usually bacteria, enter the bloodstream and attach to the inner lining of the heart (endocardium) and heart valves, resulting in inflammation. Ulceration and necrosis occur when microorganisms cover the heart valves. This usually occurs in patients with rheumatic heart disease (RHD) or degenerative heart disease; those with recent instrumentation (IV, GU, and respiratory procedures) or dental procedures; and IV drug users.

Prognosis
The prognosis depends on both the organism (as some are more virulent than others) and the degree of damage to the heart. Myocarditis may recur.

Hallmark Signs and Symptoms
- Chills/fever—due to infectious process.
- Petechiae on the palate, beneath the fingernails, Osler's nodes (painful, reddish-purple, raised areas on fingers and feet), Janeway lesions (which are non-painful erythematous or hemorrhagic lesions typically found on the palms and soles).
- Fatigue—due to infectious process.
- Murmurs—new or changing.

Common Test Results
- Blood culture and sensitivity test.
- Three sets of cultures 1 hour apart to determine the specific organism so treatment can be started.
- Echocardiogram is used to detect vegetation on valves or heart valves damaged by the microorganism, and also to determine which valves are involved.
- Transesophageal echocardiogram offers a view to detect vegetation on heart valves or view heart valves damaged by a microorganism.
- CXR to look for underlying cardiac abnormality and pulmonary infiltrate.

Treatment
Treatment depends on the underlying infectious agent. Empiric treatment should be started while waiting for culture results. Outcomes are affected by

possible valvular destruction, emboli, and growth of bacteria on the valves or endocardium.

- Administer antibiotics based on the result of culture and sensitivity test.
- Valve replacement may be necessary if damage to valves is significant.
- Bed rest to decrease demand on heart.

Nursing Diagnoses

- Decrease cardiac output
- Risk for injury
- Activity intolerance

NURSING INTERVENTION

- Monitor for signs of heart failure because of increased stress on heart due to altered valve function.
  - Breathing difficulties (dyspnea).
  - Heart rate more than 100 beats per minute (tachycardia).
  - Crackles in lungs.
  - Neck vein distention.
  - Edema, usually of extremities; may also be of sacrum in bed-bound patients.
  - Weight gain.
- Monitor for embolism—a piece of vegetation from valve may have broken off into circulation.
  - Blood in the urine (hematuria).
  - Pain with each breath due to pulmonary embolism.
- Monitor renal function.
  - Increased blood urea nitrogen (BUN).
  - Increased creatinine clearance.
  - Decreased urine output.
- Prophylactic antibiotics before, during, and after medical procedures that expose the patient's blood to microorganisms—otherwise it is easy for microorganisms to enter bloodstream and colonize the heart valves.
- **Explain to the patient:**
  - Need to complete antibiotic course.
  - Can have a relapse.
  - Call the physician, nurse practitioner, or physician assistant if the patient develops fever, chills, night sweats.

8. Heart Failure (Congestive Heart Failure)

What Went Wrong

In CHF, the heart is unable to pump sufficient blood to maintain adequate circulation. This results in a backup of blood, and the extra pressure may cause accumulation of fluid into the lungs. Usually, this is the result of one of two different mechanisms; ie, either the heart muscle is too weak to adequately push blood forward, or the heart is not able to sufficiently relax and receive enough blood returning back to the heart. Heart failure is primarily due to problems with ventricular pumping action of the cardiac muscle, which may be caused by diseases such as myocardial **infarctions** (heart attacks), endocarditis (infection in the heart), hypertension (high blood pressure), or valvular insufficiency.

When disease affects primarily the left side of the heart, the blood will back up into the lungs. When disease affects primarily the right side of the heart, the systemic circulation may be overloaded. When the heart failure becomes significant, the whole circulatory system may be compromised.

Prognosis

Medications can help the heart to pump more efficiently. Some medications are used for disease management; others are used for symptom control. Monitoring dietary intake of sodium and fluids can also help with symptom control.

Heart failure is the main complication of heart disease, produced by an abnormality of pumping function. The heart is unable to carry blood effectively to meet metabolic needs. The resulting problems include acute left ventricular dysfunction usually due to arrhythmias and myocardial infarction, and chronic failure due to fluid overload, usually in valvular heart disease.

Heart failure is a compromise of any of the following:

- Contractility of the muscle
- Heart rate
- Ventricular preload
- Ventricular afterload

While most hearts can tolerate some changes in the above items, some diseased, older hearts may not be able to do so, and this results in heart failure.

Treatment results of early disease are usually good. Long-term prognosis can be variable, depending on the severity of the disease and associated conditions.

Hallmark Signs and Symptoms

- Extra heart sounds (normal heart sounds were described in the beginning).
  - S3: Soft sound caused by vibration of the ventricular wall, resulting from rapid filling. Heard after S2 heart sound. Heard over the apex of the left ventricle, fourth intercostal space along the mid-clavicular line. Best heard when the patient lies on left side. Usually indicates heart failure.
  - S4: Vibration of valves and the ventricular walls during the second phase of ventricular filling when the atria contract. Heard before S1, in the same location as S3, usually due to a "stiff heart."
  - Murmur: Sounds of turbulence caused by blood flow through the valves. Heard anywhere around the heart.
- CHF
- Fatigue
- Syncope
- Chest pain

Early symptoms:

- Basilar rales from fluid overload
- Nocturia
- Exertional dyspnea
- Fatigue
- Positive hepatojugular reflux from liver congestion
- S3 heart sound

Moderate-stage symptoms:

- Cough
- Orthopnea
- Discomfort in right upper abdomen due to hepatomegaly
- Cardiac rales
- Edema
- Cardiomegaly

Late symptoms:

- Anasarca—generalized edema from ineffective pump function
- Frothy or pink sputum from capillary permeability

Common Test Results

- B-type natriuretic peptide—elevated levels in CHF; produced when the ventricles are stretched.
- ECG may show signs of ischemia (T-wave inversion), tachycardia, or extrasystole (extra beats).
- CBC may show anemia—Hgb less than 12 in female, less than 14 in male; hematocrit (HCT); less than three times the Hgb.
- Chemistry may show renal problems, electrolyte disturbance.
- CXR.
  - Left-sided heart failure.
    - Pulmonary congestion because of accumulation of fluid in the lungs.
    - Enlarged left ventricle (LVH) because of the increased stress on the heart to pump blood.
  - Right-sided heart failure.
    - Pulmonary congestion because of accumulation of fluid in the lungs.
    - Accumulation of fluid in the pleural cavity (pleural effusion).
  - Enlarged heart (cardiomegaly) because of the increased stress on the heart to pump blood.

Treatment

Treatment is aimed at the underlying disease, ie, ischemia, valve defects, arrhythmias. Excreting volume with diuretics, supplemental oxygen, use of medications to reduce workload of heart muscle, peripheral vascular resistance (afterload), and venous return to the heart (preload) may all be used. Dietary indiscretions may be a contributing factor, ie, too much salt, too many calories.

- Administer diuretics for symptom control resulting in patient comfort by reducing blood volume.
- Furosemide, bumetanide, metolazone, hydrochlorothiazide, spironolactone—be aware of electrolyte imbalance—these medications may alter the K+ level.

- Administer ACE inhibitors to decrease afterload.
  - captopril, enalapril, lisinopril
- Administer beta-adrenergic blocking agents, which help to raise ejection fraction and decrease ventricular size.
- Administer inotrope to strengthen myocardial contractility.
  - digoxin
- Administer vasodilator to reduce preload, relieve dyspnea.
  - nitroprusside, nitroglycerin ointment
- Administer anticoagulants in patients with severe heart failure, as they have a propensity to develop thrombus and emboli; those with concurrent atrial fibrillation will also need anticoagulation.
- Reduce fluids as fluid overload is a causative factor in CHF.
- High Fowler's position to ease breathing and enhance diaphragmatic excursion.
- Supplemental oxygen to meet increased demand of myocardium.
- Low-sodium diet to prevent additional fluid retention.
- Daily weights to promote close monitoring of fluid status.

Nursing Diagnoses

- Impaired gas exchange
- Decreased cardiac output
- Excess fluid volume

NURSING INTERVENTION

- Monitor vital signs and look for changes.
- Record fluid intake and output—weigh daily to assess for fluid overload.
- Position the patient in semi-Fowler's position to ease breathing.
- Administer oxygen as ordered because it helps to decrease workload of heart.
- **Explain to the patient:**
  - Eat foods low in sodium to avoid fluid retention. (For these patients, there is no such thing as "low-salt" cold cuts.)
  - Raise legs when sitting to lessen dependent edema.
  - Call the physician, nurse practitioner, or physician assistant if experiencing fluid retention, such as a weight gain of several pounds in 1 to 2 days.

9. Hypertension

What Went Wrong

Pressure inside blood vessels exceeds 140 mmHg **systolic** and 90 mmHg **diastolic** on more than one occasion resulting from a primary disease or no known cause. These are the classifications of HTN:

- Normal: less than 120 mmHg systolic/less than 80 mmHg diastolic
- Prehypertension: 120–139 mmHg systolic/80–89 mmHg diastolic
- Stage 1 hypertension: 140–159 mmHg systolic/90–99 mmHg diastolic
- Stage 2 hypertension: more than or equal to 160 mmHg systolic/more than or equal to 100 mmHg diastolic

Prognosis

The vast majority of patients have primary hypertension, or high blood pressure, that is not caused by other disease. Patients are typically asymptomatic and need to understand the importance of treatment to avoid long-term complications. End-organ damage can affect the heart, kidneys, brain, or eyes. Adequate control of blood pressure is possible with medications and lifestyle modification, but this needs to be maintained for the long term, often for the rest of the patient's life. Many patients will ultimately need to be on multiple medications to achieve adequate blood pressure control.

Hallmark Signs and Symptoms

- Asymptomatic
- Headache
- Dizziness

Common Test Results

- Blood pressure readings higher than 140/90 mmHg on at least three occasions.
- Ventricular hypertrophy depicted on EKG or CXR.
- Blood test to look for associated cardiovascular risks.
- High cholesterol—often associated with hypertension.
- Check electrolytes for imbalance—sodium, potassium, chloride, CO_2.

- Monitor BUN and creatinine (Cr) for renal function, a sign of impaired organ damage.
- Chemistry to check for diabetes mellitus.

Treatment

Treatment is aimed at decreasing the risk of cerebrovascular accident (CVA), CAD, heart failure, renal disease, and other long-term sequelae of hypertension. Risk factors need to be assessed.

- Smoking
- Dyslipidemia—elevated cholesterol, LDL, triglycerides, low HDL
- Diabetes
- Age more than 60
- Men and postmenopausal females
- Family history

Nonpharmacologic interventions are tried first, and then medications are prescribed.

There is a four-step treatment plan:

Step 1: Lifestyle changes

- Reduce caloric intake and exercise to reduce weight
- Low-sodium diet
- No smoking
- Reduce alcohol intake
- Reduce caffeine intake

Step 2: Begin medication

- Administer diuretics to reduce circulating blood volume.
  - furosemide, spironolactone, hydrochlorothiazide, bumetanide
- Beta-adrenergic blocking agents to lower heart rate and cardiac output.
  - propranolol, metoprolol, atenolol, carvedilol
- Calcium channel blockers to cause peripheral vasodilation, less tachycardia.
  - verapamil, diltiazem, nicardipine
- Administer ACE to inhibit the renin angiotensin aldosterone system. In diabetes, ACE inhibitors also delay the progression of renal disease.
  - enalapril, lisinopril, benazepril, captopril, fosinopril, quinapril, perindopril

Step 3: Increase dosages of currently administered medication

Step 4: Combination of agents in above classes

- Multiple drugs may be needed to control blood pressure.

Nursing Diagnoses

- Imbalanced nutrition: more than the body requires
- Knowledge deficit
- Excess fluid volume

NURSING INTERVENTION

- Monitor blood pressure with multiple readings—lying, sitting, and standing, bilateral both arms.
- Record fluid intake and output.
- Reduce stress by providing a quiet environment.
- **Explain to the patient:**
  - No smoking—smoking contributes to cardiovascular disease, raising blood pressure.
  - Change to a low-sodium and low-cholesterol diets—salt adds to elevated blood pressure in some patients by contributing to fluid retention; lower cholesterol intake lowers risk for associated hyperlipidemia.
  - Reduce alcohol intake—reduces risk for end-organ damage from alcohol intake.
  - Reduce weight—decreased risk for obesity, better BP control with better weight control.
  - Exercise.
  - Call physician, nurse practitioner, or physician assistant when BP is elevated.
  - Side effects of medications.

---

10. Hypovolemic Shock

What Went Wrong

Rapid fluid loss causes inadequate circulation resulting in inadequate perfusion of organs. Hypovolemic shock can be caused by external hemorrhage, fluids moving in the body from vessels into tissue (third spacing), or dehydration. External hemorrhage is loss of blood, plasma, fluids, and electrolytes, due to trauma, GI bleed, vomiting, or diarrhea. Third spacing can result from ascites or pancreatitis.

Prognosis

Prognosis depends on the etiology of the low volume; there may occasionally be more than one reason.

Hallmark Signs and Symptoms

- Hypotension because blood volume in the body is decreased.
- Urine output less than 25 mL/h because less blood is perfusing the kidneys, causing decreased urinary output.
- Heart rate more than 100 beats per minute (tachycardia), because the heart attempts to compensate for the decreased volume.
- Cold skin because of peripheral vasoconstriction due to decreased volume.
- Restlessness, agitation, may be seen due to poor perfusion of the brain.

Common Test Results

- Blood tests.
- CBC anemia.
- Chemistry to look at volume as depicted by the creatinine and BUN.
- Coagulation studies.
- Type and cross-match for blood transfusion.
- ABG.
  - Decrease pH—if not perfusing well, acidosis will occur.
  - Metabolic acidosis—by-products of metabolism will accumulate.
  - Increase partial pressure of arterial carbon dioxide and decrease partial pressure of arterial oxygen due to poor perfusion.

Treatment

Treatment depends on severity of symptoms. As always, maintaining open airway, breathing, circulation, and fluid resuscitation is of vital importance. After stabilization, the focus is on determining and treating the cause of the shock.

- Control bleeding—CBC, stool guaiac test (to find hidden [occult] blood in stool), assess for bleeding.
- Replace fluid—proper fluid replacement depends on the etiology of the shock; IV fluid and/or blood products are the choices.

Nursing Diagnoses

- Deficient fluid volume
- Ineffective tissue perfusion
- Decreased cardiac output

NURSING INTERVENTION

- IV using 14G catheter (16 or 18 gauge also adequate if not able to obtain 14; use largest possible).
  - Lactated Ringer's solution (which contains electrolytes) or normal saline (0.9%).
  - Blood replacement—type-specific or type O negative, which is the universal donor type.
- Monitor blood pressure every 15 minutes.
  - If systolic pressure is lower than 8 mmHg, then oxygen flow rate may be increased.
  - Monitor vital signs every 15 minutes.
- Measure urine output each hour with indwelling urinary catheter. Increase fluid rate if urine output is less than 30 mL/h. Be alert for signs of fluid overflow. These include, but are not limited to, crackles in the lungs and dyspnea.
- Assess for cool, pale, clammy skin, indicating hypovolemic shock.
- **Explain to the patient:**
  - What caused the hypovolemia and how to avoid a recurrence.
  - The purpose of the treatment.

---

11. Myocardial Infarction

What Went Wrong

Blood supply to the myocardium is interrupted for a prolonged time due to the blockage of coronary arteries. This results in insufficient oxygen reaching cardiac muscle, causing cardiac muscles to die (**necrosis**). Myocardial infarction is commonly known as a heart attack.

The area of infarction is often caused by a buildup of plaque over time (atherosclerosis). It may also be caused by a clot that develops in association with the atherosclerosis within the vessel. Patients are typically (not always) symptomatic, but some patients will not be aware of the event; they will have what is called a silent MI.

Prognosis

The outcome depends on the coronary artery that is affected. The earlier the person enters the healthcare system, the better the prognosis, because emergency measures will be available for otherwise fatal arrhythmias.

There is a better outcome for patients who receive adequate medical attention and make appropriate lifestyle changes post-myocardial infarction. Cardiac rehabilitation can help patients make these changes safely.

Hallmark Signs and Symptoms

- Chest pain that is unrelieved by rest or nitroglycerin, unlike angina.
- Pain that radiates to arms, jaw, back, and/or neck.
- Shortness of breath, especially in the elderly or women.
- Nausea or vomiting possible.
- May be asymptomatic, known as a silent MI, which is more common in diabetic patients.
- Heart rate more than 100 beats per minute (tachycardia) because of sympathetic stimulation, pain, or low cardiac output.
- Variable blood pressure.
- Anxiety.
- Restlessness.
- Feeling of impending doom.
- Pale, cool, clammy skin; sweating (diaphoresis).
- Sudden death due to arrhythmia usually occurs within first hour.

Common Test Results

- ECG.
  - T-wave inversion or hyperacute T-waves—sign of ischemia.
  - ST-segment elevated or depressed—sign of injury.
  - Significant Q-waves—sign of infarction.
- Decreased pulse pressure because of diminished cardiac output.
- Increased white blood count (WBC) due to inflammatory response to injury.
- Blood chemistry.
  - Elevated CK-MB—usually done serially, the numbers will rise along a predetermined curve to signify myocardial damage and resolution.

- Elevated troponin I- and troponin T-proteins elevated within an hour of myocardial damage.
- Less than 25 mL/h of urine output due to lack of renal blood flow.

Treatment

Treatment is focused on reversing and preventing further damage to the myocardium. Early intervention is needed to have the best possible outcome. Thrombolytic therapy is instrumental in reducing mortality. A 3-hour time window is ideal for maximizing benefit. Medications are used to enhance blood flow to the heart muscle while reducing the workload of the heart. Supplemental oxygen is used to help meet myocardial oxygen demand. Data from coronary angioplasty and percutaneous coronary intervention (stenting) of an occluded artery have been impressive. Following the acute management, the patient will have to make lifestyle changes—altering diet and exercise, stopping smoking, and so on.

- Administer oxygen, aspirin.
- Administer antiarrhythmics because arrhythmias are common, as are conduction disturbances.
  - amiodarone
  - lidocaine
  - procainamide
- Electrical cardioversion for unstable ventricular tachycardia. In cardioversion, an initial shock is administered to the heart to reestablish sinus rhythm.
- Administer antihypertensive to keep blood pressure low.
  - hydralazine
- Percutaneous revascularization.
- Administer thrombolytic therapy within 3 to 12 hours of onset because it can reestablish blood flow in an occluded artery, reduce mortality, and halt the size of the infarction.
  - alteplase
  - streptokinase
  - anistreplase
  - reteplase
- Heparin following thrombolytic therapy.

- Administer calcium channel blockers as they appear to prevent reinfarction and ischemia, only in non-Q-wave infarctions.
  - verapamil
  - diltiazem
- Administer beta-adrenergic blocking agents because they reduce the duration of ischemic pain and the incidence of ventricular fibrillation; thus decreases mortality.
  - propranolol
  - nadolol
  - metoprolol
  - carvedilol
- Administer analgesics to relieve pain, reduce pulmonary congestion, and decrease myocardial oxygen consumption.
  - morphine
- Administer nitrates to reduce ischemic pain by dilation of blood vessels; helps to lower BP.
  - nitroglycerin
- Place the patient on bed rest in CCU.
- No bathroom privileges. Provide bedside commode.
- Low-fat, low-caloric, low-cholesterol diet.

Nursing Diagnoses

- Ineffective tissue perfusion
- Decreased cardiac output

NURSING INTERVENTION

- Monitor:
  - Cardiovascular—look for changes or instability in pulse, heart sounds, murmur.
  - Respiration—look for changes, fluid in lung fields, shortness of breath.
  - ECG during attack—12-lead during any episode of pain.
  - ECG continuous monitoring for arrhythmias.
  - Vital signs—check for changes in BP, pulse quality, peripheral pulses.
  - Pulse-oximetry monitoring.

- **Explain to the patient:**
  - Change to a low-fat, low-cholesterol, low-sodium diet.
  - The difference between angina pain and myocardial infarction pain.
  - When to take nitroglycerin.
  - Medication.
  - When to call 911.
  - Smoking cessation.
  - Limit activities.
  - Need for cardiac rehabilitation.
  - Stress reduction.
  - Lifestyle changes such as increase in exercise, diet changes.

12. Myocarditis

What Went Wrong

Inflammation of the heart muscle is usually caused by infection, most often viral. Infection can also be caused by alcohol poisoning from chronic alcohol abuse, drugs, or diseases that can result in the degeneration of heart muscle. This reduces the ability of the heart to pump blood efficiently, leading to CHF.

Prognosis

Outcomes vary depending on the etiology. Improvement depends on the stresses of the causative disease. Some resolve spontaneously; others develop dilated cardiomyopathy, CHF.

Hallmark Signs and Symptoms

- Fever because of infectious process.
- Tachycardia.
- Difficulty breathing (dyspnea) because left side dysfunction leads to CHF.
- Chest pain.

- Heart sounds.
  - S3 gallop due to fluid overload.

Common Test Results

- EKG.
  - ST-segment changes because of inflammatory changes in the heart due to the irritability of the myocardium from an infectious process.
  - Endomyocardial biopsy to determine a specific organism and the presence of inflammation after infection has resolved.
  - CXR—cardiomegaly.
  - Echocardiogram to assess cardiac size and function.
  - Labs—CK, MB, and troponins because of cell injury and death.

Treatment

Treatment is directed at the causative factor(s). Occasionally treatment may include support for CHF and antiarrhythmics, if needed.

- Administer antiarrhythmics to stabilize an irritable heart.
  - amiodarone

Nursing Diagnoses

- Hyperthermia
- Decreased cardiac output
- Activity intolerance

NURSING INTERVENTION

- Temporarily limit the patient's activities to decrease stress on the heart.
- Provide bedside commode.
- Monitor for:
  - Difficulty breathing (dyspnea) because of fluid overload.
  - Heart rate more than 100 beats per minute (tachycardia) because infection or inflammation may increase the heart rate.
- No competitive sports.
- Return to normal activities slowly once physician, nurse practitioner, or physician assistant approves.

13. Pericarditis

What Went Wrong

The membrane that encloses the heart (pericardium) is inflamed. Pericarditis is either acute or chronic.

Acute pericarditis is most commonly associated with viral infections. Upper respiratory symptoms are not uncommon and can occur a few weeks prior to the onset of pericarditis. Pericarditis may be caused by any infectious agent, AMI, malignancy, autoimmune diseases, or drug reaction.

Prognosis

Outcome of acute pericarditis is often self-limited, resolving in 2 to 6 weeks. Patients are typically treated with nonsteroidal anti-inflammatory drugs (NSAIDs) to decrease the inflammation of the pericardium.

Hallmark Signs and Symptoms

Acute:

- A grating heart sound heard (pericardial friction rub) due to friction from inflammation between the layers surrounding the heart.
- Sudden sharp pain over the precordium (mid- to lower-sternum area) radiating to the neck, shoulders, back, and arm.
- Pain decreases when the patient leans forward, sits up.
- Teeth pain, anxiety, myalgia.
- Difficulty breathing (dyspnea), rapid breathing (tachypnea).
- Arrhythmias.

Chronic:

- Enlarged liver (hepatomegaly), ascites because of liver congestion.
- Increased fluid retention due to ineffective pumping.
- Pericardial friction rub.

Common Test Results

- Increase WBC and sed rate (the rate at which red blood cells settle in a test tube; a high rate indicates inflammation), thyroid studies, renal function, Rh factor, antinuclear antibody (ANA) complement.
- May see increased creatine kinase (CK), lactate dehydrogenase (LDH), liver enzyme levels.

- ECG.
- Sinus tachycardia.
- ST-segment elevation.
- Echocardiogram shows echo-free space between pericardium and the ventricular wall due to effusion, and it also shows fluid in the pericardial space.
- CXR may show fluid in spaces.

Treatment

Treatment is directed at resolving the underlying etiology.

Pericardiocentesis is done to remove fluid from the pericardial sac to relieve pressure on the heart or for diagnostic testing. A long cardiac needle is inserted near the xiphoid process, and fluid is aspirated during careful cardiac monitoring.

Pericardial biopsy:

- Administer corticosteroids to decrease inflammation of pericardium.
  - methylprednisolone
- Administer NSAID to decrease inflammation of the pericardium and provide for pain relief.
  - aspirin, indomethacin

Nursing Diagnoses

- Acute pain
- Decreased cardiac output
- Risk for activity intolerance

NURSING INTERVENTION

- Place the patient in full Fowler's position to ease breathing.
- **Explain to the patient:**
  - He/she will recover.
  - Slowly resume daily activities.
  - Plan for rest periods during the day due to fatigue.
  - Perform coughing and deep breathing exercises—patient may have been avoiding deep breathing due to discomfort.

14. Peripheral Arterial Disease

What Went Wrong

Large peripheral arteries become narrowed and restricted (**stenosis**) leading to the temporary (acute) or permanent (chronic) reduction of blood flow to tissues (**ischemia**). This is most commonly due to atherosclerosis (plaque on the inner walls of arteries), but may also be caused by a blood clot (**embolism**), or from an inflammatory process. Severe peripheral arterial occlusive disease can lead to skin ulceration and gangrene. Peripheral arterial occlusive disease is more common in patients with diabetes or hypertension, in older adults, in those with hyperlipidemia, and in those who smoke, as these conditions can predispose to diminished circulation. Vascular disease that happens in one area of the body, eg, coronary arteries, is not an isolated process. The plaque buildup caused by long-term elevated cholesterol levels will happen throughout the body. The most common area of involvement is the lower extremities.

Prognosis

Patients typically have progressive disease. It is a chronic problem, getting worse with age. Symptoms may not be present until there is a 50% or greater **occlusion** (blockage) of the vessel. Suspect disease in patients who have risk for other cardiovascular diseases. Medications can help to improve blood flow to the area, and increased activity will improve exercise tolerance and quality of life. Vascular intervention may be necessary as the disease progresses.

Hallmark Signs and Symptoms

- Femoral, popliteal arteries.
- Sudden pain in the affected area because of spontaneous muscle contractions due to the reduced oxygenation of tissue.
- Intermittent claudication—pain, numbness, and/or weakness with walking due to increased oxygen demand of the muscle during activity.
- Weak or absence of pulse in the affected area because blood flow is reduced or blocked.
- Decreased temperature distal to the blockage because of restricted blood flow.
- Pallor or patchy coloring (mottling) of the affected area because of reduced tissue oxygenation.

- Dependent rubor (increased redness when legs are lower).
- Hair loss on extremities.

Common Test Results

- Doppler ultrasonography of the affected area.
- Arteriography. Dye is injected into the affected artery enabling an outline of the artery and blockage to be seen in an x-ray.
- Ankle-brachial index (ABI) helps to determine the amount of arterial insufficiency.

Treatment

The goal of treatment is to maintain adequate blood flow to the area and avoid tissue damage. Patients are encouraged to maintain activity and reduce risk for disease, such as smoking, as well as to control blood pressure and monitor diabetes.

Medical treatment:

- Exercise
- Smoking cessation
- Decrease in lipids, depending on what the lab work shows

Surgical treatment:

- Femoropopliteal bypass graft: A vessel from another part of the body is removed and grafted to the affected artery, permitting blood to bypass the blockage.
- Percutaneous transluminal angioplasty: A catheter containing a balloon is inserted into the affected artery. The balloon is inflated, stretching the artery; this causes a healing response that breaks up plaque on the artery wall.
- Atherectomy: A catheter containing a grinding tool is inserted into the affected artery and is used to grind plaque from the artery wall.
- Embolectomy: Surgical removal of a blood clot from the affected artery.
- Thromboendarterectomy: Surgical removal of atherosclerotic tissue from the affected artery.
- Laser angioplasty: A laser-tipped catheter is inserted into the affected artery to remove the blockage.

- Stent: A metal mesh tube is inserted into the affected artery to keep the artery open.
- Amputation: Surgical removal of the affected limb that contains gangrene caused by low blood flow or complete blockage of blood to the affected limb.
- Administer antiplatelet medications to enhance blood flow to the lower extremities. This helps to get blood through the vessels and alleviates symptoms.
  - pentoxifylline
  - cilostazol
  - aspirin
  - clopidogrel
  - dipyridamole
  - ticlopidine

Nursing Diagnoses

- Fear
- Ineffective tissue perfusion
- Risk for injury

NURSING INTERVENTION

- Monitor most distal pulse to assure circulation exists.
- Compare bilateral pulses.
- Monitor temperature, color of the affected area indicating tissue perfusion.
- Support hose.
- Check capillary refill.
- Administer anticoagulant (such as heparin, warfarin) as directed.
- Administer pain medication as directed.
- Do not elevate leg or apply heat if occlusion affects the femoral or popliteal arteries.
- Elevation of the lower extremities makes it harder for the blood flow to get to the tissues.

- Avoid prolonged sitting, which increases the risk of compression to vessels (impeding blood flow to lower extremities) and increases risk of clot formation in lower extremities.
- **Explain to the patient:**
  - How to check pulses in the affected area if there is an absence of a pulse.
  - Call the physician, nurse practitioner, or physician assistant if the patient experiences numbness, paralysis, or pain.
  - Do not wear tight clothes; avoid tight knee-high hose, which constricts at the popliteal space; avoid tight waist bands; ensure wide shoe box.
  - Change his/her lifestyle to reduce the risk of peripheral arterial occlusive disease.
  - The importance of regular examinations.
  - Foot check daily for open wounds, redness.
  - Regular visits to podiatrist.
  - Regular consults to vascular MD.

15. Pulmonary Edema

What Went Wrong

Fluid builds up in the lungs due to ineffective pumping of blood by the heart as a result of left-sided heart failure, AMI, worsening of heart failure, or volume overload. The patient experiences hypoxia, which is insufficient oxygen supply to tissues, caused by decreased oxygenation of the blood. Several non-cardiac issues may lead to pulmonary edema.

Prognosis

Poor heart function results in fluid overload, which results in further diminished cardiac function, causing marked dyspnea.

Hallmark Signs and Symptoms

- Difficulty breathing even when sitting upright (because of the fluid in the lungs).
- Rapid breathing: greater than 20 breaths per minute (tachypnea), because the body is trying to get more oxygen.
- Frothy sputum with a tinge of blood due to capillary permeability.

- Cyanosis.
- Cool, clammy skin because the body is diverting blood flow from the periphery.
- Restlessness and fear due to lack of oxygenation.
- Distended jugular vein due to increased pressure within chest.
- Crackles, wheezing heard in the lungs as the air moves through the fluid.

Common Test Results

- Oxygen saturation less than 90%.
- CXR: alveolar fluid, large heart.
- Echocardiogram to determine ejection fraction percentages in the heart.
  - ABGs will show lower levels of oxygen.

Treatment

Treatment may continue at home unless a worsening change in condition merits hospitalization. Immediate treatment of heart failure, while searching for underlying correctable conditions, is necessary.

- Administer supplemental oxygen, which increases arterial pO_2. Mechanical ventilation may be necessary.
- Administer morphine, which lowers left-atrial pressure, decreases myocardial oxygen demand, lowers anxiety, and relieves pain.
- Administer diuretics to remove excess fluid.
  - furosemide, bumetanide, metolazone
- Administer cardiac glycosides to increase contractions of the heart.
  - digoxin
- Administer cardiac inotropes to strengthen the heart.
  - dobutamine
  - inamrinone
  - milrinone
- Administer nitrates to decrease BP and left ventricular filling pressures.
  - isosorbide dinitrate

Nursing Diagnoses

- Impaired gas exchange
- Anxiety
- Excess fluid volume

NURSING INTERVENTION

- Place the patient in full Fowler's position to enhance air exchange and diaphragmatic movement, sitting with legs dangling over sides of bed.
- Monitor cardiovascular function for changes in heart sounds, extra sounds, murmurs.
- Monitor respirations for changes in lung sounds, chest expansion.
- Check oxygen saturation (pulse oximetry).
- Record fluid intake and output.
- Weigh the patient daily. Call physician, nurse practitioner, or physician assistant if the patient gains 2 lb daily.
- Call physician, nurse practitioner, or physician assistant if BUN and creatinine increase.
- Record characteristics of sputum.
- **Explain to the patient:**
  - Call the physician, nurse practitioner, or physician assistant if the patient detects fluid overload; weight gain, shortness of breath, fatigue, chest pains.
  - Call 911 if in respiratory distress.
  - Decrease sodium in diet.
  - Sleep with head elevated, ie, three pillows or blocks under head of bed frame.

16. Raynaud's Disease

What Went Wrong

Blood flow to the extremities decreases as peripheral arteries narrow from vasospasm when exposed to cold or emotional stress. This results in the fingers, toes, nose, and ears blanching to a pale shade and/or turning blue and red as blood flow decreases (see Fig. 1–5). It usually occurs bilaterally, often sparing the thumbs, and begins to resolve with warming of affected areas. Raynaud's is a benign condition usually controlled by avoidance of underlying factors, ie, cold and stress. Secondary Raynaud's can be seen with other disorders, mostly inflammatory and/or connective tissue diseases. This is more common in older men, usually involves the hands, and can have other complications.

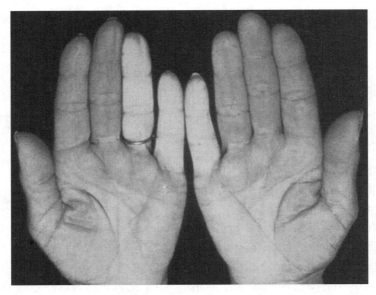

FIGURE 1-5 • Ischemic phase of attack of Raynaud's disease with marked pallor of the ring and little fingers of the left hand and little finger of the right hand.

Source: Reproduced with permission from: Goldsmith LA, Katz SI, Gilchrest BA, Paller AS, Leffell DJ, Wolff K: *Fitzpatrick's Dermatology in General Medicine*, 8th ed. New York, NY: McGraw-Hill; 2012, Fig. 170–1.

Prognosis

Prognosis for primary Raynaud's is good. Symptoms may be controlled by avoidance or by medications. In secondary Raynaud's, long-term ischemic complications may develop, such as loss of fat pads of fingers, gangrene due to diminished sensation, and propensity to develop frostbite.

Hallmark Signs and Symptoms

- Discoloration of extremities progressing from pale to blue, and then red because of decreased blood flow.
- Tingling and numbness in the extremities because of poor perfusion.

Common Test Results

- Vasospasm is detected in an arteriograph.
- Lab work to look for underlying disease process—CBC may show anemia; erythrocyte sedimentation rate (ESR), rheumatoid arthritis (RA), ANA (these autoimmune tests will be positive).

Treatment

Treatment is outpatient and consists of avoidance of aggravating factors and may need medication for primary, and treatment of underlying disorders and ischemia in secondary.

- Administer calcium channel blockers to ameliorate symptoms.
  - diltiazem
  - nifedipine
- Administer vasodilators to aid in blood flow.
- Avoid cold and stress because this may cause vasospasms.
- Avoid smoking because it causes vasoconstriction.
- Surgical removal of a part of a sympathetic nerve (sympathectomy) because it can eliminate symptoms.

Nursing Diagnoses

- Risk for injury
- Risk for peripheral neurovascular dysfunction
- Ineffective tissue perfusion

NURSING INTERVENTION

- Teach the patient to wear mittens rather than gloves when exposed to the cold because it allows for air flow around fingers to hold body heat.
- **Explain to the patient:**
  - Stop smoking.
  - Avoid cold.
  - Inspect skin regularly for cracks and treat immediately to prevent infections.
  - Use moisturizers.

17. Rheumatic Heart Disease

What Went Wrong

Rheumatic fever usually results from a prior upper respiratory infection with group A *Streptococcus*. It may lead to permanent valve disease and cardiac damage, with the mitral valve being more commonly affected.

Prognosis

Prognosis of RHD depends on the amount of damage done to the valves. When progressive valve disease occurs in the mitral valve, it is imperative to recognize the early onset of atrial fibrillation, to ensure early initiation of anticoagulation to prevent emboli.

Hallmark Signs and Symptoms

- A new murmur of insufficiency S3.
- Joint pain because of the inflammation.
- Increased temperature higher than 100.3°F because it may signify infection.
- Carditis—chest pain, heart failure, friction rub.

Common Test Results

- Increase in cardiac enzymes to look for other causes of chest pain.
- Positive C-reactive protein, ESR, which are elevated in inflammation.
- Increase in WBC because it may be of infectious origin.
- Echocardiogram to assess for damage to valves.

Treatment

Treatment of RHD is based on the severity of the valve damage. Valve replacement may be necessary. If a fibrillation (contracting of the heart) is present, ensure adequate anticoagulation with an international normalized ratio between 2 and 3. Rheumatic fever prophylaxis may be required; antibiotics are recommended for prevention of recurrent episodes.

- Administer NSAID to decrease inflammation and pain.
  - aspirin
  - indomethacin
- Administer antibiotics if an infectious process is confirmed.
  - erythromycin
  - penicillin
- Repair or replacement of heart valves due to irreparable damage.
- Antibiotic prophylaxis for unsterile procedures—usually penicillin; if allergic to penicillin, clindamycin is usually the drug of choice.
- Anticoagulation if atrial fibrillation.

Nursing Diagnoses

- Decrease cardiac output
- Activity intolerance
- Risk for infection

NURSING INTERVENTION

- Monitor for difficulty breathing (dyspnea) and hacking, nonproductive cough, because these are signs of heart failure.
- Determine if the patient is allergic to penicillin.
- Monitor for infection because rheumatic fever may recur.
  - Red, sore throat with pain when swallowing.
  - Swollen cervical lymph glands.
  - Headache.
  - Temperature higher than 100°F.
- **Explain to the patient:**
  - Anticoagulation use, interference with foods and medications, need for frequent lab monitoring.
  - Avoid contact with anyone who has a respiratory tract infection.
  - Maintain good dental hygiene.
  - Call the physician, nurse practitioner, or physician assistant if detect signs of heart failure: shortness of breath, weight gain, nonproductive cough.
  - Return to normal activities slowly.

18. Thrombophlebitis

What Went Wrong

Thrombophlebitis is the inflammation of a vein as a result of the formation of one or more blood clots (thrombus). It is usually seen in the lower extremities, calves, or pelvis (see Fig. 1–6). This may be the result of injury to the area, may be precipitated by certain medications or poor blood flow, or may be the result of a coagulation disorder.

Prognosis

Prognosis is usually good unless embolization, or moving of the clot, occurs. It may move to the lung or brain, which can be life-threatening.

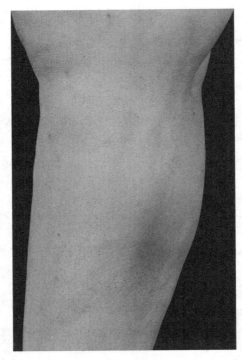

FIGURE 1–6 · Case of thrombophlebitis in the mid-calf of a 35-year-old man.

Source: Reproduced with permission from: Wolff K, Johnson RA: *Fitzpatrick's Color Atlas and Synopsis of Clinical Dermatology,* 6th ed. New York, NY: McGraw-Hill; 2009. Fig. 16–6A.

Hallmark Signs and Symptoms

- May be asymptomatic.
- Edema, tenderness, and warmth in the affected area as part of an inflammatory response.
- Palpable tender cord.
- Positive Homan's sign—pain on dorsiflexion of the ipsilateral foot—is an unreliable sign.
- Cramping because blood flow to the area is impaired due to the presence of the clot.
- If the clot dislodges from the vein and travels to the lung, other symptoms will develop.
  - Difficulty breathing (dyspnea) when the clot has traveled to the lungs.
  - Rapid breathing, more than 20 breaths per minute (tachypnea), because of a clot in the lungs.

- Chest pain in the area of clot.
- Crackle sounds in lungs in the area of clot.

Common Test Results

- Ultrasound determines if blood is flowing to the affected area.
- Photoplethysmography depicts any defects in venous filling in the affected area.
- Lab work to look for clotting disorders.

Treatment

Patients with large deep vein thrombosis (DVT), or with comorbidities (a disease coexisting with, and often impacting on, another disease present), and/or advanced age should be treated in the hospital. Treatment consists of anticoagulation to prevent further occurrences.

- Administer anti-inflammatory medication to decrease the inflammation within the vessel.
  - aspirin, indomethacin
- Administer anticoagulant medication to prevent the clot from becoming larger.
  - heparin, warfarin, dalteparin, enoxaparin, rivaroxaban, apixaban
- Limit activity initially to diminish risk of moving clot—bed rest with bathroom privileges.

Nursing Diagnoses

- Ineffective tissue perfusion
- Acute pain
- Impaired skin integrity

NURSING INTERVENTION

- Monitor breathing because changes in respiratory status can signal that a clot has dislodged and moved to the lung.
- Monitor labs because the patient is receiving anticoagulants. Monitor for therapeutic effect.
- Apply warm moist compresses over the affected area because it enhances blood flow to the area.

- **Explain to the patient:**
  - Report signs of bleeding—anticoagulant may be too much.
  - Report signs of clotting—pain in the affected area, shortness of breath—patient may have underlying clotting disorder.
  - Move about frequently when allowed—discourages chances of developing another clot.
  - Do not cross legs—avoid constriction of lower extremity vessels.
  - Do not use oral contraceptives—increases risk of clot formation.
  - Support hose.
  - Elevate affected area.

Arrhythmias

19. Atrial Fibrillation

What Went Wrong

Uncoordinated firing of electrical impulses in the wall of the atria (upper chambers of the heart) causes the heart to quiver instead of beating regularly, resulting in ineffective contractions. This is usually due to an abnormality in the electrical system of the heart. Blood is ineffectively pumped to the ventricles (lower chambers of the heart) and may result in not enough blood being pumped throughout the body. Usually the heart beats rapidly; however, this is not always the case. Atrial fibrillation (also called AF or "a fib") is the most common chronic arrhythmia and is not life-threatening on its own, but increases the patient's risk for blood clots and strokes.

Prognosis

The arrhythmia usually goes away once the cause of AF is identified and treated. If left untreated or if it returns, there is a risk of stroke and other complications.

Hallmark Signs and Symptoms

- Asymptomatic
- Irregular pulse
- Feeling faint (near syncope)
- Palpitations

- Light-headedness
- Dyspnea

Common Test Results

- Electrocardiogram will show irregularities characteristic of the disease.
  - QRS complexes are of irregular duration and structure.
  - PR interval barely noticeable.
  - Erratic, low-voltage, or absent P-waves.
- Echocardiogram to look for structural abnormalities.
- Thyroid function tests as hyperthyroidism can lead to AF.

Treatment

Treatment is directed toward restoring the regular heart rate and rhythm. If the AF is less than 72 hours old, chemical or electrocardioversion is endeavored. Electrocardioversion, or shocking the heart, often restores normal sinus rhythm. If the AF is greater than 72 hours, anticoagulation is begun as the risk of thromboembolism is great.

- Administer antiarrhythmics once the patient stabilizes—these medications may be effective in restoring a regular rhythm and also in long-term therapy.
  - amiodarone
  - diltiazem
  - verapamil
- Unstable patient: Synchronized cardioversion is a treatment that involves an electrical shock delivered to the heart, which is synchronized with the R- or S-wave of the ECG, in an attempt to restore coordinated firing of electrical impulses.
- Install a pacemaker.
- If AF is the ongoing rhythm, warfarin, aspirin, or dabigatran therapy will be initiated to reduce the risk of emboli. Also, radiofrequency ablation or cryoablation, which are catheter-based methods to ablate electrophysiological signals, may be performed to eradicate arrhythmia.

Nursing Diagnoses

- Impaired gas exchange
- Decreased cardiac output
- Ineffective tissue perfusion

NURSING INTERVENTION

- Monitor for signs of decreased blood flow to tissues or organs (hypoperfusion) because decreased cardiac output, as indicated by these symptoms, can occur as a result of AF.
  - Decreased pulse pressure.
  - Cool extremities.
  - Altered mental state.
  - Rapid resting heart rate.
  - Alternating breathing between deep and shallow.
  - Increased BUN.
- Prepare for synchronized cardioversion, if the patient is unstable.
- Assess for life-threatening arrhythmias.
- Assess for signs of drug toxicity and withhold if the patient is toxic—ie, seizures, respiratory arrest, arrhythmias.
- Limit patient's activities to reduce cardiac workload.
- **Explain to the patient:**
  - The need for warfarin therapy, as well as monitoring of INR, diet modifications, use of NSAIDs, and aspirin.
  - The importance of regular examinations to ascertain for any changes in rhythm.
  - Call the physician, nurse practitioner, or physician assistant if the patient feels light-headed or dizzy, as this can be a symptom of a change in rhythm.
  - Avoid ethanol, caffeine, and nicotine as they can trigger an arrhythmia.
  - Proper care and restrictions if the patient has a pacemaker—frequent monitoring of the pacemaker battery, who will follow up with the cardiologist, and so on. Frequency depends on the type of pacemaker and the cardiologist.

20. Asystole

What Went Wrong

Asystole is defined as no cardiac electrical activity. This causes ventricles to stop contractions, leading to no cardiac output and no blood flow. Cardiac standstill is a medical emergency. Treatment must be started immediately, while simultaneously attempting to understand the etiology of a non-beating heart. Asystole is a criterion for certifying that the patient is dead. Asystole may be caused by disruption in the electrical conduction system, causing life-threatening arrhythmias, sudden cardiac death, hypovolemia, cardiac tamponade, massive pulmonary embolism, acute myocardial infarction, metabolic disorder, or drug overdoses. In case of a drug overdose—usually pulseless electrical activity (PEA)—reverse overdose or treat.

Prognosis

Prognosis is poor unless the heart cannot be restarted. The longer asystole continues, the more tissue is lost.

Hallmark Signs and Symptoms

- No pulse
- Cyanosis
- Apnea
- No palpable blood pressure

Common Test Results

- Electrocardiogram—P-, QRS-, T-waves are barely noticeable or absent.
- ABG.
- Lab work—CBC, electrolytes, drug levels, coagulation studies.
- No atrial or ventricular rhythm on the electrocardiogram.

Treatment

Treatment consists of restarting the heart and, when that has occurred, determining the cause of the asystole. Basic life support (BLS) or cardiopulmonary resuscitation (CPR) should optimally be started within 2 minutes (once asystole is established, CPR should be initiated immediately when asystole is detected, and advanced cardiac life support [ACLS] within 8 minutes).

- Cardiopulmonary resuscitation.
- ACLS.
- Oxygen.
- Start IVs to maintain access.
- Transcutaneous pacing, where electrodes are placed on the front and back of the chest while high current is delivered to the patient to pace the ventricles.
- Endotracheal intubation.

- Administer buffering agent to correct acidosis.
  - sodium bicarbonate
- Administer antiarrhythmics to control arrhythmia.
  - atropine
  - epinephrine

Nursing Diagnoses
- Impaired gas exchange
- Decreased cardiac output
- Ineffective tissue perfusion

NURSING INTERVENTION

- Begin CPR.
- Prepare to administer medication per provider's written order or protocol.
- **Explain to the patient:**
  - If asystole exists, the patient is not conscious. Talk to family members if they are present. Refer to BLS protocol.

---

21. Ventricular Fibrillation

What Went Wrong
Electrical impulses, which trigger the ventricles to contract, fire erratically. This causes the ventricles to quiver and prevents regular effective contractions, resulting in the disruption of blood flow to the body. The usual causes are ventricular tachycardia, electrolyte disturbances, MI, electric shock, and drug toxicities.

Prognosis
Prognosis depends on how long it takes to establish a beating heart.

Hallmark Signs and Symptoms
- No pulse
- Breathing is stopped (apnea)
- No palpable blood pressure

Common Test Results

- Electrocardiogram.
  - chaotic ventricular rhythm
  - QRS irregular and wide
  - P-wave barely noticeable

Treatment

- CPR.
- ACLS.
- Defibrillation (refer to ACLS protocol).
- Endotracheal intubation to manually compress a bag to squeeze air (referred to as bag valve mask ventilation) and thus, oxygen into the lungs.
- Administer buffering agent to correct acidosis.
  - sodium bicarbonate
- Administer antiarrhythmics to control arrhythmia.
  - lidocaine
  - epinephrine
  - amiodarone
  - procainamide

Nursing Diagnoses

- Impaired gas exchange
- Decreased cardiac output
- Ineffective tissue perfusion

NURSING INTERVENTION

- Begin CPR (place on monitor, BP, P, R, pulse oximetry).
- Perform defibrillation, if certified.
- Prepare to administer medications per provider's written order or protocol.
- **Explain to the patient:**
  - Patient is more than likely noncoherent. Speak to family.
  - Call the physician, nurse practitioner, or physician assistant if the patient experiences dizziness.
  - The importance of regular examinations after rhythm has been stabilized.

22. Ventricular Tachycardia

What Went Wrong

Abnormal electrical impulses within the ventricles cause the heart to contract more than 160 beats per minute. This results in inadequate filling of the ventricles with blood between beats; subsequently, less blood is pumped throughout the body than during normal contractions.

Ventricular tachycardia (called "V tach") often occurs after acute myocardial infarction and in cardiomyopathy, CAD, mitral valve prolapse (MVP), and other myocardial diseases.

Prognosis

Prognosis depends on the duration of the arrhythmia and prompt response. Recurrent V tach signals a poor prognosis.

Hallmark Signs and Symptoms

- Unconscious.
- Apnea or diminished breathing.
- Pale, diaphoretic skin.
- Dizziness because less oxygen is reaching the brain.
- Hypotension because blood flow is increased to a rate that reduces time available to oxygenate tissues.
- Weak pulses due to poor perfusion.

Common Test Results

- ABG.
- Electrolytes.
- CBC.
- Drug levels.
- Coagulation studies.
- Electrocardiogram.
  - Unusual QRS
  - No P-wave

- Ventricular tachycardia may suddenly start and stop depending on the irritability of the heart.
- Ventricle contractions greater than 160 beats per minute.

Treatment

Treatment consists of establishing a regular rate and rhythm.

- CPR if pulse is absent (refer to ACLS: pulseless V tach requires defibrillation).
- ACLS if pulse is absent.
- Endotracheal intubation.
- Oxygen.
- Administer antiarrhythmics to control arrhythmia.
  - lidocaine
  - epinephrine
  - procainamide
  - amiodarone
- Synchronized cardioversion is an electrical discharge that is synchronized with the R- or S-wave of the QRS complex to restore coordinated firing of electrical impulses.

Nursing Diagnoses

- Impaired gas exchange
- Decreased cardiac output
- Ineffective tissue perfusion

NURSING INTERVENTION

- Begin CPR if pulse is absent.
- Prepare to administer medication per provider's written order or protocol.
- **Explain to the patient:**
  - Necessity of follow-up.
  - Call the physician, nurse practitioner, or physician assistant if the patient experiences dizziness.
  - The importance of regular examinations.

Valvular Disorders

23. Aortic Insufficiency

What Went Wrong

Leakage of the aortic valve causes blood to flow back into the left ventricle. This results in increased blood volume in the left ventricle, causing it to dilate and become hypertrophic, thus reducing blood flow from the heart. The usual cause is incompetent cusps or leaflets of the valve, from endocarditis, valve structural problems, connective tissue disorders, rheumatic heart disease, hypertension, arteriosclerosis, and other conditions.

Prognosis

Prognosis depends on the severity of the valve damage and the acuteness of the symptoms in the patient.

Hallmark Signs and Symptoms

- Difficulty breathing (dyspnea) because of ineffective pumping.
- Fatigue.
- Orthopnea.
- Palpations because the heart is irritable due to improper blood flow.

Common Test Results

- X-ray shows an enlarged left ventricle.
- Echocardiogram confirms the left ventricle is enlarged and the valve is working inefficiently.

Treatment

Treatment is based on the gravity of the symptoms of the patient.

- Aortic valve replacement or repair.
- Administer anticoagulant medication following surgery to prevent thrombus around the aortic valve.

  - heparin
  - warfarin
  - enoxaparin

Nursing Diagnoses

- Anxiety
- Decreased cardiac output
- Activity intolerance

NURSING INTERVENTION

- Place the patient in a high Fowler's position to facilitate breathing.
- Oxygen.
- Pain management.
- Monitor for:
  - Pulmonary edema because of backflow to the lungs.
  - Thrombus because a foreign object (valve) is in place and may cause clotting.
  - Arrhythmias because the heart may be irritable secondary to surgery.
- Weigh the patient daily to be aware of fluid overload.
- **Explain to the patient:**
  - Schedule rest periods during the day.
  - Restrict to low-sodium and low-fat diets.

---

24. Mitral Insufficiency

What Went Wrong

Leakage of the mitral valve causes blood to flow back from the left ventricle into the left atrium. As a result, blood might flow back into the lungs. Mitral regurgitation is due to an incompetent valve, damaged from rheumatic fever, CAD, or endocarditis.

Prognosis

The prognosis may be chronic with stabilization of symptoms, or acute, usually after myocardial infarction, leading to valve replacement.

Hallmark Signs and Symptoms

- Orthopnea due to the pressure rising into the atria, causing backflow into the lungs.
- Fatigue because of an ineffective heart.

- Systolic murmur at the apex, S3 gallop.
- Left ventricular hypertrophy—the size of the ventricle can reflect the amount of regurgitation.

Common Test Results

- Echocardiogram shows the underlying etiology of the insufficiency.
- Cardiac catheterization depicts the flow through the mitral valve and can measure the amount of regurgitation as well as pressures in the chambers.

Treatment

Patients with chronic, stable disease may be managed for years without symptoms, or their symptoms may be under control with medication. Others may require surgery, again, based on the symptoms. Ventricular damage may occur before symptoms present, so frequent monitoring is indicated.

- Administer vasodilators to reduce flow by lowering systemic vascular resistance.
- Administer anticoagulant medication following surgery to prevent thrombus around the aortic valve.
  - heparin
  - warfarin
  - enoxaparin
  - Mitral valve repair or replacement.

Nursing Diagnoses

- Anxiety
- Decreased cardiac output
- Activity intolerance

NURSING INTERVENTION

- Place the patient in a high Fowler's position to facilitate breathing.
- Monitor for:
  - Pulmonary edema because of fluid overload.

- • Thrombus because of a prosthetic valve.
  - • Arrhythmias because the heart may be irritable during and after surgery.
- Intake and output to monitor fluid balance.
- Weigh the patient daily to check fluid overload.
- **Explain to the patient:**
  - • Schedule rest periods during the day.
  - • Restrict to low-salt and low-fat diets.

25. Mitral Stenosis

What Went Wrong

In mitral stenosis, scar tissue secondary to rheumatic fever forms on the mitral valve. This causes it to narrow, increasing resistance to blood flow between the left ventricle and left atrium, which means the heart needs to pump harder to maintain blood flow.

Prognosis

Mitral valve stenosis may be asymptomatic for years, never needing attention. However, eventually symptoms may occur and progress, necessitating intervention. Medication may be enough, or surgical intervention may be necessary.

Hallmark Signs and Symptoms

- Murmur at apex.
- Difficulty breathing (dyspnea) on exertion.
- Fatigue because of a poorly functioning heart.
- Weakness because the heart is working inefficiently.
- Palpitations because the heart needs to work harder to pump blood.

Common Test Results

- Cardiac catheterization depicts the flow through the mitral valve.
- X-ray shows enlarged left atrial and left ventricle.
- ECG depicts left-atrial hypertrophy, exhibiting as broad, notched P-waves in lead II with negative deflection of the P-wave in lead V1.

Treatment

Mitral stenosis is generally a progressive disease, and treatment is directed at maintaining function. When necessary, mitral replacement is indicated. Most of these patients need endocarditis antibiotic prophylaxis, which is administering antibiotics to prevent a bacterial infection occurring before invasive procedures and dental cleaning. If atrial fibrillation occurs, anticoagulation is indicated.

- Medication to stabilize symptoms.
- Administer anticoagulant medication following surgery to prevent thrombus around the aortic valve.
  - heparin
  - warfarin
  - dalteparin
  - enoxaparin
- Mitral valve repair or replacement.

Nursing Diagnoses

- Anxiety
- Decreased cardiac output
- Activity intolerance

NURSING INTERVENTION

- Place the patient in a high Fowler's position to ease breathing.
- Monitor for:
  - Pulmonary edema because it may be a complication of surgery.
  - Thrombus because of a prosthetic valve.
  - Arrhythmias because of an irritated heart; patient may feel palpitations, anxiety.
- ABG to monitor for oxygenation, acidosis, alkalosis.
- Weigh the patient daily to determine fluid balance.
- **Explain to the patient:**
  - Be aware of signs and symptoms and to report changes in condition.
  - Schedule rest periods during the day.
  - Restrict to low-sodium and low-fat diets.

26. Mitral Valve Prolapse

What Went Wrong

The mitral valve bulges back into the left atrium, allowing blood to flow backward from the left ventricle into the left atrium. This is a common problem and is not considered a serious condition. It is often congenital.

Prognosis

Most patients with MVP are unaware they have it until symptoms start occurring. Often it is an incidental finding on an echocardiogram. A large majority of patients require no treatment other than endocarditis prophylaxis during dental and unsterile procedures. Some patients progress with their symptoms, developing arrhythmias and requiring medications. Severe MVP may require mitral valve repair or replacement.

Hallmark Signs and Symptoms

- Asymptomatic because the valve leaflets do not bulge greatly.
- Palpations because the valve is not operating properly.
- Systolic click and/or late systolic murmur.
- Chest pain.
- Fatigue.
- Syncope.
- Dyspnea.

Common Test Results

- ECG may be normal or show an atrial arrhythmia (irregular P-waves), left-atrial/ventricular enlargement (broad P-, QRS-waves).
- Chest x-ray is usually normal, unless left chambers are large (in late disease).

Treatment

Treatment of MVP is determined by the severity of the symptoms. Most patients require endocarditis antibiotic prophylaxis.

- Administer antiarrhythmic medications.
- Administer anticoagulant medication after valve replacement to prevent thrombus around the aortic valve.

- Ensure the patient understands the need for daily, lifelong anticoagulation therapy once a mechanical valve is in place.
  - heparin
  - warfarin (Coumadin)—requires frequent lab work to monitor consistency of blood.
  - dalteparin (Fragmin).
  - enoxaparin (Lovenox).
- Mitral valve repair or replacement.

Nursing Diagnoses

- Anxiety
- Decreased cardiac output
- Activity intolerance

NURSING INTERVENTION

- Place the patient in a high Fowler's position to facilitate breathing.
- After surgery, monitor for:
  - Pulmonary edema to look for blood backflowing into lungs.
  - Heart failure to assess for a poorly functioning heart.
  - Thrombus because of a prosthetic valve.
  - Arrhythmias because the heart may be irritated after surgery.
- ABG to check for adequate oxygenation and acid/base balance.
- Weigh the patient daily to assess for fluid overload.
- **Explain to the patient:**
  - Proper recovery from major surgery.
  - Schedule rest periods during the day.
  - Restrict diet to low-sodium and low-fat.

27. Tricuspid Insufficiency

What Went Wrong

Leakage in the tricuspid valve causes a backflow from the right ventricle into the right atrium. This results in increased pressure in the atrium and higher resistance to blood flowing from veins, resulting in enlargement of the right atrium. This may occur from an anatomic problem, but usually occurs from right ventricular overload (in turn caused by left ventricular overload). It may also occur due to an inferior myocardial infarction or damage from endocarditis.

Prognosis

If the underlying problem can be resolved, the insufficiency may subside. If resolution does not occur, tricuspid valve repair or replacement may be necessary.

Hallmark Signs and Symptoms

- Difficulty breathing (dyspnea) due to backflow into the lungs.
- Fatigue because the heart is working inefficiently.
- Jugular venous distention due to overload in the right atria.
- Hepatic congestion from backflow.
- S3 murmur upon inspiration.

Common Test Results

- X-ray shows enlarged right ventricle and right atrium because of volume overload.
- Echocardiogram depicts prolapsed tricuspid valve and enlarged right side of the heart.
- ECG depicts enlarged right ventricle and right atrium, characterized by broad P- and QRS-waves.

Treatment

Correct any underlying heart disease to reduce pressure on the right atrium, ventricle, and thus, the valve.

- Administer anticoagulant medication following surgery to prevent thrombus around the tricuspid valve.
  - heparin
  - warfarin
  - dalteparin
  - enoxaparin
- Tricuspid valve repair or replacement.

Nursing Diagnoses

- Anxiety
- Decreased cardiac output
- Activity intolerance

NURSING INTERVENTION

- Place the patient in a high Fowler's position to facilitate breathing.
- Monitor for:
  - Pulmonary edema because backflow to the lungs may occur.
  - Heart failure to assess cardiac function.
  - Thrombus because of a prosthetic valve.
  - Arrhythmias because the heart may be irritable.
- ABG to assess for adequate oxygenation, acid/base balance.
- Weigh the patient daily to look for fluid overload.
- **Explain to the patient:**
  - What symptoms to look for?
  - Schedule rest periods during the day.
  - Restrict to low-sodium and low-fat diets.

REVIEW QUESTIONS

1. **Which of the following dietary recommendations is the most appropriate to give a patient who has been diagnosed with CAD?**

   A. 2500 calories daily, with 45% of diet consisting of simple carbohydrates

   B. Decreased intake of sodium, animal, other fats, overall calories, and increase dietary fiber.

   C. High-protein intake with limited dairy products, decreased sodium, potassium, and phosphorus.

2. **Your patient tells you that he has chest pains when he performs strenuous work, particularly shoveling his long driveway. He is not concerned about the pain, as it always clears up if he rests for a couple of minutes. The description of his chest pain is typical of:**

   A. Stable angina.

   B. Normal aging

   C. Unstable angina.

   D. Prinzmetal's angina.

3. **The patient is experiencing chest pain and pain radiating to his arms, jaw, and back. The provider diagnosed his condition as a myocardial infarction. The patient asks what happened to him. The best response is:**

   A. You cannot tell him what has happened; he needs to wait for the provider to return and explain what is going on currently.

   B. His aortic valve was malformed at birth causing a disruption in blood flow.

   C. All patients who are overweight like him will have a heart attack.

   D. One or more arteries that supply blood to his heart are blocked, thereby preventing an adequate amount of blood from getting to his cardiac muscles.

4. **A patient diagnosed with CHF will need positive inotropic medication to improve the contractility of the cardiac muscle. Which of the following medications taken by this patient has a positive inotropic effect?**

   A. Digoxin.

   B. Nitroglycerin.

   C. Aspirin.

   D. Atorvastatin.

5. **Your patient is experiencing thrombophlebitis. Which of the following medications would you expect to administer for this condition?**

   A. Heparin.

   B. Lisinopril.

   C. Amiodarone.

   D. Furosemide.

6. **Janeway lesions are painless, erythematous, or hemorrhagic lesions found on the palms and soles. They are associated with:**

   A. CAD.

   B. Hyperlipidemia.

   C. Endocarditis.

   D. CHF.

7. **A blood pressure reading of 118/76 mmHg would be considered:**

   A. Hypertensive crisis.

   B. Stage 2 hypertension.

   C. Stage 1 hypertension.

   D. Normal.

8. **In a patient experiencing an acute episode of chest pain, you would anticipate administration of:** *(Select all that apply)*

   A. Atorvastatin.

   B. Supplemental oxygen.

C. Aspirin.

D. Nitroglycerin.

9. **Patient teaching that is specific for a person with Raynaud's disease should include:**

   A. Eating a low calorie diet with no more than 45% of the calories comprised of carbohydrates

   B. Drinking 8 to 10 eight ounce glasses of water daily.

   C. Covering the hands before going outdoors on a cold day.

   D. Avoiding animal fats and either baking or broiling all lean meat.

10. **When assessing your patient, you hear an S3 heart sound. You know this is:**

    A. A normal finding.

    B. Associated with CHF.

    C. Thrombophlebitis.

    D. Peripheral artery disease.

11. **Which of the following is an expected finding in a patient with pericarditis? (Select all that apply)**

    A. Chest pain that decreases when the patient leans forward.

    B. Pain, numbness, and/or weakness with walking due to increased oxygen demand of the muscle during activity.

    C. A pericardial friction rub on auscultation.

    D. Tachypnea with frothy sputum production.

12. **Radiofrequency ablation (or cryoablation) is an appropriate treatment for:**

    A. Aortic insufficiency.

    B. Ventricular tachycardia.

    C. Atrial fibrillation.

    D. Ventricular fibrillation.

13. **Which of the following conditions may persist in an asymptomatic patient?**

    A. Angina.

    B. Cardiogenic shock.

    C. Ventricular tachycardia.

    D. Aortic aneurysm.

14. **Which of the following medications would you expect to see on the medication list for a 26-year-old man with pericarditis?**

    A. Atorvastatin (HMG CoA reductase inhibitor or statin).

    B. Low-molecular-weight heparin (anticoagulant).

    C. Indomethacin (nonsteroidal anti-inflammatory drug).

    D. Atenolol (beta blocker).

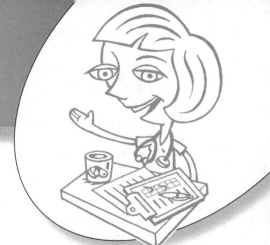

Chapter 2

Respiratory System

KEY CONCEPTS

1. Acute respiratory distress syndrome
2. Acute respiratory failure
3. Asbestosis
4. Asthma
5. Atelectasis
6. Bronchiectasis
7. Bronchitis
8. Chronic Obstructive Pulmonary Disease (COPD)
9. Cor pulmonale
10. Emphysema
11. Influenza
12. Lung cancer
13. Pleural effusion
14. Pneumonia
15. Pneumothorax
16. Pulmonary embolism
17. Respiratory acidosis
18. Severe acute respiratory syndrome
19. Tuberculosis

KEY TERMS

Acid-base balance
Alveoli
Bifurcates
Bronchi
Cilia
Crackles
Cyanosis
Dyspnea
Expiration
Fibrosis
Hypoxemia
Inspiration
Interstitium
Mesothelioma
Nasopharynx
Pulmonary edema
Rhonchi
Tachypnea

How the Respiratory System Works

The respiratory system has the following basic functions:

- Inhale/exhale air in and out of the lungs
- Exchange of oxygen and carbon dioxide
- Helping maintain acid-base balance

Ventilation moves air in (**inspiration**) and out (**expiration**) of the lungs. During inspiration, air flows in through the nose (or mouth) and passes into the **nasopharynx** (which extends from base of skull to soft palate) and hypopharynx. Air is then drawn through the pharynx, larynx, trachea, and bronchi (see Fig. 2–1). The trachea branches (**bifurcates**) right and left into smaller tubes called **bronchi**. These split into two lobular branches on the left and three lobular branches on the right lung. Then they further divide into increasingly smaller passages that terminate in alveoli. The airways are lined with mucous membranes to add moisture to the inhaled air. There is a thin layer of mucous in the airways that help to trap foreign particles, such as dust, pollen, or bacteria. **Cilia**, small, hair-like projections, help to move the mucous with the foreign material upward so it can be coughed out.

Alveoli are air-filled sacs containing membranes coated with surfactant. This surfactant helps the alveoli to expand evenly on inspiration and prevents collapse on exhalation. Carbon dioxide and oxygen are exchanged; a higher concentration of gas moves to the lower area of concentration. A higher concentration of carbon dioxide in the hemoglobin moves across the membrane

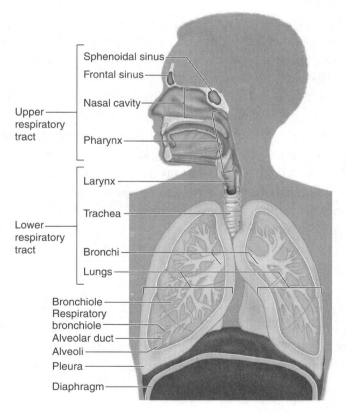

FIGURE 2−1 • Anatomy of the respiratory system.

Source: Reproduced with permission from: Mescher AL: *Junqueira's Basic Histology: Text and Atlas,* 12th ed. New York, NY: McGraw-Hill; 2010. Fig. 17–1.

into the alveoli and is expired by the lung. Higher concentration of oxygen in the alveoli crosses the membrane and attaches to the hemoglobin which is then distributed by the circulatory system throughout the body.

Lungs are contained within a pleural sac in the thoracic cavity and rely on negative pressure generated by the downward movement of the diaphragm to inflate and passively exhale as the diaphragm relaxes. The visceral pleura is close to the lungs, and the parietal pleura is close to the chest wall. There is a pleural space between these two layers, which contains a small amount of fluid to prevent friction with chest movement on inspiration and expiration.

Just the Facts

1. Acute Respiratory Distress Syndrome

What Went Wrong

Patients develop acute respiratory failure. Lungs stiffen as a result of a buildup of fluid in the lungs. Fluid builds up in the tissue of the lungs (**interstitium**) and the alveoli. This fluid and stiffness impairs the lungs' ability to move air in and out (ventilation). There is an inflammatory response in the tissues of the lungs. Damage to the surfactant within the alveoli leads to alveolar collapse, further impairing gas exchange. An attempt to repair the alveolar damage may lead to **fibrosis** (formation of excess fibrous connective tissue) within the lung. Even as the respiratory rate increases, sufficient oxygen cannot enter the circulation (**hypoxemia**). Oxygen saturation decreases. Respiratory acidosis develops, and the patient appears to have respiratory distress.

This is most commonly due to shock, sepsis, or as a result of trauma or inhalation injury. Patients may have no history of pulmonary disorders, also known as adult respiratory distress syndrome (ARDS).

Prognosis

Early recognition and treatment is critical. Even with intensive treatment, ARDS has a mortality rate of 28% to 40%. Some patients will progress into a more chronic type of ARDS which has permanent lung changes. These patients may require long-term mechanical ventilation.

Hallmark Signs and Symptoms

- Hypoxemia—insufficient level of oxygen in the blood, despite supplemental oxygen at 100%.

- Difficulty breathing (**dyspnea**)—increased need for oxygen to meet body's demand. The need for oxygen will increase as fluid builds up in the lungs and compliance worsens.
- **Pulmonary edema**—fluid buildup in the lungs.
- Breathing rate greater than 20 breaths per minute (**tachypnea**)—breathing becomes faster in an attempt to get oxygen into the body.
- Decreased breath sounds—harder to hear through fluid in alveoli; no air movement in collapsed alveoli.
- Anxiety—secondary to not getting enough oxygen.
- Rales (**crackles**) heard in the lungs—air moving through fluid in alveoli and small airways on inspiration and expiration (not heard initially).
- Wheezing (**rhonchi**)—inflammation develops or mucous is created. This narrows the airways, creating a sound as the air travels through the narrowed airway.
- Restlessness—owing to decreased oxygen levels.
- **Cyanosis** (blue or purple coloration of skin or mucous membrane due to lack of oxygenation).
- Accessory muscle use for respirations—look for retractions between ribs (intercostal) and below the sternum (substernal).

Common Test Results

- Pulse oximetry shows lowered oxygen levels below 90%.
- Arterial blood gases (ABGs) show respiratory acidosis—increased $PaCO_2$ (>45 mmHg), decreasing PaO_2 level even with supplemental oxygen.
- Chest x-ray (CXR)—both lungs show infiltrates within lung fields, "whiteout" or ground glass appearance.
- Pulmonary capillary wedge pressure (PCWP) is low to normal.

Treatment

- Bed rest.
- Endotracheal intubation.
- Mechanical ventilation with positive end-expiratory pressure (PEEP) or continuous positive airway pressure (CPAP) to help prevent diffuse atelectasis. Small tidal volumes with higher respiratory rates are used. Patients are weaned off the ventilator.

- Administer anesthetic to ease discomfort during insertion of endotracheal tube (intubation).
  - propofol/etomidate
- Combined with a neuromuscular blocking agent for intubation.
  - succinylcholine or rocuronium
- Administer a neuromuscular blocking agent—used to create a chemical paralysis when patients are on mechanical ventilation to avoid patient working against the action of the ventilator. These drugs allow respiratory muscles to rest.
  - vecuronium, cisatracurium
  - Sedation with midazolam or Ativan
- Administer diuretics to help decrease excess fluid in lungs.
  - furosemide, ethacrynic acid, bumetanide
- Administer H2 blocker or proton pump inhibitor (PPI) to decrease gastric acid. This will decrease the likelihood of developing a stress ulcer in the stomach or aspiration of gastric acid into the lung.
  - ranitidine, famotidine, nizatidine, omeprazole
- Administer PPIs to decrease gastric acid. This will decrease the likelihood of developing a stress ulcer in the stomach, or aspiration of gastric acid into the lung.
  - omeprazole, rabeprazole, esomeprazole, lansoprazole, dexlansoprazole
- Administer anticoagulant—clotting may have been causative in disease, immobility contributory to clot formation.
  - heparin
- Administer analgesic—used for comfort and to decrease myocardial oxygen demand.
  - morphine, fentanyl
- Administer steroids to decrease inflammatory response in the lung tissue.
  - hydrocortisone, methylprednisolone
- Administer exogenous surfactant.
  - beractant
- Administer antibiotics for respiratory or systemic infections.
- Ideally selected based on results of culture and sensitivity (C&S) of sputum.
- May be given to cover likely infectious organism pending results of C&S.

Nursing Diagnoses

- Ineffective breathing pattern
- Impaired gas exchange
- Ineffective tissue perfusion

NURSING INTERVENTION

- Monitor white blood cell (WBC) count.
  - Elevation of WBC with infection, inflammation.
  - Decrease in WBC in a patient who is immune-compromised or who has a viral infection.
- Monitor hemoglobin (Hgb) and hematocrit (Hct) for anemias.
- Monitor PT, PTT, and internationalized normalized ratio (INR) for coagulation abnormalities; monitor heparin dosing.
- Record intake and output of fluid.
- Monitor for signs of renal insufficiency or failure (decrease in urinary output less than 30 mL/h) and monitor blood urea nitrogen (BUN) and creatinine.
- Monitor for possible fluid overload—more fluid intake than output. Patient may end up in heart failure, compounding the fluid building up in the lungs.
- Weigh the patient daily—inability to handle excess fluids, causing third spacing of fluids into interstitial spaces, increasing weight and causing edema.
- Change position at least every 2 hours to prevent pressure buildup, causing skin breakdown.
- Avoid overexerting the patient during treatment—patient will tire easily and will have problems with increased oxygen demands. Also provide rest periods during activities.
- **Explain to the patient:**
  - The importance of coughing and deep-breathing exercises—after coming off the ventilator the patient needs to circulate adequate air in and out of the lungs. Coughing helps to rid the lungs of any remaining fluid.
  - How to identify the signs of respiratory distress, any sign that symptoms may be returning: shortness of breath, coughing, wheezing, rapid breathing, cyanosis, restlessness, or anxiety.

2. Asbestosis

What Went Wrong

Asbestos fibers enter the lungs, causing inflammation in the bronchioles and in the walls of the alveoli. After inhalation, the fibers settle into the lung tissue. Fibrosis often develops and pleural plaques form in some patients. Scar tissue within the lungs prevents normal expansion and contraction with respiration. These changes within the lung result in a restrictive lung disease. The damage to the lung causes impairment in breathing and air exchange.

Prognosis

It may take a decade or longer from the time of exposure before symptoms begin to develop. Some patients have worked in occupations known for asbestosis exposure (mining, shipyards, fireproofing, and construction before the mid-1970s), for 10 or 15 years prior to symptom development. There is an increased risk of lung cancer (**mesothelioma**) in patients with history of asbestosis exposure, especially if the patient has also smoked. Mesothelioma may develop 2 to 4 decades postexposure. About three-fourths of the patients with mesothelioma will die of the disease.

Hallmark Signs and Symptoms

- Difficulty breathing (dyspnea) on exertion and at rest due to changes in the lung tissue. This becomes more pronounced over time.
- Chest pain or tightness as a result of changes within the lung tissue and restrictive air movement.
- Dry cough due to irritation within the lungs.
- Frequent respiratory infections because of changes within the lung, increasing susceptibility to infection.
- Respiration greater than 20 breaths per minute (tachypnea) owing to decreased vital capacity.
- Rales or crackles when listening to breath sounds.
- Cough.
- Chest pain due to restrictive lung disease.
- Clubbing of fingers owing to decreased tissue oxygenation.

Common Test Results

- CXR: Lungs show linear opacities and/or irregular opacities. Opacities are increased tissue density on the lung indicating fibrosis or pleural plaque.
- CT scan shows opacities indicating increased tissue density of fibrosis or pleural plaque.
- ABG shows decreased oxygen owing to restrictive pattern of respiration.

- Pulse oximetry shows lower than normal levels.
- Pulmonary function test (PFT) shows a restrictive pattern, decreased vital capacity.

Treatment

There is neither specific treatment for asbestosis nor a cure.

- Flu (annually) and pneumococcal vaccines to reduce chance of illness.
- Oxygen therapy (1-2 L/min) to ease breathing discomfort by increasing levels of available oxygen to meet body's needs.
- Administer antibiotics for exacerbations of respiratory symptoms—to treat infectious process based on results of C&S study or empirically.
- Lung transplant.

Nursing Diagnoses

- Fatigue
- Impaired gas exchange
- Imbalanced nutrition: less than the body requires

NURSING INTERVENTION

- Administer chest percussion and vibration to loosen and expel secretions.
- Increase fluids to help loosen mucus in lungs.
- Administer aerosolized medications to help remove mucus.
- **Explain to the patient:**
  - How to avoid infections (reduced exposure to others with an infection and vaccines administered according to physician's orders).
  - Proper use of oxygen therapy.

3. Asthma

What Went Wrong

The airways become obstructed from either inflammation of the lining of the airways or constriction of the bronchial smooth muscles (bronchospasm). A known allergen, for example, pollen—is inhaled, causing activation of antibodies that recognize the allergen (see Fig. 2–2). Mast cells and histamine are activated, initiating a local inflammatory response. Prostaglandins enhance the effect of histamine. Leukotrienes also respond, enhancing the inflammatory

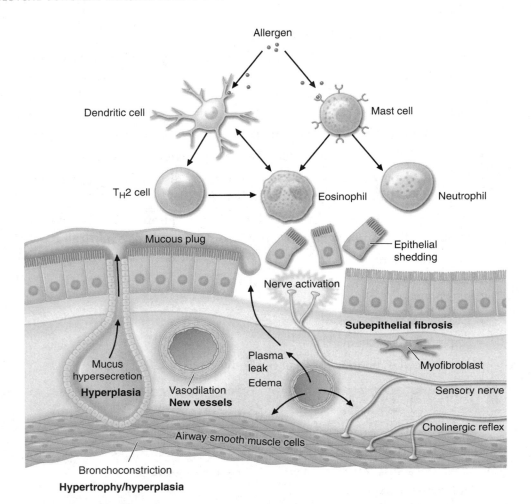

FIGURE 2–2 · The pathophysiology of asthma is complex with participation of several interacting inflammatory cells, which result in acute and chronic inflammatory effects on the airway.

Source: Reproduced with permission from: Longo DL, Fauci AS, Kasper DL, Jameson JL, Loscalzo J: *Harrison's Principles of Internal Medicine*, 18th ed. New York, NY: McGraw-Hill; 2012. Fig. 254–3.

response. White blood cells responding to the area release inflammatory mediators.

A stimulus causes an inflammatory reaction, increasing the size of the bronchial linings, this resulting in restriction of the airways. There may be a bronchial smooth muscle reaction at the same time. There are two kinds of asthma:

- Extrinsic asthma, also known as atopic, caused by allergens such as pollen, animal dander, mold, or dust. Often accompanied by allergic rhinitis and eczema; this may run in families.

- Intrinsic asthma, also known as nonatopic, caused by a nonallergic factor such as following a respiratory tract infection, exposure to cold air, changes in air humidity, or respiratory irritants.

- Common triggers for asthma exacerbation include pollens, mold, animal dander, dust, chemicals (such as fragrances), smoke, aspirin, exercise, weather changes, or upper respiratory infection.

Prognosis

Triggers for the asthmatic patient can often be identified and avoided. Patients can learn to check peak flow levels and manage symptoms in conjunction with their caregiver. Well-controlled asthma typically has temporary, reversible exacerbations that can be controlled with medications, often in an outpatient setting. With frequent attacks, a mild exposure to a known trigger will often be sufficient to exacerbate an attack. Patients who do not respond to medications or who use medications improperly may die during an asthma attack.

Hallmark Signs and Symptoms

- Wheezing initially present on expiration continues throughout respiratory cycle as inflammation progresses. Air has difficulty moving through the narrowed airways, making noise. Not all asthmatics will have wheezing. (Not all wheezing is because of asthma.)

- Asymptomatic between asthma attacks. Symptoms resolve when there is no inflammation present.

- Shortness of breath as patient experiences symptoms of narrowed airways.

- Difficulty breathing (dyspnea) as airways narrow due to inflammation. This is typically progressive as inflammation increases.

- Respiration greater than 20 breaths per minute (tachypnea) as the body attempts to get more oxygen into the lungs to meet physiologic needs.

- Use of accessory muscles to breathe as the body tries harder to get more air into the lungs.

- Tightness in the chest owing to narrowing of the airways (bronchoconstriction).

- Cough.

- Tachycardia—heart rate greater than 100, as the body attempts to get more oxygen to the tissues.
- Decreased alertness due to hypoxia (low oxygen levels).
- Cyanosis if oxygen levels drop.
- Anxiety related to shortness of breath.

Common Test Results

- Decreased oxygen and increased carbon dioxide present in ABG due to inability to move adequate air, which results in inadequate gas exchange.
- Decreased force on expiration (either forced expiratory volume in the first second [FEV_1] or peak expiratory rate flow [PERF]) during attack shown in PFT. Narrowed airways make it more difficult for the patient to exhale, prolonging time of exhalation and decreasing force of exhalation. Patients can check expiratory effort at home on a peak flow meter.
- Hyperinflated lungs shown in CXR because of air trapping.
- Pulse oximetry shows diminished oxygen saturation.
- CBC—elevated eosinophils.
- Sputum—positive for eosinophils.

Treatment

The focus of treatment is to return the respiration to normal, deliver adequate oxygen, and limit the number of recurrences. Patient education should focus on understanding the disease, its management, and when emergency care may be necessary.

- Administer supplemental oxygen to help meet body's needs during exacerbation.
- Identify and remove allergens and known triggers to avoid causing an asthma attack.
- Give patient 3 L/day of fluid to help liquefy any secretions.
- Administer short-acting $beta_2$-adrenergic blocking agents (rescue medications) to bronchodilate.
  - albuterol, pirbuterol, metaproterenol, terbutaline, levalbuterol
  - Administer long-acting $beta_2$-adrenergic blocking agents to manage symptoms day to day; keep airways open, not for acute symptoms.
  - salmeterol, formoterol

- Administer leukotriene modulators to reduce local inflammatory response in lung to reduce exacerbations; given daily and do not have immediate effect on symptoms.
  - zafirlukast, zileuton, montelukast
- Administer anticholinergic drugs.
  - ipratropium inhaler, tiotropium HandiHaler
- Administer antacid, H2 blocker, or PPI to decrease the amount of acid in the stomach, reducing the possibility of ulcers due to stress of disease or medication effects.
  - antacids: aluminum hydroxide/magnesium hydroxide, calcium carbonate
  - H2 blockers: ranitidine, famotidine, nizatidine, cimetidine
  - PPI: omeprazole, lansoprazole, esomeprazole, rabeprazole, pantoprazole
- Administer mast cell stabilizer to retain an early component of the initial response to allergens, which will prevent further reactions from occurring; this is not for acute symptoms. This is useful for pretreatment for allergen exposure or chronic use to improve control of symptoms.
  - cromolyn, nedocromil
- Administer steroids to decrease inflammation, which will help open airways; these are not for acute symptoms.
  - hydrocortisone, methylprednisolone intravenously
  - beclomethasone, triamcinolone, fluticasone, budesonide, flunisolide, mometasone inhalers
  - prednisolone, prednisone orally
- Administer methylxanthines to assist with bronchodilation, often used when other medications are not effective.
  - aminophylline, theophylline
- Administer omalizumab (inhibits binding of IgE to mast cells) via subcutaneous injection to reduce frequency of allergic asthma exacerbation in patients not controlled by steroids. Anaphylaxis has been seen with use of this medication. It should only be given in a healthcare provider office (not for home use).

Nursing Diagnoses

- Impaired gas exchange
- Ineffective airway clearance
- Ineffective tissue perfusion

> ## NURSING INTERVENTION
>
> - Monitor respiration: patient's respiration can continue to deteriorate; look at respiratory rate, effort, use of accessory muscles, skin color, breath sounds.
> - Monitor for decrease in alertness or irritability which may be seen in hypoxia.
> - Place patient in high Fowler's position to ease respirations.
> - Monitor vital signs: look for changes in BP, tachycardia, tachypnea.
> - **Explain to the patient:**
>   - How to use a peak flow meter.
>   - How to properly use the metered dose inhaler or dry powder, and in which order to take inhaled medication.
>   - Avoid exposure to allergen.
>   - How to recognize the early signs of asthma.
>   - How to perform coughing and deep-breathing exercises.
>   - When to contact their healthcare provider.
>   - When to go to the emergency room or call 911.

4. Atelectasis

What Went Wrong

A portion of the lung does not expand completely, decreasing the lung's capacity to exchange gases, which often results in decreased oxygenation of blood. Obstruction of part of the airway will cause collapse distal to the area that is blocked. Obstruction can be from a mucous plug inside the airway, or a tumor or fluid within the pleural space may be pressing on the airway from the outside. Postoperatively, patients are at risk for atelectasis due to pain, immobility, medications for pain or anesthesia, and lack of deep breathing.

Prognosis

Prognosis depends on the cause and the size of the involved area.

Hallmark Signs and Symptoms

- Difficulty breathing (dyspnea) owing to the lack of expansion of part of the lung.
- Chest pain because of airless state of area of lung.
- Anxiety because of decrease in oxygenation.

- Increased respiratory rate (tachypnea) in an attempt to increase available oxygen.
- Heart rate above 100 beats per minute (tachycardia) as body tries to increase available oxygen.
- Sweating (diaphoresis) as a result of increased work of respirations.
- Cyanosis due to decreased oxygen level.
- Hypoxemia because of lack of gas exchange in the affected area.
- Decreased breath sounds due to lack of air movement in the area of collapse.
- Accessory muscle use with respiration as the body tries to get more oxygen.

Common Test Results

- Shadows on CXR indicate collapsed area of the lung. The airless state in this area of the lung creates a more dense appearance on the x-ray.
- CT scan will show an area of atelectasis.
- Bronchoscopy can help identify cause or clear mucus plug.

Treatment

Treatment is focused on reinflation of the involved area of the lung, removing the cause of obstruction, and the delivery of adequate oxygen. The extent of the treatment depends on the area of the lung involved and the cause.

- Administer oxygen to meet body's demand.
  - Chest PT and postural drainage to loosen mucus
- Administer mucolytics to help loosen or thin secretions.
  - acetylcysteine, inhaled
  - guaifenesin, oral
- Administer bronchodilators to open airways.
  - albuterol
  - levalbuterol

Nursing Diagnoses

- Impaired gas exchange
- Risk for infection
- Ineffective tissue perfusion

> ## NURSING INTERVENTION
>
> - Cough and deep-breathing exercise every 2 hours to prevent a further area of atelectasis.
> - Instruct the patient to use the incentive spirometer every 2 hours to encourage deep breathing and monitor progress.
> - Provide humidified air.
> - Monitor breath sounds for abnormalities such as diminished sounds.
> - Monitor mechanical ventilation if needed. If a large area of the lung is affected, respiratory support may be needed.
> - **Explain to the patient:**
>   - How to perform coughing and deep-breathing exercises.
>   - Proper use of incentive spirometer.

5. Bronchiectasis

What Went Wrong

Bronchi and bronchioles become abnormally and permanently dilated, caused by infection and inflammation. This results in excessive production of mucus that obstructs the bronchi. There is some obstruction of the airways and a chronic infection. The changes within the lung can be localized or generalized. The lung may develop areas of atelectasis where thick mucus obstructs the smaller airways, making the mucous difficult to expel. This results in inflammation and infection of the airways and leads to bronchiectasis.

Prognosis

Early diagnosis and appropriate treatment of infections are essential for management. Postural drainage and chest physical therapy aid in movement of mucous from the airways. Cystic fibrosis accounts for about a third of all the bronchiectasis cases in the United States. The difficulty in breathing is caused by excess mucus.

Hallmark Signs and Symptoms

- Difficult breathing (dyspnea) owing to the mucous production and irritation within the airways.
- Productive, foul-smelling, odorous cough, because of thick, difficult-to-expel, tenacious mucous often with bacterial colonization.

- Cough may be worse when lying down.
- Recurrent bronchial infections.
- Hemoptysis (blood-tinged or bloody mucous).
- Loss of weight because patients are not eating well, due to respiratory changes and foul-smelling mucous with cough. Increased respiratory effort requires more calories to meet requirements.
- Crackles or rhonchi on inspiration due to mucous buildup.
- Anemia of chronic disease.
- Cyanosis.
- Clubbing of the fingers.

Common Test Results

- Culture and sensitivity of sputum to identify bacteria and appropriate antibiotics.
- Shadows in the affected area of the lungs on the CXR.
- CT scan or high-resolution CT will show areas of bronchiectasis.
- Decreased lung vital capacity on PFT.
- Alpha-1 antitrypsin blood test may be done to diagnose a deficiency (may be seen in early onset of chronic obstructive pulmonary disease—COPD).

Treatment

Treatment is focused on getting enough oxygen to meet current needs of the patient, expel mucous, and treat infections.

- Supplemental oxygen to help meet body's needs.
- Postural drainage to assist with drainage of secretions.
- Chest PT to loosen secretions.
- Remove excessive secretions during a bronchoscopy.
- Administer bronchodilators to help keep airways open.
  - albuterol, levalbuterol
- Administer antibiotics to treat infection.
  - Selected based on the results of a culture and sensitivity study
- Surgical resection of lung may be recommended.

Nursing Diagnoses

- Ineffective airway clearance
- Imbalanced nutrition: less than what the body requires
- Impaired gas exchange

NURSING INTERVENTION

- Monitor respiratory rate, effort, breath sounds, skin color, and use of accessory muscles.
- Perform chest percussion to help loosen secretions.
- **Explain to the patient:**
  - That family member can perform chest PT.
  - How to do postural drainage. Reinforce information given by respiratory therapist.
  - How to administer oxygen.
  - How to properly administer medications.

---

6. Bronchitis

What Went Wrong

Increased mucus production, caused by infection and airborne irritants that block airways in the lungs, results in the decreased ability to exchange gases. There are two forms of bronchitis: acute bronchitis (where blockage of the airways is reversible) and chronic bronchitis (where blockage is not reversible). Patients with acute bronchitis are symptomatic typically for 7 to 10 days often due to viral (but sometimes bacterial) infection. Patients with chronic bronchitis will have symptoms of a chronic productive cough for at least 3 consecutive months in 2 consecutive years. There is increased mucus production, inflammatory changes, and, ultimately, fibrosis in the airway walls (see Fig. 2–3). The patient with chronic bronchitis has an increased incidence of respiratory infection.

Prognosis

Patients with acute bronchitis who have a resolution of symptoms and respiratory status will return to normal condition. Chronic bronchitis is classified as COPD, which is often linked to smoking and has a progressive pattern. Shortness of breath is initially present due to exertion, and eventually is present even at rest. Patients with chronic bronchitis often develop right-sided heart failure

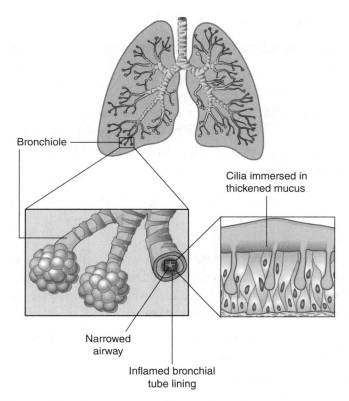

Bronchiole

Cilia immersed in
thickened mucus

Narrowed
airway

Inflamed bronchial
tube lining

FIGURE 2–3 · Inflamed bronchiole with increased mucus production.

and peripheral or dependent edema. Patients will have acute exacerbations of
chronic bronchitis.

Hallmark Signs and Symptoms

- Cough due to mucous production and irritation of airways.
- Shortness of breath.
- Fever in acute episodes because of infection.
- Accessory muscles are used for breathing—as respiratory effort increases,
  additional muscles are necessary to assist.
- Productive cough owing to irritation of airways. Mucus is a protective
  reaction of the respiratory system.
- Weight gain secondary to edema in chronic bronchitis is because of right-
  sided heart failure.
- Wheezing due to inflammation within the airways.

Common Test Results

- Shadows in the affected area of the lungs on the CXR present during infection.
- PFT shows:
  - Forced vital capacity (FVC) changes because more time is needed to forcibly exhale an amount of air after a maximal inhalation.
  - FEV_1 is decreased because more time is needed for exhalation.
  - Residual volume (RV) is increased due to air trapping.
- Decreased oxygen and increased carbon dioxide in arterial blood gas.

Treatment

Acute bronchitis is treated in the short term with symptomatic treatment, and antibiotics are needed only when a bacterial infection is present. Chronic bronchitis is treated with a combination of medications to keep the airways open, reduce inflammation within airways, and prevent complications or exacerbations.

- Administer beta$_2$-agonists by inhaler or nebulizer to dilate the bronchi.
  - terbutaline, albuterol, levalbuterol
  - formoterol, salmeterol
- Administer anticholinergics which allow for relaxation of bronchial smooth muscle.
  - ipratropium, tiotropium inhaler
- Administer steroids to decrease inflammation within the airways.
  - hydrocortisone, methylprednisolone systemically
  - beclomethasone, triamcinolone, fluticasone, budesonide, flunisolide inhalers
  - prednisolone, prednisone orally
- Administer methylxanthines to enhance bronchodilation.
  - aminophylline
  - theophylline (Theo-Dur)
- Administer diuretics to reduce fluid retention in patients who develop right-sided heart failure.
  - furosemide, bumetanide
- Administer expectorant to help liquefy secretions.
  - guaifenesin

- Administer antibiotics in acute exacerbation of chronic bronchitis.
  - selected by culture and sensitivity study or given empirically
- Administer antacid, H2 blocker, or PPI to decrease the amount of acid in stomach, reducing possible ulcer formation due to stress of disease or medication effects.
  - antacids: aluminum hydroxide/magnesium hydroxide, calcium carbonate
  - H2 blockers: ranitidine, famotidine, nizatidine, cimetidine
  - PPI: omeprazole, lansoprazole, esomeprazole, rabeprazole, pantoprazole
- Administer vaccines to decrease chances of infection.
  - influenza (annually)
  - pneumonia
- Give 3 L of fluid every day to help liquefy secretions.
- Oxygen: 2 L per minute via nasal canula to help meet body's needs; low flow rates help reduce dyspnea while avoiding CO_2 retention in chronic bronchitis.
- Increase protein, calories, and vitamin C in diet to meet body's needs.
- Administer the incentive spirometer or flutter valve to encourage coughing and expelling of mucus.
- Nocturnal negative pressure ventilation used for hypercapnic (elevated CO_2 levels) patients.

Nursing Diagnoses

- Ineffective airway clearance
- Activity intolerance
- Ineffective breathing pattern

NURSING INTERVENTION

- Monitor respirations looking at rate, effort, use of accessory muscles, skin color; listen to breath sounds.
- Place patient in high Fowler's position to ease respiration.
- Weigh the patient daily. Excess fluid due to heart failure will increase weight. Notify physician, NP, or PA of weight gain of 2 lb or more in 24 hours.
- Have the patient perform the turning, coughing, and deep-breathing exercises to enhance lung expansion and expel mucous.

- Monitor sputum for changes in color or amount, which may signal infection in patients with chronic bronchitis.
- Monitor intake and output.
- Increase fluids to keep mucous thinner and easier to expel.
- **Explain to the patient:**
  - How to administer oxygen.

7. Chronic Obstructive Pulmonary Disease (COPD)

What Went Wrong

Obstruction in the lungs makes it difficult to empty air from the lungs leading to shortness of breath and decrease oxygenation of blood. As a result, the patient works hard to breathe and feels tried due to exhaustion and decrease oxygen levels. COPD is a general term associated with other chronic obstructive pulmonary disorders that include chronic bronchitis and emphysema. Asthma is not considered COPD although some patients may also be diagnosed with asthma. In chronic bronchitis swelling and mucus produced in the bronchial block the airway. In emphysema the alveoli lose elasticity and are unable to stretch leading to trapped air (hyperinflation) that block the air from emptying the lungs. COPD is commonly caused by cigarette smoke, genetics and exposure to dust, chemicals, and air pollution.

Prognosis

COPD is a chronic dysfunction of the lungs that will not resolve although ongoing treatment may occasionally improve symptoms for a period of time. Shortness of breath and fatigue will never go away; however, consistent treatment helps patients manage COPD enabling them to perform activities of daily living.

Hallmark Signs and Symptoms

- Cough that produces substantial amounts of mucous.
- Shortness of breath due to airway obstruction.
- Wheezing due to inflammation within the airways.
- Chest tightness.
- Accessory muscles are used for breathing—as respiratory effort increases, additional muscles are necessary to assist.

Common Test Results

- Pulmonary Function Test (PFT) shows:
  - FVC changes because more time is needed to forcibly exhale an amount of air after a maximal inhalation.
  - FEV_1 is decreased because more time is needed for exhalation.
  - RV is increased due to air trapping.
- Decreased oxygen and increased carbon dioxide in arterial blood gas.

Treatment

COPD is treated with a combination of medications to keep the airways open, reduce inflammation within airways, and prevent complications or exacerbations.

- Administer $beta_2$-agonists by an inhaler or a nebulizer to dilate the bronchi.
  - terbutaline, albuterol, levalbuterol
  - formoterol, salmeterol
- Administer anticholinergics that allow for relaxation of bronchial smooth muscle.
  - ipratropium, tiotropium inhaler
- Administer steroids to decrease inflammation within the airways.
  - hydrocortisone, methylprednisolone systemically
  - beclomethasone, triamcinolone, fluticasone, budesonide, flunisolide inhalers
  - prednisolone, prednisone orally
- Administer methylxanthines to enhance bronchodilation.
  - aminophylline
  - theophylline (Theo-Dur)
- Administer diuretics to reduce fluid retention in patients who develop right-sided heart failure.
  - furosemide, bumetanide
- Administer expectorant to help liquefy secretions.
  - guaifenesin
- Administer antacid, H2 blocker, or PPI to decrease the amount of acid in stomach, reducing possible ulcer formation due to stress of disease or medication effects.

- antacids: aluminum hydroxide/magnesium hydroxide, calcium carbonate
  - H2 blockers: ranitidine, famotidine, nizatidine, cimetidine
  - PPI: omeprazole, lansoprazole, esomeprazole, rabeprazole, pantoprazole
- Administer vaccines to decrease chances of infection.
  - influenza (annually)
  - pneumonia
- Give 3 L of fluid every day to help liquefy secretions.
- Oxygen: 2 L/min via nasal canula to help meet body's needs; low flow rates help reduce dyspnea while avoiding CO_2 retention in chronic bronchitis.
- Increase protein, calories, and vitamin C in diet to meet body's needs.
- Administer the incentive spirometer or flutter valve to encourage coughing and expelling of mucus.
- Nocturnal negative pressure ventilation used for hypercapnic (elevated CO_2 levels) patients.

Nursing Diagnoses

- Ineffective airway clearance
- Activity intolerance
- Ineffective breathing pattern

NURSING INTERVENTION

- Monitor respirations looking at rate, effort, use of accessory muscles, skin color; listen to breath sounds.
- Place patient in high Fowler's position to ease respiration.
- Weigh the patient daily. Excess fluid due to heart failure will increase weight. Notify physician, NP, or PA of weight gain of 2 lb or more in 24 hours.
- Have the patient perform the turning, coughing, and deep-breathing exercises to enhance lung expansion and expel mucous.
- Monitor sputum for changes in color or amount, which may signal infection in patients with chronic bronchitis.
- Monitor intake and output.
- Increase fluids to keep mucous thinner and easier to expel.
- **Explain to the patient:**
  - How to administer oxygen.

8. Cor Pulmonale

What Went Wrong

In cor pulmonale, the structure and function of the right ventricle are compromised due to prolonged pulmonary artery hypertension. This may be caused by COPD, obstruction of the airflow into and out of the lungs. The heart tries to compensate, resulting in right-sided heart failure.

The patient has heart failure owing to a primary lung disorder, which causes pulmonary hypertension and enlargement of the right ventricle. Patients will have symptoms of both the underlying pulmonary disorder and the right-sided heart failure. COPD includes chronic bronchitis and emphysema.

Prognosis

Management of both the underlying lung disease and the heart failure is necessary to alleviate the symptoms for the patient. Medical management may provide significant relief of symptoms for the patient. Exacerbations of the underlying disease process are still likely. Progression of the disease state is possible, requiring adjustment in medications or making further lifestyle modifications.

Hallmark Signs and Symptoms

- Cyanosis.
- Fatigue due to hypoxia and heart failure.
  - Syncope (fainting) due to exertion.
- Wheezing because of underlying lung condition such as COPD or emphysema.
- Difficulty breathing (dyspnea) on exertion and when lying down (orthopnea) due to increased oxygen needs with movement and increased respiratory effort of the diaphragm when lying down.
- Productive cough due to underlying respiratory condition.
- Edema due to right-sided heart failure; fluid buildup will be in dependent areas.
- Weight gain due to fluid retention.
- Respiration greater than 20 breaths per minute (tachypnea); rate increases to meet body's oxygen needs.

- Increased heart rate above 100 beats per minute (tachycardia) as the body attempts to compensate for hypoxia and carry more oxygen.
  - Jugular venous distention owing to increased right-sided pressures within the heart.

Common Test Results

- Enlarged pulmonary arteries and right ventricle shown on a CXR.
- Enlarged right ventricle shown on echocardiography as a result of pulmonary hypertension.
- Increased right ventricular and pulmonary artery pressures in a pulmonary artery catheterization. The right ventricle is pumping against greater-than-normal resistance within the pulmonary artery when supplying blood to the lungs.
- Decreased oxygen and increased carbon dioxide in ABG due to underlying lung disease.
- Pulse oximetry shows decreased oxygen saturation.
- Increased hemoglobin to compensate for hypoxia.
  - Brain natriuretic peptide (BNP) may be elevated, indicating heart failure.

Treatment

- Bed rest or decreased activity.
- Oxygen therapy at 2 L/min (low flow rate) to help meet body's needs. The COPD patient cannot tolerate a high flow of oxygen.
- Administer endothelin receptor antagonist for pulmonary artery hypertension to slow progression of disease.
  - ambrisentan
  - bosentan
- Administer prostaglandins to block platelet production, thus reducing chance of blood clots.
  - prostacyclin
- Administer phosphodiesterase (PDE) inhibitor to relax the vessels within the lungs.
  - sildenafil (Revatio)
- Administer calcium channel blockers to vasodilate.
  - diltiazem, nifedipine, nicardipine, amlodipine

- Administer medications to vasodilate the pulmonary artery.
  - diazoxide, hydralazine, nitroprusside
- Administer angiotensin-converting enzyme inhibitor.
  - captopril, enalapril, lisinopril, quinapril
- Administer anticoagulant to reduce risk of clot formation.
  - heparin
- Administer diuretic to remove excess fluid.
  - furosemide, bumetanide
- Administer cardiac glycoside for symptom relief of heart failure.
  - digoxin
- Reduce sodium in the diet to reduce fluid retention.
- Reduce fluid intake to reduce fluid retention.
- Administer vaccine.
  - Flu (annual)
  - Pneumococcal

Nursing Diagnoses

- Excessive fluid volume
- Impaired gas exchange
- Activity intolerance

NURSING INTERVENTION

- Limit fluid to 2 L/day.
- Monitor digoxin level to avoid toxic effect.
- Check pulse before administering cardiac glycoside. A side effect of the drug is slowing of the heart rate. Hold medication and contact the physician as needed.
- Monitor serum potassium levels; ACE inhibitors and some diuretics can cause potassium retention.
- Monitor respiratory status for rate, effort, use of accessory muscle, skin color, and breath sounds.
- **Explain to the patient:**
  - How to administer oxygen therapy.
  - Medication management.
  - Avoid traveling to high altitudes.
  - Importance of smoking cessation.

9. Emphysema

What Went Wrong

Chronic inflammation reduces the flexibility of the walls of alveoli, resulting in over-distention of the alveolar walls. This causes air to be trapped in the lungs, impeding gas exchange. The alveoli are overfilled with air (resulting in minimal or nonexistent air movement), which impairs the ability to exchange carbon dioxide for oxygen. Structural changes in the lung result in air trapping within the alveoli. Smoking is often linked to development of emphysema. A less frequent cause is an inherited alpha$_1$-antitrypsin deficiency.

Prognosis

Symptoms often begin insidiously and are progressive. There is no cure for emphysema. Medications can help manage the symptoms and prolong the progression of disease. Shortness of breath is initially associated with exertion, then presents at rest. These patients are more susceptible to lung infections. Supplemental oxygen becomes necessary at first for exacerbations, then for daily use. Periodic exacerbations requiring hospitalization are not unusual. Quality of life is diminished. Emphysema is the fourth leading cause of death in the United States.

Hallmark Signs and Symptoms

- Difficulty breathing (dyspnea) or shortness of breath (most common symptom) due to air trapping, which retains carbon dioxide and reduces alveolar gas exchange.
  - Cough due to mucus production from airway irritation
  - Decreasing exercise tolerance
- Barrel chest develops over time as more air is trapped within the distal airways. The anteroposterior diameter (distance between front and back of the chest) increases, giving the chest a more barrel-like appearance.
- Use of accessory muscles to breathe as the respiratory effort increases. The number of muscles used to inhale will increase in an effort to get enough oxygen into the body.
- Loss of weight as extra calories is needed to maintain respiration. Increased effort of breathing also detracts from eating.
- Patients prefer a seated position which allows for greater chest expansion.

- "Pursed lip" breathing (which increases the pressure within the distal airways) in an attempt to empty trapped air.

Common Test Results

- Increased residual volume shown in PFT due to air trapping.
- Decreased oxygen and increased carbon dioxide in ABG as gas exchange is impaired owing to air trapping; more pronounced as disease progresses.
- CXR shows overinflation of lungs and flattening of the diaphragm.

Treatment

Treatment will vary depending on the stage of the emphysema. As the disease progresses, the treatment will change. Medications to control symptoms and keep airways open, use of supplemental oxygen, and smoking cessation are the mainstays of treatment.

- Administer beta$_2$-agonists to bronchodilate (fast acting) by an inhaler or a nebulizer.
  - terbutaline, albuterol, levalbuterol
- Administer long-acting bronchodilating medications by a metered dose inhaler or a dry powder inhaler.
  - formoterol, salmeterol
- Administer anticholinergics that allow relaxation of bronchial smooth muscle.
  - ipratropium, tiotropium inhaler
- Administer methylxanthines to dilate the bronchi. These are typically used in conjunction with other medications, not for acute effect.
  - aminophylline
  - theophylline
- Administer steroids to decrease inflammation within the airways.
  - hydrocortisone, methylprednisolone systemically
  - beclomethasone, triamcinolone, fluticasone, budesonide, flunisolide inhalers
  - prednisolone, prednisone orally
- Administer antacid, H2 blocker, or PPI to decrease the amount of acid in stomach, reducing possible ulcer formation due to stress of the disease or medication effects.

- antacids: aluminum hydroxide/magnesium hydroxide, calcium carbonate
- H2 blockers: ranitidine, famotidine, nizatidine, cimetidine
- PPI: omeprazole, lansoprazole, esomeprazole, rabeprazole, pantoprazole
- Administer expectorant—to loosen secretions.
  - guaifenesin
- Administer diuretics to decrease fluid retention in patients that are developing right-sided heart failure secondary to lung disease.
  - furosemide, bumetanide
- Administer vaccines—to prevent respiratory infections.
  - influenza (annually)
  - pneumonia
- Administer antibiotics.
- Selection based on results of culture and sensitivity study or given empirically
- Administer alpha$_1$-antitrypsin therapy for patients with deficiency.
- Administer oxygen, 2 L/min, to help meet body's oxygen needs while avoiding CO_2 retention.
- Give patient 3 L of fluids every day to help liquefy secretions.
- Nocturnal negative pressure ventilation for hypercapnic (elevated CO_2 levels) patients.
  - Pulmonary rehabilitation.
  - Incentive spirometer or flutter valve.
  - Bilateral lung volume reduction surgery, which will allow for improved lung expansion.
  - Lung transplant surgery.
  - Need for ongoing antirejection drugs posttransplant.

Nursing Diagnoses

- Impaired gas exchange
- Fatigue
- Risk for infection

> ## NURSING INTERVENTION
>
> - Monitor the patient's sputum for color, amount, or changes in characteristics, which may indicate infection.
> - Place patient in high Fowler's position, which eases respiratory effort.
> - Administer low-flow oxygen, which increases oxygen supply to patient without compromising respiratory drive.
> - Monitor intake and output of fluids.
> - **Explain to the patient:**
>   - The importance of turning, coughing, and deep-breathing exercises.
>   - How to administer oxygen therapy.
>   - Avoid exposure to irritants and people with infections.
> - Teach patient how to use:
>   - The incentive spirometer to encourage deep breathing and enhance coughing and expelling of mucous.
>   - The flutter valve to increase expiration force.

10. Influenza

What Went Wrong

Influenza is a viral infection affecting the respiratory tract that spreads through droplets. The virus can be inhaled or picked up from surfaces through direct contact. Infection can settle into either the upper or the lower respiratory tract. The virus causes damage to the upper layers of cells. The natural defenses of the respiratory tract are compromised and it is easier for bacteria to attach to the underlying respiratory tissues. H1N1 (a different strain of flu) infection can cause illness that ranges from fairly mild to severe.

Prognosis

Influenza symptoms typically run their course within about a week. Current medications help to decrease the length and severity of symptoms associated with influenza. Some patients will develop secondary infections, such as sinusitis or viral or bacterial pneumonia following influenza. Patients with pneumonia have an increased risk of mortality from influenza. Patients with comorbidities are also more likely to develop serious complications from both traditional influenza infection and from H1N1 infection.

Hallmark Signs and Symptoms

- Symptoms have an abrupt onset
- Nonproductive cough
- Chills and sweats
- Fatigue and malaise
- Fever over 101°F
- Headache
- Muscle aches (myalgia)
- Watery, nasal discharge
- Sore throat

Common Test Results

- Nasopharyngeal viral culture
- Rapid diagnostic kit

Treatment

Symptomatic treatment to increase patient comfort and medications to shorten the duration and intensity of symptoms are the focus of patient treatment. Medications need to be started early in the symptoms.

- Administer antipyretics for comfort.
  - acetaminophen
- Administer antiviral medications.
  - zanamivir, oseltamivir
- amantadine, rimantadine

Nursing Diagnoses

- Risk for injury
- Impaired gas exchange
- Hyperthermia

NURSING INTERVENTION

- Administer fluids and electrolytes to replace what is being lost due to sweating and insensible loss from elevated temperature.
- Monitor vital signs.

- Monitor respiratory status for rate, effort, use of accessory muscles, skin color, and breath sounds.
  - Teach patient to cover their mouth and nose when coughing or sneezing.
  - Encourage hand washing.

11. Lung Cancer

What Went Wrong

Lung cancer is the abnormal, uncontrolled cell growth in lung tissues, resulting in a tumor. A tumor in the lung may be primary, when it develops in lung tissue, or secondary, when it spreads (metastasizes) from cancer in other areas of the body, such as the liver, brain, or kidneys. There are two major categories of lung cancer—small cell (about 15% to 20% of lung cancers) and non-small cell (more common). Repetitive exposure to inhaled irritants increases a person's risk for lung cancer. Cigarette smoke, occupational exposures, air pollution containing benzopyrenes and hydrocarbons have all been shown to increase risk. Exposure to inhaled irritants such as coal, gasoline, diesel exhaust, uranium, beryllium, nickel chromates, or radon gas is linked to increased cases of lung cancer. Cigarettes' smoke (as the smoker or through secondhand smoke) is the primary cause of lung cancer.

- Small cell:
  - Oat cell—fast-growing, early metastasis often found centrally, in or near the bronchus
- Non-small cell:
  - Adenocarcinoma—moderate growth rate, early metastasis often found in outer (peripheral) areas of lung
  - Squamous cell—slow-growing, late metastasis often found more centrally, near a bronchus
  - Large cell—fast-growing, early metastasis

Prognosis

Lung cancer is the leading cause of death. More people die of lung cancer each year than the combined total of breast, colon, and prostate cancer deaths. Many patients with lung cancer are diagnosed at a later stage, leading to the long-term (5-year) survival rate of less than 20%. Earlier diagnosis is more beneficial for treatment and outcome. The longer the cancer has been in the lungs, the greater the likelihood of metastasis to other areas.

Hallmark Signs and Symptoms

- Chronic coughing due to irritation from mass. Presence of mucus or exudate may not be until later in disease.
- Coughing up blood (hemoptysis).
- Fatigue.
- Weight loss due to the caloric needs of the tumor, taking away from the needs of the body.
- Anorexia.
- Difficulty breathing (dyspnea) caused by damaged lung tissue. The patient begins to have respiratory problems later in the disease.
- Chest pains as mass presses on surrounding tissue; may not be until late in disease.
- Sputum production.
- Pleural effusion.
  - Wheezing due to narrowing of airways as tumor presses on airway.

Common Test Results

- Mass in lung shown on CXR.
- CT scan shows mass, lymph node involvement.
- Bronchoscopy may show cancer cells on bronchoscopic washings and may reveal tumor site.
- Sputum cytology–cancer cells seen in sputum.
- Biopsy will show cell type.
  - Thoracentesis—removal of pleural fluid for analysis
  - Fine needle aspiration—needle biopsy through chest wall for peripheral tumors.
  - Thoracoscopy (fiberoptic tube inserted through chest wall), thoracotomy (surgical incision), or mediastinoscopy (fiberoptic tube inserted through chest wall at top of sternum)—tissue biopsy from lung for tumors that are located deep within the chest.
- Bone scan or CT scan shows metastasis of the disease.

Treatment

Treatment is focused on resolution of the tumor. Surgical removal is appropriate for some patients, but not always necessary. Chemotherapy and radiation are both methods that are used to destroy the cancerous cells. Oxygen therapy is used to aid in meeting the current needs of the body, but not all patients will require supplemental oxygen therapy. Attention to nutrition is important to meet the demands of the body. Pain control is an integral component of care in any type of cancer treatment. Appropriate pain management needs to be individualized for the patient.

- Surgical removal of the affected area of the lung (wedge resection, segmental resection, lobectomy) or total lung (pneumonectomy).
- Radiation therapy to decrease tumor size.
- Chemotherapy often with a combination of drugs, depending on the cell type.
  - May see relapse after treatment.
- Targeted therapy (currently not first-line treatment).
  - Gefitinib—an anilinoquinazoline that targets non-small cell lung cancers that have not responded to chemotherapy.
- Oxygen therapy to supplement the needs of the body.
- High-protein, high-calorie diet to meet the needs of the body.
- Administer antiemetics to combat side effects of chemotherapy.
  - ondansetron, prochlorperazine
- Administer analgesics for pain control.
  - morphine, fentanyl

Nursing Diagnoses

- Anxiety
- Activity intolerance
- Impaired gas exchange

NURSING INTERVENTION

- Monitor respiratory status, looking at rate, effort, use of accessory muscles, and skin color; auscultate breath sounds.
- Monitor pain and administer analgesics appropriately.
- Monitor vital signs for changes, elevated pulse, elevated respiration, change in BP, and elevated temperature, which may signal infection.

- Monitor pulse oximetry for decrease in oxygenation levels.
- Assist patient with turning, coughing, and deep-breathing exercises.
- Place patient in semi-Fowler's position to ease respiratory effort.
- **Explain to the patient:**
  - The importance of taking rest periods.

12. Pleural Effusion

What Went Wrong

Abnormal accumulation of fluid develops within the pleural space between the parietal and visceral pleura covering the lungs. The fluid may be serous fluid, blood (hemothorax), or pus (empyema). Fluid builds up when the development of the fluid exceeds the body's ability to remove the fluid. Excess fluid inhibits full expansion of the lung. A large area of fluid buildup will displace the lung tissue, compromising air exchange in the area. As fluid builds up and takes the place of lung tissue, it may push the collapsing lung past the middle (mediastinum) of the chest. This displaces the central structures, compromising the air exchange of the other lung as well. Causes of pleural effusion are varied and include congestive heart failure, renal failure, malignancy, lupus erythematosus, pulmonary infarction, infection, or trauma. It can also occur as a postoperative complication.

Prognosis

Prognosis varies depending on the cause and the amount of fluid present. Once fluid is removed, patient is monitored to see if fluid builds up again. The fluid may need to be removed periodically, depending on the cause.

Hallmark Signs and Symptoms

- Chest pain due to the presence of inflammation of the pleura in the area; not always present.
- Difficulty breathing (dyspnea) because of diminished chest expansion in the area.
- Decreased breath sounds on auscultation over the area due to the presence of fluid.
- Dullness on percussion over the affected area owing to the presence of fluid.

- Fever due to infection with empyema.
- Increased pulse (tachycardia) and respirations (tachypnea); decreased BP because of blood loss with hemothorax.
- Low oxygen saturation on pulse oximeter.

Common Test Results

- CXR shows pleural effusion.
- Chest CT scan shows pleural effusion.
- Chest ultrasound shows pleural effusion.
- Thoracentesis (removal of fluid with a needle from the pleural space) shows type of fluid.

Treatment

Fluid removal is performed either as a onetime procedure or with a chest tube, to continuously allow for drainage of the fluid until the tube is removed. Supplemental oxygen may be needed to help meet the body's needs.

- Thoracentesis to remove the fluid.
- Chest tube to remove larger amounts of drainage over time.
- Oxygen as needed.
  - Administer diuretics for fluid resulting from heart failure.
- Administer antibiotics for empyema.
  - Selected according to results of culture and sensitivity study

Nursing Diagnoses

- Impaired gas exchange
- Risk for infection
- Pain

NURSING INTERVENTION

- Administer supplemental oxygen therapy to help meet body's needs.
- Monitor for changes in vital signs.
- Have the patient perform turning, coughing, deep-breathing exercises to enhance lung expansion.

- Monitor chest tube drainage for color, amount, and changes in drainage.
- Assure patency of chest tube to make sure the tube is draining properly.
- **Explain to the patient:**
  - Disease process.
  - Need for coughing and deep breathing.

13. Pneumonia

What Went Wrong

Pneumonia may be due to a variety of microorganisms and can be community-acquired or hospital-acquired (nosocomial). A patient can inhale bacteria, viruses, parasites, or irritating agents, or a patient can aspirate liquids or foods. He or she can also develop increased mucus production and thickening of alveolar fluid as a result of impaired gas exchange. All of these can lead to inflammation of the lower airways.

Organisms commonly associated with pneumonia include *Staphylococcus aureus, Streptococcus pneumonia (most common), Haemophilus influenzae*—infection with these organisms results in a typical pneumonia.

Mycoplasma pneumoniae, Legionella pneumoniae, Chlamydia pneumoniae (parasite)—infection with these organisms may have an atypical (or walking) pneumonia presentation and are more common in young adults. Some strains of *Pseudomonas aeruginosa* have increasing resistance to bacteria. It is a concern in patients with cystic fibrosis, *Pneumocystis jiroveci* may be seen in patients with immunocompromised chronic lung disease. Patients may also develop pneumonia due to viral infection. Common causative viruses are influenza, adenovirus, parainfluenza, and respiratory syncytial virus.

Prognosis

Prognosis will vary depending on patient's age, preexisting lung disease, infecting organism, and response to antibiotics. Patients at risk for pneumonia are: older patients; those with respiratory disease; patients with comorbid conditions such as heart, liver, or kidney disease; and patients who develop complications (such as atelectasis or pleural effusion). Patients at greater risk for complications from pneumonia will be treated within the hospital, while those at lower risk may be treated at home. Patients with respiratory rates over 30 breaths per minute, tachycardia, altered mental status, or hypotension also are considered at higher risk.

Patients without other coexisting conditions, who do not appear to have the higher-risk symptoms listed above, can usually be safely treated as outpatients. Patients with comorbidities (higher-risk coexisting symptoms) or who appear ill are usually treated in the hospital. Some require critical care treatments and must be closely monitored. There is still a significant mortality rate from pneumonia, despite the recognition of pneumonia and use of antibiotics.

Hallmark Signs and Symptoms

- Shortness of breath due to inflammation within the lungs, impairing gas exchange.
- Difficulty breathing (dyspnea) owing to inflammation and mucus within the lungs.
- Fever because of infectious process.
- Chills due to increased temperature.
- Cough due to mucous production and irritation of the airways.
- Crackles owing to fluid within the alveolar space and smaller airways.
- Rhonchi because of mucus in airways; wheezing due to inflammation within the larger airways.
- Discolored, possibly blood-tinged, sputum due to irritation in the airways or microorganisms causing infection.
- Tachycardia and tachypnea as the body attempts to meet the demand for oxygen.
- Pain on respiration because of pleuritic inflammation, pleural effusion, or atelectasis development.
- Headache, muscle aches (myalgia), joint pains, or nausea may be present depending on the infecting organism, and are more typical of an atypical pneumonia.

Common Test Results

- Shadows on CXR, indicating infiltration, may be in a lobar or segmental pattern or more scattered depending on the causative organism.
- Culture and sensitivity of the sputum to identify the infective agent and the appropriate antibiotics.
- Elevated WBC (leukocytosis) showing sign of bacterial infection.
- Low oxygen saturation on pulse oximetry.
- ABG may show low oxygen and elevated carbon dioxide levels.

Treatment

Supplemental oxygen is given to help meet the body's needs. Antibiotics are given for the most likely organism (empirically) until the sputum culture results are returned. Patients may need bronchodilators to help open the airways.

- Administer oxygen as needed.
- For bacterial infections, administer antibiotics such as macrolides (azithromycin, clarithromycin), fluoroquinolones (levofloxacin, moxifloxacin), beta-lactams (amoxicillin/clavulanate, cefotaxime, ceftriaxone, cefuroxime axetil, cefpodoxime, ampicillin/sulbactam), tetracyclines (doxycycline), or ketolide (telithromycin).
- Administer antipyretics when fever is higher than 101°F for patient comfort.
  - acetaminophen, ibuprofen
- Administer bronchodilators to keep airways open, enhance airflow if needed.
  - albuterol, metaproterenol, levalbuterol via nebulizer or metered dose inhaler
- Increase fluid intake to help loosen secretions and prevent dehydration.
- Instruct the patient on how to use the incentive spirometer to encourage deep breathing; monitor progress.

Nursing Diagnoses

- Risk for aspiration
- Impaired ventilation
- Ineffective airway clearance

NURSING INTERVENTION

- Monitor respiration for rate, effort, use of accessory muscles, skin color, and breath sounds.
- Record fluid intake and output for differences, signs of dehydration.
- Record sputum characteristics for changes in color, amount, and consistency.
- Properly dispose of sputum.
- **Explain to the patient:**
  - Take adequate fluids—3 L every day—to prevent excess fluid loss through the respiratory system with exhalation.
  - Use of incentive spirometer.

14. Pneumothorax

What Went Wrong

The pleural sac surrounding the lung normally contains a small amount of fluid to prevent friction as the lungs expand and relax during the respiratory cycle. When air is allowed to enter the pleural space between the lung and the chest wall, a pneumothorax develops. This air pocket takes up space that is normally occupied by lung tissue, causing an area of the lung to partially collapse. If there is a penetrating chest wound, the patient may have an open pneumothorax, also known as a sucking chest wound (for the sound it makes during breathing). A closed pneumothorax may be caused by blunt trauma, postcentral line insertion, or post-thoracentesis. Spontaneous pneumothorax may be secondary to another disease or occur on its own. As the air accumulates, there may be a partial or complete collapse of the lung—the more air that accumulates, the greater the area of collapse. If there is a large enough amount of air trapped between the pleural layers, the tension within the area increases. This increase in tension results in pushing the mediastinum toward the unaffected lung, causing it to partially collapse and compromising venous return to the heart. This is a tension pneumothorax.

Prognosis

Prognosis will vary depending on causes and size of pneumothorax. Any pneumothorax that enlarges or progresses to a tension pneumothorax is a greater risk for the patient. Tension pneumothorax presents a life-threatening situation. A small area of pneumothorax may be monitored without intervention while a larger area requires treatment for resolution of the problem.

Hallmark Signs and Symptoms

- Sharp chest pain, made worse by activity, moving, coughing, and breathing.
- Shortness of breath due to inability to fully expand the lungs during inspiration.
- Absent breath sounds over the affected area because of the presence of air between lungs and chest wall.
- Subcutaneous emphysema (presence of air in the tissue beneath the skin)—a crackling feeling beneath the skin on palpation over the area.

- Tachycardia (increased heart rate) and tachypnea (increased respiratory rate) as body attempts to meet needs.
- Mediastinal shift and tracheal deviation toward the unaffected side with tension pneumothorax.

Common Test Results

- Shadows on CXR, indicating a collapsed lung.
- Increased carbon dioxide shown in ABG.
- Low oxygen saturation on pulse oximetry.

Treatment

Once identified, a pneumothorax can be treated and completely resolved. A tension pneumothorax can become a life-threatening condition. Careful monitoring and early intervention is critical for these patients. A small area may resolve without intervention, but the patient will still be monitored until resolution.

- Bed rest.
- Supplemental oxygen if needed.
- Chest tube connected to suction to re-expand lung if needed.
- Administer analgesic if needed.
  - morphine

Nursing Diagnoses

- Acute pain
- Ineffective breathing
- Impaired gas exchange

NURSING INTERVENTION

- Place patient in high Fowler's or semi-Fowler's position to ease respiratory effort.
- Monitor chest tube for drainage amount and characteristics of output. Note changes.
- Monitor vital signs for changes.
- Monitor respirations for rate, effort, use of accessory muscles, skin color, and breath sounds.

- Teach turning, coughing, and deep-breathing exercises.
- **Explain to the patient:**
  - Disease process.
  - Importance of coughing and deep breathing.

15. Pulmonary Embolism

What Went Wrong

Blood flow is obstructed in the lungs by thrombus (blood clot), air, or fat emboli that become stuck in an artery, causing impaired gas exchange. Patients may be predisposed to clot formation, have pooling of blood, or damage to vessel walls, or take certain medications that increase the risk of thrombus formation. Thrombi are commonly found in vessels in lower extremities. When a thrombus loosens and travels in the peripheral circulation, it is called an embolus. The embolus travels through the right side of the heart and is sent to the lungs where it lodges in one of the arteries. Depending on the size of the artery that the embolus lodges in, a section of lung will have no blood supply and alveolar function will suffer. As blood supply to an area of the lung diminishes, alveoli collapse, causing atelectasis.

There is increased risk for developing a pulmonary embolism in the postoperative period, with prolonged immobility, cancer, pregnancy, exogenous estrogen use, smoking, obesity, or dehydration.

Prognosis

A small area of atelectasis will allow for resolution and return to normal function of the rest of the lung tissue. A large embolus at or near the main pulmonary artery may be fatal. Patients may need to take ongoing anticoagulants if they have repeat episodes or emboli or have an underlying clotting disorder.

Hallmark Signs and Symptoms

- Sudden difficulty breathing (dyspnea) happens when the clot suddenly lodges in the artery.
- Heart rate greater than 100 beats per minute (tachycardia).
- Respiration greater than 20 breaths per minutes (tachypnea) as the body attempts to get more oxygen.
- Chest pain due to clot presence and area of atelectasis.

- Coughing with blood-tinged sputum (hemoptysis).
- Crackles (rales) heard near area of clot.

Common Test Results

- CXR may show dilated pulmonary artery or pleural effusion.
- Lung scan shows ventilation-perfusion mismatch.
- Helical CT scan will show clot in pulmonary arteries.
- Pulmonary angiography will show the presence of clot.
- ABG may show decreased oxygen (PaO_2) and carbon dioxide ($PaCO_2$), depending on the size of the clot.
- D-dimer will be positive when a thromboembolic event has occurred. Other causes will elevate the D-dimer also.
- Lower extremity duplex-venous ultrasound is often done to test for the presence of thrombus.
- MRI may be used in pregnant women to diagnose pulmonary embolism.

Treatment

Treatment is aimed at meeting the body's oxygen needs, preventing the clot from enlarging or moving, and preventing other clots from forming.

- Supplemental oxygen therapy.
- Administer thrombolytics to enhance breakdown of existing clot.
  - recombinant tissue plasminogen activator, urokinase, alteplase
- Administer anticoagulants to prevent further clot formation.
  - heparin, low-molecular-weight heparin, fondaparinux, warfarin
  - Low-molecular-weight heparins are recommended for use in pregnancy.
- Administer analgesic for pain control and to decrease myocardial oxygen demand.
- morphine
- Surgical insertion of a vena cava filter in select patients to catch clots that travel from lower extremities up through inferior vena cava toward lung.
- Bed rest to prevent thrombus from breaking free from lower extremities.
- Surgical removal of the embolus may be necessary in some cases.

Nursing Diagnoses

- Impaired gas exchange
- Ineffective tissue perfusion
- Anxiety

NURSING INTERVENTION

- Monitor cardiovascular status for heart rate, rhythm, heart sounds, and pulse deficit.
- Monitor ABG for changes and decrease in oxygenation.
- Monitor pulse oximetry for oxygen saturation.
- Place patient in high Fowler's position.
- Have the patient perform turning, coughing, and deep-breathing exercises to enhance air movement.
- Monitor respiration for rate, effort, use of accessory muscles, skin color, and lung sounds.
- **Explain to the patient:**
  - To avoid sitting and standing for too long to decrease chance of clot formation.
  - Not to cross legs to avoid constriction of vessels in the lower extremities, decreasing the chances of clot formation.
  - How to identify side effects from using anticoagulants, such as bleeding or bruising.
  - That pulmonary embolism is an adverse effect of using hormonal contraceptives, and a different (nonhormonal) form of birth control needs to be used in the future.

---

16. Respiratory Acidosis

What Went Wrong

Hypoventilation, asphyxia, or central nervous system disorders cause a disturbance in the **acid-base balance** of the patient's blood, resulting in increased carbon dioxide in the blood (hypercapnia). The increase in carbon dioxide in the blood combines with water; this combination releases hydrogen and bicarbonate ions. The brain stem is stimulated and increases the respiratory drive to blow off carbon dioxide. Over time, the sustained elevated arterial carbon dioxide level causes the kidneys to attempt to compensate by retaining bicarbonate and sodium and excreting hydrogen ions.

Prognosis

Respiratory acidosis may be due to an acute or chronic respiratory condition. Respiratory failure results in severe acidosis. The more rapid onset of acidosis does not allow time for the kidneys to compensate. Healthy patients usually can increase the amount of CO_2 that the lungs are getting rid of to assist in lowering the blood levels of CO_2. Patients with underlying respiratory disorders will not be able to rid the body of the excess CO_2 in this way.

Hallmark Signs and Symptoms

- Hypoxemia
- Cardiac arrhythmia or tachycardia due to hypoxemia from hypoventilation
- BP changes depending on underlying cause
- Headache because of hypoxemia
- Difficulty breathing (dyspnea) owing to hypoxemia
- Confusion and restlessness due to hypoxemia
- Irritability because of hypoxemia

Common Test Results

- Carbon dioxide (CO_2) more than 50 mmHg shown in arterial blood gas.
- pH of blood less than 7.35 shows acidosis in arterial blood gas.

Treatment

Treatment is focused on restoring appropriate ventilation, returning carbon dioxide and pH levels to normal.

- Give supplemental oxygen, monitoring flow rate to avoid excess oxygen to those who have chronic pulmonary conditions. The chronic nature of the respiratory acidosis in these patients may have caused the internal respiratory control to adjust in response to a decrease in oxygen level rather than an increase in carbon dioxide level, which is always higher than normal.
- Administer bronchodilators to open constricted airways.
  - albuterol, metaproterenol, levalbuterol
- Administer medications to correct underlying disorder.
- Administer antibiotics ordered as a result of the sensitivity test.
- Mechanical ventilation if necessary to support breathing.
- Treat underlying cause.

Nursing Diagnoses

- Ineffective breathing
- Fear
- Impaired gas exchange

NURSING INTERVENTION

- Monitor respiration for rate, effort, use of accessory muscles, skin color, mucous production, and breath sounds.
- Monitor blood chemistry—potassium, CO_2, chloride.
- **Explain to the patient:**
  - How to administer oxygen therapy.
  - How to perform turning, coughing, and deep-breathing exercises.

---

17. Acute Respiratory Failure

What Went Wrong

The lungs are unable to adequately exchange oxygen and carbon dioxide because of insufficient ventilation. The body is not able to maintain enough oxygen or the body may not get rid of enough carbon dioxide. A respiratory illness can deteriorate into acute respiratory failure. Central nervous system depression (due to trauma or medication) or disease can also lead to acute respiratory failure.

Prognosis

Patients with respiratory failure are not getting enough oxygen. This may be a sudden event or a decompensation of a chronic respiratory condition such as emphysema or chronic bronchitis. Supplemental oxygen and bronchodilating medications are used to enhance airflow to the lungs. The underlying cause needs to be identified and corrected to reverse the problem and return the patient to normal respiratory status.

Hallmark Signs and Symptoms

- Accessory muscles used to breathe as body works harder to move air
- Difficulty breathing (dyspnea) or shortness of breath due to lack of oxygen
  - Air hunger—the subjective feeling that the patient is not getting enough air

- Difficulty breathing when lying down (orthopnea) owing to increased work of breathing in this position; diaphragm has to work harder; posterior chest wall does not expand well
- Fatigue due to work of breathing and lack of oxygenation
- Coughing may be because of inflammation, bronchospasm, fluid, or underlying lung condition
- Blood in sputum (hemoptysis) due to irritation of airways
- Respiration greater than 20 breaths per minute (tachypnea) in attempt to get more air and oxygen into lungs
- Sweating (diaphoresis) as body works harder to move air, using more muscles
- Cyanosis because of hypoxemia
- Anxiety due to air hunger and lack of oxygenation
- Rales (crackles) heard in the lungs if fluid builds up in alveoli and smaller airways
- Wheezing (rhonchi) owing to inflammation within airways
- Diminished breath sounds due to decreased air movement

Common Test Results

- ABG.
  - Decreased oxygen PaO_2 less than 60 mmHg without underlying lung disease
  - Elevated carbon dioxide ($PaCO_2$) more than 50 mmHg without underlying lung disease
  - Arterial oxygen saturation (SaO_2) less than 90%
  - pH less than 7.30 (respiratory acidosis)
- Pulse oximetry shows low oxygen saturation.
- Increased WBC count due to infection.

Treatment

- Oxygen therapy to meet body's needs through nasal canula or mask.
- Administer bronchodilators to enhance airflow through airways in lungs.
  - albuterol, levalbuterol, metaproterenol, terbutaline

- Administer anticholinergics to treat bronchospasm.
  - ipratropium
- Intubation to maintain patent airway and assist mechanical ventilation.
- Administer anesthetic to ease intubation.
  - propofol/etomidate in conjunction with a neuromuscular blocking agent (such as succinylcholine or rocuronium) to create a chemical paralysis which will decrease the likelihood of coughing or gagging during intubation
- Mechanical ventilation to support respiratory effort.
- Administer neuromuscular blocking agent to ease mechanical ventilation so the patient would not fight ventilator.
  - vecuronium, atracurium
- Administer steroids to decrease inflammatory response within lungs.
  - hydrocortisone, methylprednisolone, prednisone
- Administer anticoagulant to reduce risk of clot formation.
  - heparin, warfarin
- Administer analgesic for discomfort and to decrease myocardial oxygen demand.
  - morphine, fentanyl
- Administer histamine-2 blockers or PPI to reduce chances of stress-induced gastric ulcer.
  - famotidine, ranitidine, nizatidine, cimetidine
  - omeprazole, esomeprazole, lansoprazole, rabeprazole, pantoprazole
- Administer antibiotics to treat infection (or may be preventative).
  - Selected according to results of culture and sensitivity study

Nursing Diagnoses

- Ineffective breathing pattern
- Ineffective airway clearance
- Anxiety

NURSING INTERVENTION

- Monitor respiratory status for rate, effort, use of accessory muscles, sputum production, and breath sounds.

- Monitor pulse oximetry to check oxygen saturation levels.
- Monitor sputum for changes in color and amount.
- Monitor vital signs for changes.
- Place patient in high Fowler's or semi-Fowler's position on bed rest to ease respiratory effort by allowing optimal diaphragmatic excursion.
- Monitor ventilator settings if appropriate.
- Change patient position every 2 hours to decrease chance of skin breakdown.
- Monitor intake and output of fluids to check for balance.
- **Explain to the patient:**
  - The importance of doing coughing and deep-breathing exercises to fully expand lungs and enhance the expelling of mucous.
  - How to identify the signs of respiratory distress.

18. Severe Acute Respiratory Syndrome

What Went Wrong

This is a potentially life-threatening viral infection, caused by severe acute respiratory syndrome (SARS)-associated *Coronavirus*. The virus replicates in the respiratory system and gastrointestinal tract. After a patient is infected, the cells are destroyed as the virus reproduces. The cell destruction occurs primarily in the lungs, with alveolar damage being most notable. Chronic hepatitis B infection or diabetes also increase the risk of death. Patients may need intensive care treatment and mechanical ventilation.

Prognosis

Severe acute respiratory syndrome is a serious infection. The outbreak in 2002–2003 resulted in the death of almost 6% of infected patients in North America and almost 10% worldwide. In older patients, there is a higher rate of mortality, approximately half of those over age 65 die from the illness.

Hallmark Signs and Symptoms

- Prior history of exposure to person with SARS.
- Flu-like symptoms (fever, chills, headache, muscle aches, loss of appetite) as virus replicates within the patient. This stage may last up to a week.
- Lower respiratory tract symptoms such as dry cough, shortness of breath, progressing hypoxia. This stage may begin in 3 days after the onset.
- Respiratory failure is possible.

Common Test Results

- CXR is normal in the initial stages; then it shows areas of infiltration that encompass greater areas of the lung as the disease progresses.
- Pulse oximetry will show low oxygen levels.
- White blood cell counts, lymphocytes, and platelet counts are low.
- Creatine kinase, lactate dehydrogenase, aspartate aminotransferase (AST), and alanine aminotransferase (ALT) will be elevated.
- Antibodies may be identified using indirect fluorescent assay or enzyme-linked immunosorbent assay (ELISA) after infection.

Treatment

There is no confirmed treatment plan for SARS.

- Hospitalization, often in intensive care, and isolation
- Mechanical ventilation may be necessary
- Pulse oximetry

Nursing Diagnosis

- Ineffective breathing pattern
- Impaired gas exchange
- Ineffective tissue perfusion

NURSING INTERVENTION

- Monitor respiratory status.
- Maintain isolation.

19. Tuberculosis

What Went Wrong

Tuberculosis (TB) is an infectious disease spread by airborne route. Infection is caused by inhalation of droplets that contain the tuberculosis bacteria, *Mycobacterium tuberculosis* (see Fig. 2–4). An infected person can spread the small airborne particles through coughing, sneezing, or talking. Close contact with those affected people increases the chances of transmission. Once inhaled, the organism typically settles into the lung, but can infect any organ in the body. The organism has an outer capsule.

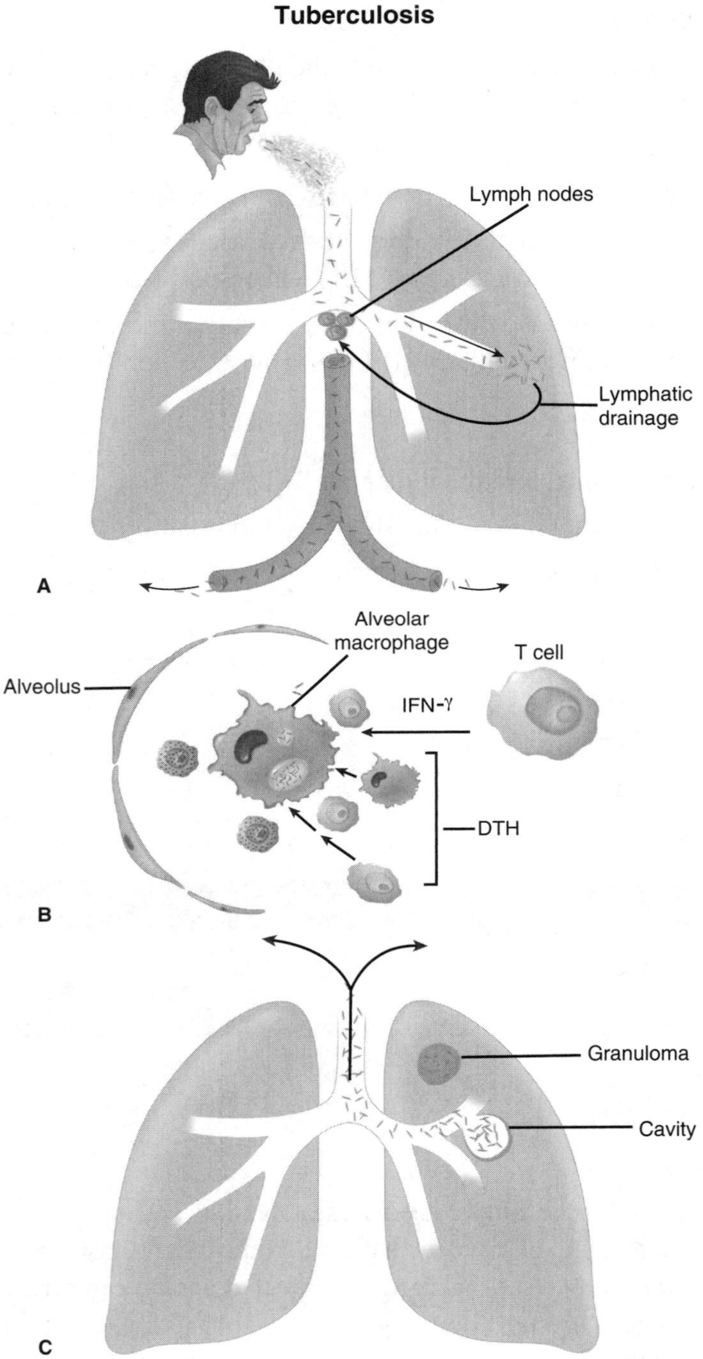

Tuberculosis

FIGURE 2-4 · The primary pathway of tuberculosis infection.

Source: Reproduced with permission from: Ryan KJ, Ray CG: *Sherris Medical Microbiology*, 5th ed. New York, NY: McGraw-Hill, 2010. Fig. 27–4.

Primary TB occurs when the patient is initially infected with the *Mycobacterium*. After being inhaled into the lung, the organism causes a localized reaction. As the body's immune system responds to the infection, surrounding lung tissue is also damaged. The body's immune response to the bacteria creates a granulomatous lesion. Inside this lesion, necrosis (tissue death) occurs. There may also be development of granulomas along the channels of lymph nodes at the same time. These areas create a Ghon's complex, which is a combination of the area initially infected by the airborne bacillus called the Ghon's focus and a lymphatic lesion. The majority of people with newly acquired infections and an adequate immune system will develop latent infection, as the body walls off the infecting organism within these granulomas. The patient will have positive tuberculin skin test but no symptoms of disease. CXR may show granuloma or calcification at this time. Disease is not active in these patients at this point and will not be transmitted until there is some manifestation of the disease. In patients with inadequate immune response, the tuberculosis will be progressive, lung tissue destruction will continue, and other areas of the lung will also be affected.

In secondary TB, the disease is reactivated at a later stage. The patient may be reinfected from droplets, or from a prior primary lesion. Since the patient has previously been infected with TB, the immune response is to rapidly wall off the infection. Cavitation of these areas occurs as the organism travels along the airways.

Exposure to TB occurs when a person has contact with a person suspected or confirmed of having TB. These patients do not have positive skin test, signs or symptoms of disease, or CXR changes. They may or may not have disease.

TB disease is confirmed when a person has its signs and symptoms. The CXR typically has abnormalities in the apical aspects of the lung fields. In HIV patients other areas may also be affected.

Prognosis

Some patients develop drug-resistant TB, making treatment more difficult. The drug-resistant TB may be resistant at the time of initial infection, or may develop as a result of medications during treatment. This occurs either because the treatment was not adequate or not taken appropriately.

Hallmark Signs and Symptoms

- Weight loss and anorexia
- Night sweats

- Fever, possibly low-grade, due to infection
- Productive cough with discolored, blood-tinged sputum
- Shortness of breath owing to lung changes
- Malaise and fatigue because of active illness affecting lungs

Common Test Results

- Positive Mantoux (purified protein derivative [PPD]) skin test shows exposure to tuberculosis due to development of cell-mediated immunity; typically takes between 2 and 10 weeks from time of exposure.
- CXR may show areas of granuloma or cavitation.
- Sputum test identifies *M tuberculosis* bacteria.
  - Acid-fast staining done to initially screen for TB—bacillus will hold stain.
  - Culture confirms the diagnosis but is slow-growing.
  - Interferon-gamma release assays (IGRAs) (blood test) for confirmation of active TB.

Does not give a false-positive with a history of BCG vaccine. Drug susceptibility testing.

Treatment

Patients with active TB are initially placed on respiratory isolation as inpatients to reduce the risk of spreading the organism by droplet infection or aerosolization. Medications are initiated to treat TB and prevent transmission to others. Treatment may be initiated for active disease or for those without active disease who have had recent exposure. Combination therapy is typically used to decrease the likelihood of drug-resistant organisms. Initial treatment times generally range from 6 to 12 months. Longer treatment plans may be necessary for those with HIV infection or drug-resistant strains of TB. Some patient populations are monitored closely for compliance with direct observation of drug treatment. Patient teaching is important for medication protocol compliance and monitoring for side effects. Repeat sputum cultures are typically taken to see that the treatment for active disease is effective.

- Administer antitubercular medications to treat and prevent transmission.
  - isoniazid, rifampin, pyrazinamide, ethambutol, streptomycin

- Respiratory isolation for in-hospital care—the bacteria is spread by droplet.
- Increase protein, carbohydrates, and vitamin C diets for patients.

Nursing Diagnoses

- Fatigue
- Ineffective airway clearance

NURSING INTERVENTION

- Monitor respiration for rate, effort, use of accessory muscles, and skin color changes.
- Increase fluid intake to help liquefy any secretions.
- Record fluid intake and output.
- **Explain to the patient:**
  - How to prevent spreading the disease.
  - The importance of finishing all prescribed medication.
  - Plan for rest periods during the day.

REVIEW QUESTIONS

1. **A 25-year-old nonsmoker who is normally in good health reports having a bad cough for the past 3 weeks. He has crackles and rhonchi, and shows the physician a small clear plastic container that has discolored, blood-tinged sputum that he produced this morning. What would the physician want to rule out?**

   A. Lung cancer.

   B. The flu.

   C. Pneumonia.

   D. Asthma.

2. **The patient hospitalized with bronchitis is concerned that she might have chronic bronchitis. She asks the physician to explain the difference between acute and chronic bronchitis. What is the best response?**

   A. Acute bronchitis lasts for 3 consecutive months and is reversible.

   B. Acute bronchitis lasts 7 to 10 days.

   C. Chronic bronchitis lasts 3 consecutive months in 2 consecutive years, resulting in blockage of the airways and cannot be reversed. Acute bronchitis is caused by a viral or bacterial infection and lasts about 10 days. Blockage of the airways is reversible in acute bronchitis.

   D. The physician needs to explain the differences during his rounds.

3. **The physician has scheduled a thoracentesis. The patient asks why there is so much fluid in the pleural space. The best response is:**

   A. An error occurred and the patient was administered too much IV medication.

   B. The patient's body is unable to remove fluid, resulting in a buildup of fluid in the pleural space around lungs.

   C. This is the result of oxygen therapy.

   D. This is a normal side effect of bumetanide, which is the medication ordered by physician.

4. **A patient reports sudden difficulty breathing with tachypnea and tachycardia and localized chest pain. The physician suspects a pulmonary embolism. What test would you expect the physician to order?**

   A. Helical CT scan.

   B. EKG.

   C. ECC.

   D. Vital capacity.

5. **Following an asthmatic attack, a mother asks the physician how to prevent another asthmatic attack. The physician should:**

   A. Tell her that asthmatic attacks cannot be prevented.

   B. Help the mother identify triggers that cause asthmatic attacks and show her how to avoid them.

   C. Change her medication.

   D. Immediately move her family to a dry climate.

6. **The patient is apprehensive about undergoing bronchoscopy. He cannot imagine having anything inserted into his throat. What is the best response?**

   A. The physician performs this procedure hundreds of times a week.

   B. The physician had it performed 3 years ago and he/she was fine.

   C. The thought of this procedure seems to be disturbing the patient. He/she will be asleep during this procedure. The physician should visit the patient again and answer any questions that he/she has regarding the procedure.

   D. The patient would not feel a thing. He/she will be fine.

7. **A patient who has successfully been treated for a pulmonary embolism is about to be discharged. How can he lower the risk of experiencing another pulmonary embolism?**

   A. Avoid sitting and standing for too long and do not cross legs.

   B. Take vitamin K with heparin.

   C. Avoid confined spaces.

   D. Jog 5 miles each day.

8. **The physician orders a PFT. The patient asks you how the test is performed. The best response is:**

   A. A tube is inserted into lungs while the patient is asleep to expand his/her lungs to their full capacity.

   B. The patient breathes through a mouthpiece into a spirometer until all air in lungs is expelled. Then the patient will take a deep breath through the mouthpiece. This is done three times and a computer calculates the capacity of lungs.

   C. The patient breathes into a spirometer to measure lung capacity.

   D. A computer is used to measure volume and vital capacity.

9. **The patient presents with difficulty breathing and a barrel chest. He is diagnosed with emphysema. The patient asks why increasing oxygen therapy does not relieve his difficulty breathing. The best response is:**

   A. Difficulty breathing is due to air trapped in lungs, reducing the lungs' ability to exchange oxygen and carbon dioxide. Increasing oxygen does not resolve the trapped air.

   B. The patient must lie on his/her right side for oxygen therapy to work properly.

   C. The patient's barrel chest has decreased, causing lungs to overexpand.

   D. The patient must take deeper breaths when receiving oxygen therapy.

   E. Asthma.

10. **The patient returns from the operating room. Why would the physician monitor the patient for atelectasis?**

    A. All postoperative patients are at risk for infection.

    B. Postoperative patients might have received too much oxygen during surgery.

    C. Immobility, anesthesia, and lack of deep breathing place the patient at risk for atelectasis.

    D. Postoperative patients do not receive enough oxygen during surgery.

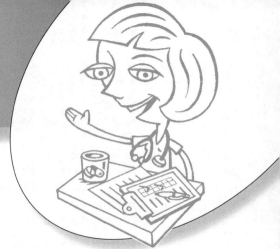

Chapter 3

Immune System

LEARNING OBJECTIVES

At the end of this chapter, the student will be able to:

- Identify normal anatomy and physiology related to the immune system
- Discuss the disease-causing pathologic changes within the immune system
- List four signs or symptoms of specific immunologic disease or injury
- Recognize expected nursing and medical management of immunologic injury or disease

KEY CONCEPTS

1. Acquired immunodeficiency syndrome
2. Anaphylaxis
3. Ankylosing spondylitis
4. Epstein-Barr virus/Chronic fatigue syndrome
5. Kaposi's sarcoma
6. Lyme disease
7. Lymphoma
8. Mononucleosis
9. Rheumatoid arthritis
10. Scleroderma
11. Septic shock
12. Systemic lupus erythematosus

KEY TERMS

Allergies
Anaphylaxis
Antigen
Autoimmune disorders
B cells
Exudation
Histamines
Human immunodeficiency virus (HIV)

Hypersensitivity reactions
Immunodeficiency disorders
Lymphocytes
Reed-Sternberg cells
T cells
Tryptase
Urticaria
Western blot

How the Immune System Works

Normal functioning of the immune system protects the body against the invasion of outside organisms. A variety of organisms are capable of this; however, not all are harmful. The cells of the immune system recognize organisms that invade the body, then isolate and destroy them. At times, the immune system is not able to adequately function in this capacity. This results in infection, **immunodeficiency disorders**, **autoimmune disorders**, **allergies**, and **hypersensitivity reactions**.

Lymphocytes are the primary cells of the immune system. Lymphocytes are divided into B cells and T cells (see Fig. 3–1). **B cells** provide a humoral

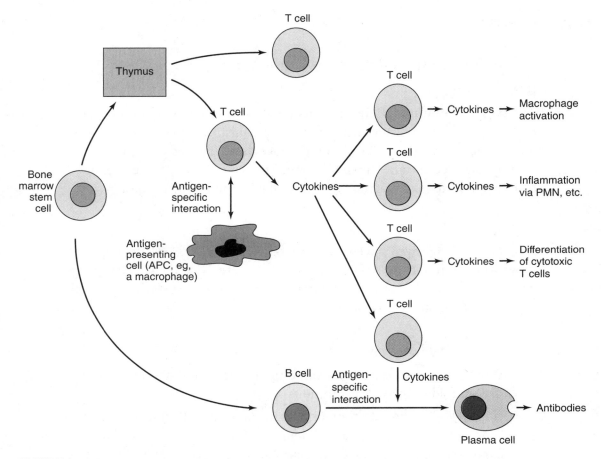

FIGURE 3−1 · Schematic diagram of the cellular interactions in the immune response.

Source: Reproduced with permission from: Brooks GF, Carroll KC, Butel JS, Morse SA, Mietzner TA: *Jawetz, Melnick, & Adelberg's Medical Microbiology*, 25th ed. New York, NY: McGraw-Hill; 2010, Fig. 8–2.

immune response, since they produce an antigen-specific antibody (an **antigen** is a foreign protein or chemical marker present on the outer membrane surrounding an invading cell). **T cells** provide a cellular immune response. Mature T cells are composed of CD4 and CD8 cells. CD8 cells are responsible for destroying foreign and viral inhabited cells, and they suppress immunologic functions. CD4 cells, also known as helper T cells, stimulate immune functions, such as B cells and macrophages. A macrophage is a cell whose functions include ingesting foreign body or invading cells.

Just the Facts

1. Acquired Immunodeficiency Syndrome

What Went Wrong

The **human immunodeficiency virus (HIV)** causes malfunction of T cells that protect the body from invading microorganisms. When it enters a cell, HIV replicates, causing the cell to reproduce more infected cells. It also frequently causes cell death. The CD4 lymphocyte is most often affected, followed by B lymphocytes and macrophages. It results in immunodeficiency.

Prognosis

Prognosis has improved since HIV was discovered in 1981. Fewer patients are progressing from HIV to AIDS, and both classes are living longer. New drugs and therapies are decreasing the number of deaths. Patients are living with fewer disabilities and comorbidities.

Hallmark Signs and Symptoms

- Anorexia—secondary to gastrointestinal (GI) manifestations, oral disease, and side effects of medications
- Fatigue—cells dying at an abnormal rate; opportunistic infections due to a poorly functioning immune system
- Night sweats—immune system–triggered response
- Fever—may be owing to a concurrent infection related to a low white blood cell (WBC) count
- Malnutrition—because of poor appetite and nutrition, nausea and vomiting, and most often from a secondary infection; decreased protein synthesis

Common Test Results

- Less than 200 T cells per microliter—the CD4 lymphocyte is the most commonly used count; less than 200 cells per microliter signals the process from HIV to AIDS, and thus it increases the risk for malignancies and advancing infection.
- Positive HIV antibody titer—95% positive 6 weeks after contact. Often used with the **Western blot** to confirm diagnosis.
- Positive Western blot—confirms positive HIV test.

Treatment

- High-calorie and high-protein diets to combat wasting and weight loss.
- Administer antibiotics to combat opportunistic infections.
  - trimethoprim/sulfamethoxazole
- Administer antiviral medication to suppress HIV replication, causing support of the immune system and fewer opportunistic infections.
- Nucleoside analogs (have antiviral activity).
  - didanosine
  - zidovudine
  - stavudine
  - zalcitabine
- Nucleotide analog.
  - tenofovir
- Protease inhibitors (suppress HIV replication).
  - Fortovase
  - ritonavir
  - indinavir
  - nelfinavir
- Nonnucleoside reverse transcriptase inhibitors (stop reverse transcriptase at a different site).
  - nevirapine
  - delavirdine
  - efavirenz
- Administer antiemetic to combat nausea.
  - prochlorperazine
- Administer antifungal medication to combat fungal infections, which are often opportunistic.
  - fluconazole

Nursing Diagnoses

- Hopelessness
- Social isolation
- Ineffective protection

NURSING INTERVENTION

- Maintain activity as tolerated and schedule rest periods to maintain physical functioning.
- Avoid exposure to blood to prevent the spread of the virus.
- **Explain to the patient:**
  - Use of condoms to prevent the spread of the virus.

2. Anaphylaxis

What Went Wrong

Anaphylaxis occurs when an allergen, usually food or medication, enters the body causing the release of **histamines**, which result in capillaries dilating and smooth muscle contracting (see Fig. 3–2). This results in edema, respiratory distress, hypotension, and skin changes, leading to an allergic reaction. Lesser degrees of extreme allergy are **urticaria** (hives) and angioedema (swelling caused by **exudation**, or escape of fluid, cells, and cellular debris from blood vessels).

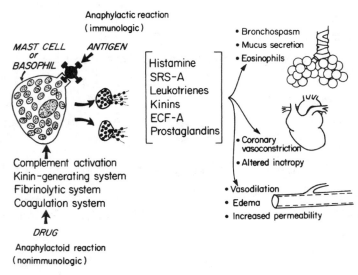

FIGURE 3–2 • Pathophysiologic changes that occur in anaphylaxis, as an allergen enters the body (top) and combines with immunoglobulin E antibodies on the surface of mast cells and basophils. The mast cells and basophils degranulate, releasing mediators such as histamine. The release of these substances is associated with some of the signs and symptoms of anaphylaxis, including bronchospasm; pharyngeal, glottic, and pulmonary edema; vasodilation; hypotension; decreased cardiac contractility and arrhythmias; subcutaneous edema; and urticaria.

Source: Reproduced with permission from: Hall JB, Schmidt GA, Wood LDH: *Principles of Critical Care*, 3rd ed. New York, NY: McGraw-Hill; 2005, Fig. 106–1.

Prognosis

Prognosis may be guarded, depending on how severe the reaction is and how quickly treatment is rendered. Patients need to be monitored for 1 to 2 days after treatment and cautioned about reexposure to the offending item.

Hallmark Signs and Symptoms

- Shortness of breath due to swelling of the larynx
- Hypotension and shock owing to generalized vasodilation
- Sneezing—a common occurrence to an allergen
- Anxiety secondary to difficulty in breathing
- Rales (crackles) heard in the lungs—because of fluid in the lungs
- Wheezing (rhonchi) due to bronchospasm

Common Test Results

Tryptase levels are from mast cells that increase in anaphylaxis. After the acute episode is over, allergy skin testing is recommended.

Treatment

- Administer emergency medications.
  - epinephrine to open airways and to reduce bronchospasm
  - corticosteroids to reduce symptoms
  - antihistamines to mitigate symptoms
- Administer circulatory volume expanders to treat hypotension caused by vasodilation.
  - saline
  - plasma
  - IV fluids
- Administer vasopressors to counteract vasodilation and to increase blood pressure.
  - norepinephrine
  - dopamine
- Oxygen therapy to support breathing.
- Insert endotracheal tube to maintain airway.

Nursing Diagnoses

- Decrease cardiac output
- Risk for suffocation
- Anxiety

NURSING INTERVENTION

- Maintain airway to facilitate breathing.
- Monitor for hoarseness and difficulty breathing to check for symptoms of decreased respiration.
- **Explain to the patient:**
  - Avoid exposure to allergens to prevent future occurrences.
  - Seek medical help immediately if exposed to allergens to prevent anaphylaxis.

---

3. Ankylosing Spondylitis

What Went Wrong

Ankylosing spondylitis (AS) is a progressive form of arthritis that affects less than 1% of the population. Joints between the spine and pelvis become inflamed, as do some of the ligaments, resulting in instability of the joints. Heredity factors play an important role in the development of AS. The disease is strongly associated with the presence of histocompatibility antigen HLA-B27 on the chromosomes of affected individuals. It begins in the sacroiliac joints and spreads up the spine.

Prognosis

The course of the disease may vary in each case and from individual to individual. Some have episodes of transient back pain while others have more chronic severe back pain that leads to varying degrees of spinal stiffness over time. The disease is characterized by acute painful exacerbations and remissions.

Hallmark Signs and Symptoms

- Severe lower back pain after a period of inactivity because of inflammation and stiffness.
- Reduced motion of the lumbar area of the spine due to the pain of inflammation.

Common Test Results

- Spinal x-ray: joints show the characteristic bamboo spine that is a late sign. Early x-rays may show arthritic erosion.
- Blood serum contains the HLA-B27 antigen, which is present in about 90% of those with AS.
- Elevated erythrocyte sedimentation rate (ESR).

Treatment

Nonpharmacologic measures include patient education, family education, genetic counseling, positioning, extension exercises, and physical therapy. The primary goals are to relieve pain, decrease inflammation, begin strengthening exercises, and maintain good posture and function. Medications take an empiric approach. If one nonsteroidal anti-inflammatory drug (NSAID) is not effective for that particular patient, another is tried. Corticosteroids should not be utilized for long-term treatment due to the systemic effects.

- Stretching exercises—to maintain flexibility.
- Back brace—to maintain posture.
- Administer NSAID—to decrease inflammation and for the analgesic effect.
  - aspirin
  - ibuprofen
  - indomethacin
  - sulfasalazine
  - sulindac
- Physical therapy.

Nursing Diagnoses

- Activity intolerance
- Impaired physical mobility
- Chronic pain

NURSING INTERVENTION

- Administer intermittent heat to the lumbar area of the spine for symptom relief.
- Massage the lumbar area of the spine for symptom relief.
- Provide comfort to the patient.

> - **Explain to the patient:**
>   - It is best to sit in a high-backed chair for posture.
>   - Repeated attempts to maintain erect posture.

4. Epstein-Barr Virus/Chronic Fatigue Syndrome

What Went Wrong

Chronic fatigue syndrome (CFS) is a chronic, multisymptom, multisystem syndrome in a previously healthy adult. It results from any of five so far known viruses: Epstein-Barr virus (EBV), cytomegalovirus (CMV), coxsackievirus B, adenovirus type I, and human herpesvirus 6. In an unknown way, the viruses disturb the immune system that is then unable to adequately fight off the virus.

Prognosis

The prognosis varies as the disease waxes and wanes. Remissions and exacerbations may be frequent. By adulthood, most of the population in the United States will test positive for EB virus.

Hallmark Signs and Symptoms

- Persistent fatigue unrelieved by rest.
- Impairment of memory and concentration.
- Myalgias, arthralgias, headache, change in sleep, malaise, depression, and labile mood.
- Insomnia is a common occurrence.

Common Test Results

Since CFS is a diagnosis of exclusion, testing is done to rule out other etiologies for the symptoms. These may include complete blood count (CBC), metabolic panel, thyroid studies, HIV, ESR, rheumatoid factor, Lyme, EBV, and CMV titers.

Treatment

Treatment is empirical and based on symptoms. Treating and eliminating other diagnoses is imperative. Frequent rest periods and adequate nutrition are necessary. Pharmacologic treatment may include NSAIDs and analgesics. As there is a higher prevalence of past and present psychiatric diagnoses in patients with

CFS, an evaluation may be indicated. Psychotherapy may help. Physical therapy is often indicated, and routine exercising has been found to be helpful.

Nursing Diagnoses

- Activity intolerance
- Fatigue
- Chronic pain

NURSING INTERVENTION

- Provide supportive care.
- Encourage fluids and adequate nutrition.
- Rest.
- Offer psychotherapy.
- Exercise regimen.

5. Kaposi's Sarcoma

What Went Wrong

Kaposi's sarcoma (KS) is an overgrowth of blood vessels, which leads to malignant tumors and cancer of lymphatic tissue and skin, and is commonly found in patients with AIDS. It is usually seen in cases of advanced AIDS.

Prognosis

Kaposi's sarcoma is often associated with AIDS. The treatment of AIDS with antiretrovirals usually helps the symptoms of KS.

Hallmark Signs and Symptoms

- Red, brown, and purple lesions on the buccal mucosa, lips, gums, tongue, and palates because it is a malignancy affecting the skin and mucosa.
- Difficulty breathing (dyspnea) if the malignancy invades the pulmonary system.

Common Test Results

- Biopsy to look for the HIV virus and B lymphocytes
- CT scan to determine metastasis of the lesion to ascertain the severity of the disease

Treatment

The treatment for KS is often specific for the individual lesion, using radiation. Treatment for AIDS will also ameliorate, to some degree, the effects of AIDS.

- Radiation in the affected tissue to shrink and treat tumors. Laser surgery may be utilized to remove some lesions.
- Administer antiemetic medication to counter effects of chemotherapy and radiation.
  - trimethobenzamide
- Administer chemotherapy medication to slow or halt the disease.
  - doxorubicin
  - etoposide
  - vinblastine
  - vincristine

Nursing Diagnoses

- Disturbed body image
- Ineffective protection
- Risk for infection

NURSING INTERVENTION

- Monitor skin for lesions to determine new lesions and/or metastasis.
- Daily weighing to determine changes in weight from baseline.
- **Explain to the patient:**
  - The need for dietary changes, such as a high-protein, high-calorie diet.
  - How to conserve energy.
  - Hospice care.

---

6. Lyme Disease

What Went Wrong

A bite from a deer tick causes the bacteria (a spirochete) *Borrelia burgdorferi*, to be transmitted into the human bloodstream. The patient presents with fever, myalgias, the classic bull's eye rash, and erythema chronicum migrans up to 3 weeks following the bite.

Prognosis

Early treatment generally leads to a better outcome. Lingering constitutional symptoms occasionally occur.

Hallmark Signs and Symptoms

- Fever
- Generalized aches
- Headache
- Rash at site of the bite (patient may not recall bite)

Common Test Results

- IgM antibody is elevated.
- Lyme titers may be drawn.

Treatment

- doxycycline, 100 mg bid (twice a day) × 14 to 21 days
- aqueous penicillin G, 20 million units
- ceftriaxone, 4 g per day IM or IV

Nursing Diagnoses

- Impaired skin integrity
- Impaired physical mobility

NURSING INTERVENTION

- Cover all exposed skin while outside.
- Use appropriate insect repellant.
- Inspect arms and legs for ticks when coming in from outside.
- Inspect pets.
- Educate on proper way to remove tick.

7. Lymphoma

What Went Wrong

Functionless and damaged cells of the lymphatic system undergo overgrowth, decreasing the effectiveness of the lymphatic system. There are two main types of lymphoma, characterized by painless lymph node swelling:

- Hodgkin's disease (see Fig. 3–3) is malignant lymphoma characterized by the presence of **Reed-Sternberg cells**. There are four stages of Hodgkin's disease:
  - Stage I—Reed-Sternberg cells appear in one lymph node region.
  - Stage II—Reed-Sternberg cells appear in multiple lymph node regions on the same side of the diaphragm.
  - Stage III—Reed-Sternberg cells appear in multiple lymph node regions on both sides of the diaphragm.
  - Stage IV—Reed-Sternberg cells appear throughout the body.
- Non-Hodgkin's lymphoma (NHL) is cancer of the B lymphocytes and is characterized by the absence of Reed-Sternberg cells.

The lymphomas are caused by a disruption of cells during differentiation. Diagnosis is made on lymph node biopsy.

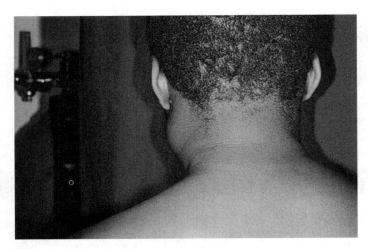

FIGURE 3–3 • A 13-year-old adolescent boy with enlarged lymph nodes extended over both posterior and anterior triangles of the neck. A lymph node biopsy confirmed the diagnosis of Hodgkin's lymphoma.

Source: Reproduced with permission from: Tintinalli JE, Stapczynski JS, Ma OJ, Cline DM, Cydulka RK, Meckler GD: *Tintinalli's Emergency Medicine: A Comprehensive Study Guide,* 7th ed. New York, NY: McGraw-Hill; 2011, Fig. 136–2.

Prognosis

Prognosis depends on what stage the patient was in upon diagnosis, and on response to treatment. Survival is generally less than 10 years for non-Hodgkin's and may be more for Hodgkin's, with an optimistic staging.

Hallmark Signs and Symptoms

- B symptoms (night sweats, fever, and weight loss)
- Enlarged, painless lymph nodes in the cervical region, mesentery, abdomen, and pelvis

Common Test Results

- Lymph node biopsy contains Reed-Sternberg cells, which typify Hodgkin's disease.
- Bone marrow biopsy contains follicular type cells (non-Hodgkin's lymphoma).

Treatment

Treatment depends on the staging, which is based on the number of involved lymph nodes, the number of cavities, and bone marrow involvement.

- Radiation in the affected tissue to shrink the nodes.
- Administer Hodgkin's disease medication.
  - vincristine
  - doxorubicin
  - bleomycin
  - dacarbazine
- Administer non-Hodgkin's lymphoma medication.
  - cyclophosphamide
  - vincristine
  - doxorubicin
  - rituximab
  - prednisone
  - radiation

Nursing Diagnoses

- Impaired tissue integrity
- Risk for infection
- Ineffective protection

NURSING INTERVENTION

- Monitor vital signs to determine variations from baseline.
- Monitor for complications such as new palpable lymph nodes and fever.
- Increase fluid intake.
- Increase calories, protein, iron, calcium, vitamins, and minerals to counteract weight loss.
- Administer prescribed antiemetic medication for nausea.
- Monitor laboratory results for blood counts in response to chemotherapy.
- **Explain to the patient:**
  - Consult with physician before using over-the-counter medication.

---

8. Mononucleosis

Mononucleosis is a viral syndrome consisting of sore throat, enlarged lymph glands, and fevers. It is usually caused by the Epstein-Barr virus, but sometimes other viruses are the cause. Occasionally, a rash may be seen. The spleen is sometimes enlarged due to sequestration of cells during the immune response.

What Went Wrong

A virus is transmitted from contact to contact. Often, a secondary bacterial infection, *Streptococcus*, is found.

Prognosis

Prognosis is good. Since it is a disease of young people, recovery is generally uncomplicated.

Hallmark Sign and Symptoms

- General malaise
- Fever
- Myalgias

- Headache
- Sore throat

Common Test Results

- Monospot or a positive heterophil antibody test is used to identify the Epstein-Barr virus.
- CBC, chemistry.
- Throat culture for *Streptococcus*.

Treatment

Treatment is supportive with rest and over-the-counter medications for symptom resolution.

- Penicillin or erythromycin for coexistent streptococcal throat, if present.

Nursing Diagnoses

- Fatigue
- Activity intolerance
- Impaired physical mobility

NURSING INTERVENTION

- Encourage adequate rest.
- Assure fluids and nutritional intake.
- Monitor fever and vital signs.
- Throat culture, if indicated.
- Analgesics.

---

9. Rheumatoid Arthritis

What Went Wrong

Antibodies from the bloodstream move into the synovial lining of joints, causing joints to swell. The swelling affects the functionality of tendons, bones, and ligaments that move the joint, resulting in pain with movement. Etiology is unknown, although genetics plays a part. The usual age of onset is 20 to 40 years, and it affects about 2% of the population. Inflammation and nodules around joints are common, usually involving the wrists, hands, knees, and feet.

Prognosis

Prognosis is variable. Some patients go into remission and need only moderate treatment. Others progress with decreased functioning, with cardiac, renal, and respiratory disease. Life expectancy is greatly lessened for this group.

Hallmark Signs and Symptoms

- Morning stiffness in joints due to the inflammation
- Enlarged joints from swelling
- Pain when moving due to the stiffness
- Limited range of motion (ROM) because of the inflammation and pain
- Fever, malaise, and weight loss

Common Test Results

- Rheumatoid factor is positive in blood test.
- Positive antinuclear antibody (ANA).
- Positive ESR.
- Gamma globulins.
- X-rays show changes in the affected joints.

Treatment

Reduction of pain and inflammation is the goal of treatment, along with preserving range of motion of the joint. Treatment is divided into nonpharmacologic and pharmacologic methods.

- Administer NSAID medication to decrease inflammation and pain.
  - ibuprofen
  - indomethacin
  - flurbiprofen
  - naproxen
  - sulindac
  - diflunisal

- Administer disease-modifying antirheumatic drugs (DMARDs).
  - methotrexate is an antimetabolite
- Tumor necrosis factor 1 (TNF1) increases lymphocytes and leukocytes found in the joint fluids.
  - etanercept
  - infliximab
  - adalimumab
  - antimalarials
  - hydroxychloroquine
- Administer corticosteroids.
  - prednisone
- Administer antacids to coat the stomach.
  - magnesium hydroxide
  - aluminium hydroxide
- Physical therapy and occupational therapy to maintain ADL and independence.
- Cold and heat therapy for pain relief, anti-inflammatory effect, to help muscles and joints.
- Splints to maintain joints in positions that are most used.
- Exercises to maintain flexibility and ROM.

Nursing Diagnoses

- Chronic pain
- Activity intolerance
- Disturbed body image

NURSING INTERVENTION

- Assist the patient in placing a splint on affected joint.
- Weight loss to place less stress on joints.
- **Explain to the patient:**
  - Get a full night's sleep.
  - Avoid the cold.
  - Reduce stress.

10. Scleroderma

What Went Wrong

Antibodies attack connective tissues in an autoimmune response. This results in scar tissue (fibrosis) forming on skin, organs, GI tract, blood vessels, and muscles, causing systemic sclerosis.

It is a chronic disease of unknown etiology, usually seen in 30- to 50-year-olds.

Prognosis

Scleroderma is a progressive disease causing early death, especially in those patients with diffuse disease. Organ damage indicates an earlier demise; those with limited organ involvement have longer life expectancies.

Hallmark Signs and Symptoms

- Stiffness and pain due to the fibrosis
- Skin thickens
- Edema, malaise, and fever

Common Test Results

- Positive antinuclear antibody.
- Dermis appears thickened in skin biopsy.

Treatment

Treatment is based on treating the patient's symptoms to ensure comfort. No known medications are able to stop the disease. Various medications may be used to treat the symptoms of the affected organs caused by scleroderma.

- Physical therapy to maintain joint mobility

Nursing Diagnoses

- Impaired physical mobility
- Impaired skin integrity
- Pain

NURSING INTERVENTION

- Monitor for increasing blood pressure, which is the leading cause of death to scleroderma patients due to the renal effects of the disease.
- **Explain to the patient:**
  - That there is no cure for scleroderma, but it may go into remission and then relapse.
  - Schedule rest periods during activities.
  - Avoid the cold.

11. Septic Shock

What Went Wrong

Septic shock starts with bacteremia, usually gram-negative bacteria infecting the blood. The sources are usually genitourinary system, GI tract, and lungs. The infection may be underlying for some time before shock develops. Once the cascade from bacteremia to septic shock starts, it may be difficult to halt the process. Shock may occur more quickly in patients who are elderly, immune-compromised, or with other comorbidities. In response to a bacterial infection, TNF-alpha and other inflammatory chemicals are released into the blood, causing an increase in the blood leaking from vessels into both the infected and noninfected tissues (vascular permeability).

Prognosis

Prognosis depends on the general state of the patient, on the type of bacteria, how quickly a definitive diagnosis is made, and the originating source(s) of the bacteremia. Mortality rates vary from 40% to 80%.

Hallmark Signs and Symptoms

- Nausea and vomiting from the source of the infection
- Temperature over 101°F due to infection
- Hypotension because of fluid displacement, vasodilation
- Tachycardia from fever and infection
- Tachypnea from fever and infection
- Lactic acidosis results from poor oxygenation

Common Test Results

- WBC 15,000 to 30,000—indicates infection.
- Decreased platelet count—blood coagulopathies are common in shock.
- Abnormal prothrombin time (PT) and partial thromboplastin time (PTT)—blood coagulopathies.

Treatment

Treatment result depends on the individual. Varying responses are due to the variable immune and inflammatory responses of each patient and their comorbidities. Treatment depends on identifying the organism, the source of the bacteremia, the appropriate antibiotic, and maintaining normal vital signs.

- Antibiotic specific for the type of bacteria present
- Fluid resuscitation

Nursing Diagnoses

- Decreased cardiac output
- Deficient fluid volume
- Skin integrity

NURSING INTERVENTION

- Monitor vital signs, especially fever.
- Monitor fluid intake and output to assess for fluid overload and hydration status.
- Monitor coagulation factors.

12. Systemic Lupus Erythematosus

What Went Wrong

Systemic lupus erythematosus (SLE) is a chronic inflammatory immune disorder affecting the skin and other body organs. Antibodies to DNA and RNA cause an autoimmune inflammatory response, resulting in swelling and pain. It is most common in young women and has a strong genetic factor. The etiology is not known.

Prognosis

Prognosis is good but is consistent with many remissions and exacerbations. Most patients do quite well on a course of medications, but some progress rapidly with severe organ involvement and, subsequently, death. Certain medications may produce lupus-like symptoms in patients. A review of medications is indicated before a diagnosis is made.

Hallmark Signs and Symptoms

- Butterfly rash on face due to deposition of immunoglobulin and complement in the skin
- Fatigue may be because of anemia
- Anemia owing to inflammation
- Fever, malaise
- Joint pain

Common Test Results

- Positive antinuclear antibody test—antibodies are present in the blood.
- Positive rheumatoid factor.
- CBC may show anemia due to hemolysis of RBCs, low WBC, and low platelets.
- Positive Sm antibodies, cardiolipin antibodies, or double-stranded DNA.
- Urine tests may reveal excess protein or cellular casts if the kidneys are affected.

Treatment

Treatment of SLE is supportive. The drugs used should match the stage the patient is in at the time. Treatment of systemic signs is dependent on the organ system involved.

- Administer NSAIDs to decrease the inflammation and give analgesic effects.
  - ibuprofen
  - flurbiprofen

- indomethacin
- sulindac
- naproxen
- diclofenac
- Antimalarials—used to treat joint manifestations and skin rashes.
  - hydroxychloroquine
- Administer immunosuppressants in patients who are unresponsive to corticosteroids.
  - azathioprine
  - cyclophosphamide
  - mycophenolate
  - leflunomide
  - methotrexate
  - benlimumab
- Administer analgesic.
  - NSAIDs
  - aspirin
  - acetaminophen
  - tramadol

Nursing Diagnoses

- Impaired mobility
- Disturbed body image
- Ineffective protection
- Chronic pain

NURSING INTERVENTION

- Avoid sunlight.
- Cover butterfly rash with cosmetics.
- Reduce stress.
- Monitor for infections.

REVIEW QUESTIONS

1. **The primary mode of treatment for ankylosing spondylitis is:**
   A. Relaxed posture for comfort.
   B. Strict bed rest.
   C. Physical therapy.
   D. Respiratory therapy.

2. **When assessing a patient for anaphylaxis, be alert for:**
   A. Chest pain and indigestion.
   B. Hives and dyspnea.
   C. Hypertension and blurred vision.
   D. Headache and photophobia.

3. **The best treatment for mononucleosis is:**
   A. Antibiotics.
   B. Physical therapy.
   C. NSAIDs.
   D. Rest and fluids.

4. **A cell whose functions include ingesting foreign or invading cells is a (an):**
   A. T cell.
   B. B cell.
   C. Macrophage.
   D. Erythrocyte.

5. **Which of the following would have the highest priority in septic shock?**
   A. Monitoring temperature.
   B. Monitoring airway, breathing, circulation (ABC).
   C. Monitoring pupillary reaction.
   D. Monitoring ANA and RF levels.

6. **Patients with rheumatoid arthritis typically have pain:**
   A. With activity.
   B. Upon awakening.
   C. Late in the evening.
   D. All day without remission.

7. **During exacerbations of SLE, patients are often treated with:**
   A. Antiemetics.
   B. Antineoplastics.

C. Corticosteroids.

D. Antibiotics.

8. **A confirmatory lab test for HIV includes:**

A. Western blot.

B. Low WBC.

C. Comprehensive metabolic panel.

D. Enzyme-linked immunosorbent assay (ELISA).

9. **In a patient with a CD4 count less than 200, the most important nursing assessment would include:**

A. Bowel movements.

B. Urinary output.

C. Fever.

D. Blood pressure.

10. **The joints most commonly involved with rheumatoid arthritis include:**

A. Symmetrical involvement of major joints.

B. Small joints of hands and feet.

C. Spine, from the sacrum upward to cervical.

D. Slightly movable joints of the axial skeleton.

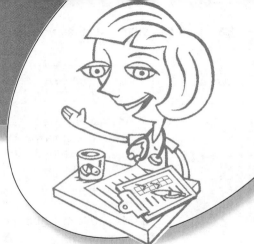

Chapter 4

Hematologic System

At the end of this chapter, the student will be able to:

- Identify normal anatomy and physiology related to the hematologic system
- Discuss the disease-causing pathologic changes within the hematologic system
- List four signs or symptoms of specific hematologic disease or injury
- Recognize expected nursing and medical treatment of hematologic injury or disease

KEY CONCEPTS

1. Anemia
2. Aplastic anemia (pancytopenia)
3. Deep Vien Thrombosis
4. Disseminated intravascular coagulation
5. Hemophilia
6. Idiopathic thrombocytopenic purpura
7. Iron Deficiency anemia
8. Leukemia
9. Multiple myeloma
10. Polycythemia vera
11. Pernicious anemia
12. Sickle cell anemia
13. Von Willebrand disease

KEY TERMS

Clotting factors
Ecchymosis
Epistaxis
Hematocrit
Hemoglobin
Hemolysis
Leukopenia
Lymphocytes
Macrophages

Microemboli
Partial thromboplastin time (PTT)
Petechiae
Prothrombin
Prothrombin time (PT)
Purpura
Stem cells
Thrombocytopenia

How the Hematologic System Works

The hematologic system refers to the blood and blood-forming organs. The formation of red blood cells (RBCs), white blood cells (WBCs), and platelets begins in the bone marrow (see Fig. 4–1). **Stem cells** are produced in the bone marrow. Initially, these cells are not differentiated and may become RBCs, WBCs, or platelets. In the next stage of development, the stem cell becomes committed to a particular precursor cell, to become either a myeloid or lymphoid type of cell and will differentiate into a particular cell type in the presence of a specific growth factor.

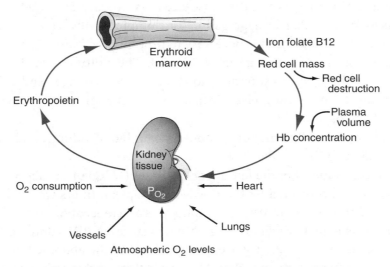

FIGURE 4–1 • Diagram of the physiologic regulation of RBC production called erythropoiesis.
Source: Reproduced with permission from: Longo DL, Fauci AS, Kasper DL, Hauser SL, Jameson JL, Loscalzo J: *Harrison's Principles of Internal Medicine*, 18th ed. New York, NY: McGraw-Hill; 2012. Fig. 57–1.

Erythropoietin is a hormone that is produced in the kidneys and controls the production of RBCs within the bone marrow. RBC production is ongoing as an individual RBC has an expected lifespan of about 120 days. RBCs contain hemoglobin which is a protein that transports oxygen from the lungs to the cells of the body. Alterations in normal body function can change the production of RBCs. For example, the body may attempt to create an increased number of RBCs in the presence of hypoxia or in those individuals living at high altitude in an attempt to improve the oxygen-carrying capability of the blood. Individuals lacking in certain nutrients may not be able to adequately meet the demand for RBC production as iron, vitamin B12, and folic acid are necessary for production of RBCs. The body initially produces reticulocytes which are immature RBCs and will mature within 48 hours of release into the bloodstream.

White blood cells or leukocytes protect the body from infection and are composed of granulocytes, monocytes, and **lymphocytes**. Granulocytes and monocytes remove bacteria and other foreign particles by phagocytosis. There are various kinds of lymphocytes; B cells (which produce antibodies to attack invading microorganisms, such as bacteria or viruses) and T cells (which destroy the body's own cells that are infected or cancerous).

Blood typically clots when there has been damage to a blood vessel. Platelets initially adhere to the disrupted edges of the vessel in a process called aggregation. This triggers a clotting cascade. These initial platelets attract more platelets to the area. Platelet aggregation (or clumping) will create a temporary plug at the site of injury and is necessary to prevent blood loss. Fibrin strands come to the area and create an insoluble clot. The clotting cascade has two components: intrinsic (responding to direct vessel damage) and extrinsic (responding to everything else—inflammation, malignancy, extravascular damage, hypoxia, etc.).

Plasma comprises the majority, about 55%, of blood volume, and the cells comprise about 45% (see Fig. 4–2).

The spleen is found in the left upper quadrant (LUQ) of the abdomen and is normally well protected by the ribcage. The spleen filters whole blood. It removes old and imperfect WBCs (lymphocytes and **macrophages**) and RBCs. The spleen also breaks down **hemoglobin** and stores of RBCs and platelets.

The liver is found in the right upper quadrant of the abdomen and is the main production site for many of the **clotting factors**, including **prothrombin**. Normal liver function is important for vitamin K production in the intestinal tract. Vitamin K is necessary for clotting factors VII, IX, X, and prothrombin.

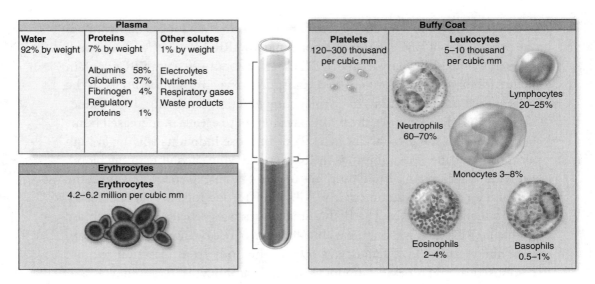

FIGURE 4–2 · Composition of whole blood. A tube of blood after centrifugation (center) has about 43% of its volume represented by erythrocytes (RBCs) in the bottom half of the tube, a volume called the hematocrit. Between the sedimented erythrocytes and the supernatant light-colored plasma is a thin layer of leukocytes and platelets called the buffy coat. The average concentrations of erythrocytes, platelets, and leukocytes in normal blood are included here, along with the percentage each type of leukocyte represents in the buffy coat. A cubic millimeter of blood is equivalent to a microliter (μL).

Source: Reproduced with permission from: Mescher AL: *Junqueira's Basic Histology: Text and Atlas,* 12th ed. New York, NY: McGraw-Hill; 2010. Fig. 12–1.

Just the Facts

1. Anemia

What Went Wrong

A low hemoglobin or RBC count results in a decreased oxygen-carrying capability of the blood. This may be owing to blood loss, damage to the RBCs due to altered hemoglobin or destruction (**hemolysis**), nutritional deficiency (iron, vitamin B12, folic acid), lack of RBC production, or bone marrow failure. Some patients have a family history of anemia due to genetic transmission, such as thalassemia or sickle cell. Mild anemia is fairly common during pregnancy and in chronic disease states.

Prognosis

Anemia is a symptom of something else happening. The cause of the anemia needs to be determined in order to correct the anemia and its symptoms.

Hallmark Signs and Symptoms

- Fatigue due to lower hemoglobin levels causing hypoxia from less oxygen being available to the tissues of the body.
- Weakness because of hypoxia.
- Difficulty concentrating.
- Pallor owing to less oxygen being available to the surface tissues.
- Tachycardia as the body attempts to compensate for less available oxygen by beating more rapidly to increase blood supply.
- Systolic murmur may develop due to increased turbulence of blood flow with significant anemia.
- Dyspnea or shortness of breath because of hypoxia as the body attempts to get more oxygen.
- Angina as the myocardium is not getting enough oxygen.
- Headache, light-headedness due to hypoxia.
- Bone pain because of increased erythropoiesis as the body attempts to correct anemia.
- Jaundice in hemolytic anemia owing to increased levels of bilirubin as RBCs break down.

Common Test Results

- Hemoglobin level is low.
- **Hematocrit** level is low.
- RBC count is low.
- Mean corpuscular volume (MCV) shows size of cell—normal (normocytic), microcytic (low), or macrocytic (high).
- Mean corpuscular hemoglobin (MCH) shows color of cell—normal (normochromic), hypochromic (low).
- Red cell distribution width (RDW) elevated—shows the variation of the cell sizes; there is greater variation in a cell size when the body is attempting to compensate for anemia.
- Reticulocyte count elevated when RBC cell production is increased to compensate for the anemia.

Treatment

Correction of the underlying cause is necessary. Treatment may include dietary modifications and supplementations (such as iron or vitamin B12), corticosteroids (to suppress the immune system), erythropoietin (to stimulate the bone marrow to produce cells), or blood transfusions. See specific anemias to follow.

Nursing Diagnoses

- Fatigue
- Activity intolerance

NURSING INTERVENTION

- Check vital signs for changes.
- Monitor CBC—hemoglobin, RBC, MCV, MCH, RDW.
- Plan nursing care based on patient tolerance of activity.
- Monitor for angina.

2. Aplastic Anemia (Pancytopenia)

What Went Wrong

The bone marrow stops producing a sufficient amount of new RBCs, WBCs, and platelets, thereby increasing the risk of infection and hemorrhage. The red cells remaining in circulation are normal in size and color. This may be due to chemical exposure, high-dose radiation exposure, or exposure to toxins (such as pesticides, arsenic, or benzene). Cancer treatments such as radiation therapy and chemotherapeutic agents may suppress bone marrow function, which results in anemia (low RBC), **thrombocytopenia** (low platelets), and **leukopenia** (low WBC). Disorders such as rheumatoid arthritis (RA), Epstein-Barr virus, hepatitis, cytomegalovirus, HIV infection, and parvovirus may cause anemia. The cause may also be unknown or idiopathic.

Prognosis
The bone marrow dysfunction may be slow-onset or sudden. The lifespan of the RBCs is longer than the platelets and WBCs, so the anemia may show up later than the effects of losing the other cells. Some exposures to toxic agents or medications are severe and potentially fatal in susceptible individuals. Patients with severe aplastic anemia typically need hospital care. In some individuals with severe aplastic anemia, the disease will be fatal.

Hallmark Signs and Symptoms
- Fatigue due to hypoxemia
- Weakness owing to tissue hypoxia
- Shortness of breath as oxygen-carrying capability is diminished
- Pallor because of lack of oxygen reaching superficial tissues due to anemia
- Arrhythmias, murmurs, or heart failure as the cardiovascular system has difficulty with decreased oxygen supply
- Infections due to low WBC production, causing decreased ability to fight infection
- Fever because of infection
- Bruising (**ecchymosis**) and tiny subcutaneous (SC) hemorrhages (**petechiae**) due to a decrease in platelets, altering clotting ability
- Bleeding from mucous membranes (GI tract, mouth, nose, vagina)

Common Test Results
- Low hemoglobin—decreases oxygen-carrying capabilities.
- Low hematocrit—fewer RBCs within circulation.
- Low RBC count.
- Thrombocytopenia—low platelet count.
- Leukopenia—low WBC.

- Reticulocyte count low—no immature cells available for release into circulation.
- Positive fecal occult blood test.
- Decreased cell counts in bone marrow biopsy as the body stops producing.
- Bone marrow aspiration to determine components of bone marrow.

Treatment

- Administer hematopoietic growth factor to correct anemia in patients with low erythropoietin levels.
  - erythropoietin, epoetin alfa (recombinant human erythropoietin), by SC injection or IV
- Administer human granulocyte colony-stimulating factor (G-CSF) to correct low WBC levels.
  - filgrastim by SC injection or IV
  - granulocyte-macrophage colony-stimulating factor (GM-CSF) sargramostim by IV infusion
- Packed RBC transfusions when anemia is symptomatic.
- Platelet transfusion for severe bleeding.
- Administer antithymocyte globulin that is an immunosuppressant which contains antibodies against human T cells. This is often the treatment of choice for elderly patients.
- Bone marrow transplant replaces functioning stem cells.
- Administer corticosteroids.
- Splenectomy when the spleen is enlarged and destroying RBCs.

Nursing Diagnoses

- Risk for infection
- Activity intolerance
- Risk for deficient fluid volume

NURSING INTERVENTION

- Monitor vital signs for changes.
- Record intake and output of fluids.

- Protect the patient from falls.
- Avoid IM injections due to altered clotting ability.
- **Explain to the patient:**
  - Do not take aspirin due to the effect on platelet aggregation (clotting ability).
  - Plan to take rest periods during activities because of fatigue.
  - Only use an electric razor to decrease the risk of bleeding owing to decreased platelet count.
  - Call your physician, nurse practitioner, or physician assistant for signs of bleeding or bruising.

3. Iron Deficiency Anemia

What Went Wrong

A lower-than-normal amount of iron in blood results in low formation of hemoglobin and a decreased ability of the blood to carry oxygen. Iron stores are typically depleted first, followed by serum iron levels. Iron deficiency may be due to blood loss, dietary deficiency, or increased demand owing to pregnancy or lactation. As RBCs age, the body breaks them down and the iron is released. This iron is reused to produce new blood cells. A small amount of iron is lost daily through the gastrointestinal (GI) tract, necessitating dietary replacement. When RBCs are produced without a sufficient amount of iron, the cells are smaller and paler than usual.

Prognosis

Iron deficiency anemia is a very common type of anemia. Typically, patients respond to oral supplementation of iron. Occasionally, a patient will have problems absorbing iron from the intestinal tract. These patients will need parenteral supplementation. Once iron stores are replaced, the anemia should correct and hemoglobin levels return to normal. Some patients may need life-long supplementation, depending on the cause of the deficiency.

Hallmark Signs and Symptoms

- Weakness because of anemia and tissue hypoxia
- Pallor due to a decreased amount of oxygen getting to surface tissues
- Fatigue owing to anemia and hypoxemia
- Koilonychia—thin, concave nails raised at edges, also called spoon nails
- Tachycardia and tachypnea on exertion due to increased demand for oxygen

Common Test Results

- Decrease in serum hemoglobin as fewer RBCs are made.
- Serum ferritin is low.
- MCV initially normal until iron stores are depleted, and then low—microcytic anemia as the RBCs produced are smaller than usual due to decreased level of available iron.
- MCH initially normal, and then low—hypochromic anemia.
- Serum iron level is low.
- Serum iron-binding capacity is increased.
- Transferrin saturation decreases.
- Peripheral blood smear shows poikilocytosis (RBCs of different shapes).
- Platelet count may increase.

Treatment

Iron replacement therapy is continued to correct the deficiency and replace the lost stores of iron in the body. The typical timeframe for oral therapy is to continue for 3 to 6 months after the anemia has been corrected. If oral treatment is not adequate, parenteral treatment may be necessary. There have been documented incidents of anaphylactic reactions to iron dextran. Patients new to this treatment typically have a smaller test dose initially, prior to the initiation of treatments.

- Administer iron to replace what has been lost to return stores to normal levels.
  - Oral replacement in split doses (3 times a day).
    - ferrous sulfate
    - ferrous gluconate
    - ferrous fumarate
  - Parenteral iron replacement for those who cannot tolerate or do not respond to oral therapy, have gastrointestinal illness, or continued bleeding.
    - ferric carboxymaltose given IV
    - iron dextran given deep IM using the Z-track method
    - iron sodium gluconate given IV
    - iron sucrose complex given IV

- Increase dietary intake of iron, such as lean red meat, organ meats, oysters, iron-fortified cereals, dried fruit or beans, poultry, salmon, tuna, canned sardines, whole grains, dark green leafy vegetables, and whole grains

Nursing Diagnoses

- Imbalanced nutrition, less than what body requires
- Activity intolerance

NURSING INTERVENTION

- Monitor intake and output.
- Monitor vital signs for tachycardia or tachypnea.
- Monitor for reactions to parenteral iron therapy.
- **Explain to the patient:**
  - Check for bleeding.
  - Increase iron in diet.
  - Teach dietary sources of iron, including dark green leafy vegetables, edamame, peas, dried beans, dried fruit, tofu, oatmeal, dark chocolate, liver, oysters, octopus, clams, mussels, sardines, lean red meat, lamb, pork, poultry, venison, iron-fortified foods (cereals).
  - Avoid taking iron supplements with antacids as this will interfere with the absorption of the iron. Antacids may be taken 2 hours prior or 4 hours after the iron supplement.

---

4. Pernicious Anemia

What Went Wrong

The body is unable to absorb vitamin B12, which is needed to produce RBC, resulting in a decreased RBC count. More common in people of northern European descent, the anemia typically develops in adulthood. Family history and autoimmune diseases increase the risk of developing the disease. An intrinsic factor is normally secreted by the parietal cells of the gastric mucosa, and it is necessary to allow intestinal absorption of vitamin B12. Destruction of the gastric mucosa due to an autoimmune response results in loss of parietal cells within the stomach. The ability of vitamin B12 to bind with the intrinsic factor is lost, decreasing the amount that is absorbed. Vitamin B12 is commonly found in meat, poultry, shellfish, eggs, and dairy products. Typical onset is between the ages of 40 and 60.

Prognosis

Ongoing replacement of vitamin B12 is necessary to correct the deficit and alleviate symptoms that may have developed. Without treatment, the neurologic effects will continue, ultimately leading to dementia. Patients have an increased risk of gastric polyps, gastric cancer, and gastric carcinoid tumors.

Hallmark Signs and Symptoms

- Asymptomatic initially
- Pallor due to anemia
- Weakness and fatigue owing to anemia
- Tingling in hands and feet—"stocking-glove paresthesia"—because of bilateral demyelination of dorsal and lateral columns of spinal cord nerves
- Diminished vibratory and position sense
- Poor balance due to the effect on cerebral function
- Dementia appears later in the disease
- Atrophic glossitis—beefy red tongue
- Nausea may lead to anorexia and weight loss
- Shortness of breath on exertion as disease progresses
- Premature graying of hair

Common Test Results

- Decreased hemoglobin due to decreased production of RBCs.
- Increased MCV—macrocytic anemia.
- Intrinsic factor antibodies—positive.
  - Parietal cell antibodies positive
  - Cobalamin level is low
  - Elevated fasting gastrin level
  - Decreased pepsinogen level
- A decreased amount of hydrochloric acid in the stomach (hypochlorhydria) due to changes within the parietal cells of the gastric mucosa.
- Positive Romberg's test owing to ataxia and neurologic changes.
- Diminished sensation when testing for vibration, position sense, or proprioception of extremities.

- Gastric biopsy shows atrophic gastritis.
- False + Pap test – vitamin B12 alters appearance of epithelial cells.

Treatment

Lifelong repletion of vitamin B12 will correct the anemia and improve the neurologic changes that have occurred. Initially, the patient is given weekly injections of B12 to combat the deficiency. The injections eventually become monthly for lifelong maintenance. Oral supplementation is not effective in these patients because they cannot adequately absorb vitamin B12 due to insufficient intrinsic factor.

- Administer vitamin B12 by IM injection.
- Transfusion of packed RBC if anemia is severe.

Nursing Diagnoses

- Impaired gas exchange
- Imbalanced nutrition, less than what body requires
- Risk for injury

NURSING INTERVENTION

- Prevent injuries.
- **Explain to the patient:**
  - Use soft toothbrush due to oral changes.
  - Avoid activities that could lead to injury because of paresthesias or changes in balance.
  - Inspect feet each day for injury due to paresthesia.

---

5. Sickle Cell Anemia

What Went Wrong

This is an autosomal recessive disorder in which an abnormal gene causes damage to the RBC membrane. The abnormal hemoglobin within the RBC is called hemoglobin S. Dehydration or drying of the RBC makes it more vulnerable to sickling (forming a crescent-like shape), as do hypoxemia and acidosis. Hemolytic anemia results as RBCs are destroyed due to the damage to the outer membrane. The sickled cells can also clump together, causing difficulty getting through the smaller vessels.

Prognosis

Sickle cell anemia will become a chronic multisystem disease. Causes of death in these patients are usually related to organ failure. Patients may also inherit a single gene for sickle cell. These patients may develop sickle cell trait, in which symptoms would only be present in the setting of extreme circumstances (vigorous exercise at high altitude, especially with rapid ascent).

Hallmark Signs and Symptoms

- Acute pain (especially back, chest, and long bones) from vascular occlusion of the small vessels as the sickled cells clump
- Fever as the body responds to acute sickling episode and accompanying provoking event
- Painful, swollen joints due to vaso-occlusive crisis (VOCOR)
- Fatigue because of chronic anemia
- Stroke (cerebrovascular accident) owing to the vaso-occlusive process
- Enlarged liver (hepatomegaly)
- Enlarged heart and systolic murmur

Common Test Results

- Low RBC count due to chronic hemolytic anemia; the RBCs have a shorter lifespan.
- Elevated WBCs.
- Increased reticulocytes.
- Presence of Howell-Jolly bodies and target cells.
- Sickle cells appear in blood smear.
- Indirect bilirubin level elevated.
- Hemoglobin electrophoresis shows majority hemoglobin S (80% to 98%).

Treatment

During acute episodes, pain control, hydration, and oxygenation are the focus of treatment. The underlying cause that sent the patient into crisis will also need to be treated concurrently.

- Administer analgesics to alleviate the pain associated with the vaso-occlusive process.
- Rapid introduction of opioids for severe pain

- Warm compresses on joint.
- Blood transfusion of packed RBCs when anemia indicates.
- Supplemental oxygen if hypoxic.
- Adequate hydration, using IV fluids.
- Treat infections.

Hydroxyurea therapy recommended for adults with three or more crises in the past year, daily pain impacting quality of life, recurrent acute chest syndrome, or severe symptomatic chronic anemia.

Nursing Diagnoses

- Fatigue
- Acute pain
- Impaired gas exchange

NURSING INTERVENTION

- Increase fluid intake.
- Monitor IV fluids.
- Monitor pain control and frequently reassess pain levels.
- Record fluid intake and output to monitor renal function.
- Administer supplemental oxygen to increase available oxygen.
- **Explain to the patient:**
  - Avoid the cold.
  - No cold compresses.
  - Plan for rest periods during the day.

---

6. Deep Vein Thrombosis

What Went Wrong

Thrombophlebitis, or the formation of a clot within the vein, commonly occurs within the deep veins in the legs and may also occur in the arms (see Fig. 4–3). Initially, platelets and white cells clump together, sticking to the inside of the vessel wall. As blood flows over the area, other cells may deposit onto the area, making the thrombus larger. Compression of blood flow, which will increase the venous pressure or sluggishness of the blood flow, can increase the risk of clot formation. Immobility, obesity, or hormonal changes such as pregnancy can all

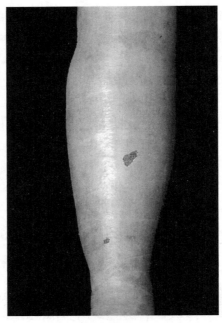

FIGURE 4-3 · Patient with deep vein thrombosis (DVT). The leg is swollen, pale, with a blotchy cyanotic discoloration, and is painful. The episode occurred after abdominal surgery (the circular marks are from a compression bandage).

Source: Reproduced with permission from: Wolff K, Johnson RA: *Fitzpatrick's Color Atlas and Synopsis of Clinical Dermatology*, 6th ed. New York, NY: McGraw-Hill; 2009. Fig. 16–6B.

contribute to increased risk. It is most common over the age of 60 years. There is an increased risk with bed rest, recent surgery, cancer, smoking, fractures (especially involving lower extremities), heart failure, obesity, or estrogen use.

Prognosis

The clot may develop without any outward signs for some time. It may also be due to another disease process or medication that affects clotting abilities. A small piece of the clot may break free to become an embolus and travel elsewhere in the body. This embolus may lodge in a vessel in the lung (a pulmonary embolism), causing acute respiratory symptoms, possibly even death.

Hallmark Signs and Symptoms

- Some patients will be asymptomatic.
- Unilateral leg (or arm) pain or tenderness (calf, thigh, groin, upper or lower arm) depending on location of thrombosis.
- Unilateral swelling (edema) of leg (or arm) due to vascular occlusion.

- Positive Homan's sign (pain on dorsiflexion of foot) seen in minority of patients with deep vein thrombosis (DVT).
- Warmth and redness over the site.

Common Test Results

- Doppler flow studies.
- Venous duplex ultrasound.
- Impedance plethysmography looks at venous outflow; better at diagnosis in thigh than in calf.
- Venography uses contrast dye to visualize the thrombus; not commonly done due to need for dye and other available tests.
- MRI directs thrombus imaging useful for inferior vena cava and pelvic vein locations.
- PT, PTT, INR, and CBC with platelet count as baseline.
- D-dimer to test for hypercoagulable state.

Treatment

Most patients undergo medical treatment and rest. Preventive measures are instituted for future occurrences. Patients with repeat occurrences may have an umbrella filter implanted.

- Bed rest with elevation of extremity.
- Warm, moist soaks of the area.
- Monitor **PT**, **PTT**, and INR.
- Weight-dosed heparin IV.
- Low-molecular-weight heparin.
- Warfarin—at therapeutic levels for 2 days, then stop heparin, and continue for 3 months.
- Thrombolytic therapy to dissolve clot with drugs such as recombinant tissue plasminogen activator (t-PA).
- An umbrella filter is inserted into the inferior vena cava for patients with recurring lower extremity DVT.
- Thrombectomy is the surgical removal of the thrombus.
- Antiembolic (elastic) stockings.
- Low-risk patients with DVT can be safely treated in an outpatient setting with low-molecular-weight heparin.

Nursing Diagnoses

- Impaired physical mobility
- Risk for acute pain

NURSING INTERVENTION

- Monitor vital signs for changes.
- Monitor for signs of pulmonary embolism, shortness of breath, chest pain, tachycardia (rapid heart rate), tachypnea (rapid respirations), and diaphoresis (sweating).
- Avoid massaging the area to lessen the possibility of dislodging the clot.
- Intermittent warm, moist soaks. Assess skin between changes.
- Follow weight-dosed heparin protocol.
- Monitor lab results: PT, PTT, INR, and CBC with platelets.
- Low-molecular-weight heparin (enoxaparin, dalteparin).
- Take warfarin orally.
- Monitor for signs of bleeding or bruising.
- **Explain to the patient:**
  - Report signs of bleeding or bruising to physician, nurse practitioner, or physician assistant.
  - Avoid injury.
  - Use an electric razor and soft toothbrush; avoid flossing between teeth.
  - Observe diet restrictions, and to check with healthcare provider or pharmacist about interactions of any medications, if on warfarin as outpatient.
  - Take warfarin as directed.
  - Continue to have blood tests to monitor anticoagulant therapy.
  - Call 911 or go to ER if there is chest pain, difficulty breathing, and hemoptysis.
  - Duration of treatment with anticoagulants is likely to be between 3 and 12 months.

7. Disseminated Intravascular Coagulation

What Went Wrong

Blood coagulates through the entire body within the vascular compartment. This depletes platelets and the body's ability to coagulate, resulting in an increased risk of hemorrhage. It occurs as a complication of some other condition. The coagulation sequence is activated causing many microthrombi to develop throughout the body. The clots that form are the result of coagulation proteins and platelets, resulting in the risk of bleeding or severe hemorrhage. It is often due to obstetric complications, post-trauma, sepsis, cancer, or shock.

Prognosis

The prognosis varies depending on the underlying disease process and the ability to reverse the coagulopathy.

Hallmark Signs and Symptoms

- Unexpected bleeding (**epistaxis**, mucous membranes)—oozing from puncture sites (venipuncture, IVs, surgical wounds).
- Petechiae as clotting factors are lost.
- **Purpura** as clotting factors are lost.
- Internal bleeding as clotting factors are lost.
- Severe hemorrhage as clotting factors are lost.
- Uncontrolled postpartum bleeding.
- Tissue hypoxia from **microemboli** (small blood clots in the bloodstream).
- Hemolytic anemia, as cells are destroyed trying to pass through partially blocked vessels.
- Thrombosis may lead to organ failure.

Common Test Results

- PT prolonged (may be normal in early disease or chronic disease).
- PTT normal or prolonged.
- Thrombin time may be elevated due to consumption of fibrinogen.
- Platelet count low—thrombocytopenia.
- Blood smear will show schistocytes (fragmented red blood cells)
- Fibrin degradation products elevated (may be normal in early disease).
  - D-dimer is likely to be elevated (best single test).

Treatment

Treatment needs to decrease coagulation ability (to prevent further clot development) and replace clotting components (to prevent further bleeding). Other interventions may be necessary depending on the locations of clot development and any compromise of body system function due to clot formation.

- Transfusion.
  - Packed RBC to replace what has been lost due to bleeding.
  - Fresh frozen plasma—replaces coagulation factor deficiency.
  - Platelets—replaces needed cells.
  - Cryoprecipitate—replaces fibrinogen.
- Administer anticoagulant drugs to decrease coagulation; not done in all patients.
  - heparin
- Bed rest
- Supplemental oxygen

Nursing Diagnoses

- Ineffective tissue perfusion
- Risk for deficient fluid volume
- Risk for bleeding

NURSING INTERVENTION

- Monitor for bleeding from obvious sites (wounds, suture lines, venipuncture, etc.) and occult sites (GI, urine).
- Avoid cleaning clots from exposed areas—may start bleeding from the site and not have sufficient clotting factors to stop.
- **Explain to the patient:**
  - Avoid situations that might cause bleeding—use an electric razor, soft toothbrush, avoid flossing between teeth.

---

8. Hemophilia

What Went Wrong

The patient is missing a coagulation factor that is essential for normal blood clotting and as a result the blood does not clot when the patient bleeds (see Fig. 4–4). It is an X-linked recessive inherited disorder, passed on so that it presents symptoms in males, and rarely in females. Hemophilia A is the result of insufficient clotting factor VIII. Hemophilia B is the result of insufficient

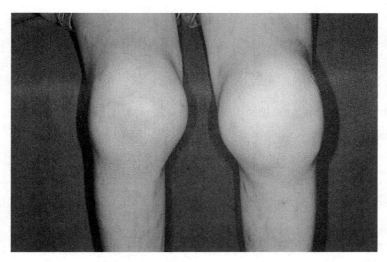

FIGURE 4–4 • A 9-year-old male child with hemophilia A presented with swelling of both knees.
Source: Reproduced with permission from: Shah BR, Lucchesi M: *Atlas of Pediatric Emergency Medicine*, 2nd ed. New York, NY: McGraw-Hill; 2013. Fig. 11–9A.

clotting factor IX and is also known as Christmas disease. Hemophilia A and B are typically diagnosed in young children, often before the age of 2 years. Hemophilia C is due to insufficient clotting factor XI, it typically has mild symptoms and may not be diagnosed as early.

Prognosis
The most common sites of bleeding are into the joints, muscles, or from the GI tract. Mild forms of the disease will only cause bleeding after surgery or trauma, whereas severe forms of the disease will cause bleeding without any prior cause.

Hallmark Signs and Symptoms
- Unexplained bleeding or bruising
- Unusual bleeding after minor trauma (vaccinations, dental cleanings, etc.)
- Unexplained epistaxis (nosebleeds)
- Tender joints due to bleeding
- Swelling of knees, ankles, hips, and elbows because of bleeding
- Blood in stool (tarry stool) owing to GI blood loss
- Blood in the urine (hematuria)

Common Test Results

- CBC normal.
- PTT prolonged.
- PT normal.
- Bleeding time is prolonged.
- Fibrinogen level is normal.
- Decrease in clotting factor VIII found in blood serum in hemophilia A.
- Decrease in clotting factor IX found in blood serum in hemophilia B.
- Decrease in clotting factor XI found in blood serum in hemophilia C.

Treatment

- Avoid aspirin.
- Plasma-derived or recombinant factor concentrates.
- For hemophilia A administer factor VIII concentrates.
- For hemophilia B administer factor IX concentrates.
- Epsilon aminocaproic acid to prevent clots from breaking down.
- DDAVP for patients with mild deficiency to enhance the release of stored factor VIII.
- DDAVP can be administered by intravenous infusion or via nasal spray.

Nursing Diagnoses

- Acute pain
- Impaired gas exchange
- Risk for bleeding

NURSING INTERVENTION

- Avoid IM injections.
- No aspirin.
- To stop bleeding:
  - Elevate site.
  - Apply direct pressure to the site.

- **Explain to the patient:**
  - Wear a medical alert identification.
  - Contact physician, nurse practitioner, or physician assistant for any injury.
  - Avoid situations where injury might occur.

9. Idiopathic Thrombocytopenic Purpura

What Went Wrong

Idiopathic thrombocytopenic purpura (ITP) is an autoimmune disorder in which antibodies to the patient's own platelets are developed. Antibodies attach to the platelets which are then destroyed within the spleen. Normal clotting is affected due to loss of platelets. ITP in adults is typically more common in women and may become chronic in adults.

Prognosis

Problems for the patient are most likely the result of bleeding due to inadequate platelets. Spontaneous bleeding may occur when platelet count drops below 10,000 platelets per microfilter (normal 150,000 to 450,000 platelets per microfilter). In mild cases, watchful waiting is appropriate with periodic monitoring and blood tests for platelet counts. Prednisone can control the majority of cases of ITP. Remission is common.

Hallmark Signs and Symptoms

- Bleeding in mucous membranes or skin due to low platelet count.
  - epistaxis
  - oral bleeding
  - purpura
  - petechiae
  - Menorrhagia (heavy menstrual bleeding)

Common Test Results

- Thrombocytopenia—low platelet count. Some patients will have a platelet count below 20,000 platelets per microfilter.
- Mild anemia—usually secondary to bleeding.
- PT is normal.
- PTT is normal.

- Bleeding time is prolonged.
- Blood smear to confirm the number of platelets
- Antibodies are detected.
- Bone marrow aspiration (not recommended at initial diagnosis) shows increased megakaryocytes (immature platelets).

Treatment

The use of prednisone in patients with ITP is to decrease the body's immune response, in this case the action on the antibody-tagged platelets. Initially, the use of prednisone will also help to enhance vascular stability. High-dose therapy needs to be tapered down. Long-term maintenance doses of prednisone are not recommended due to the potential side effects of the medication (elevated blood sugar, cataract formation, osteoporosis, infection). Splenectomy provides complete or partial remission.

- Prednisone—bleeding will stop even before platelet count begins to rise.
- High-dose IV immunoglobulin (gamma globulin or IVIG).
- Danazol (synthetic steroid) administration.
- Immunosuppressive therapy.
  - rituximab (monitor for hypotension, fever, sore throat, rash)
- Stem cell transplantation.
- Splenectomy (not commonly done).

Nursing Diagnoses

- Risk for infection
- Disturbed body image
- Risk for ineffective individual coping
- Risk for bleeding

NURSING INTERVENTION

- Monitor vital signs for changes.
- Monitor for signs of bleeding or bruising.
- Decrease chance of bleeding.
- Use soft toothbrushes, no flossing, only electric razors.
- Protect from potential infection, sick visitors, etc.
- Encourage patient to discuss feelings about illness.
- Avoid aspirin and nonsteroidal anti-inflammatory drugs (NSAIDs).

10. Leukemia

What Went Wrong

Replacement of bone marrow by abnormal, cancerous cells results in unregulated proliferation of immature WBCs entering the circulatory system. These immature WBCs do not function properly, grow faster than normal, and do not stop growing. The abnormal cells crowd out the normal cells. These leukemic cells may also enter the liver, spleen, or lymph nodes, causing these areas to enlarge. Leukemia is classified according to the type of cell it is derived from, lymphocytic or myelocytic, and as either acute or chronic. Lymphocytic leukemias involve immature lymphocytes originating in the bone marrow and typically infiltrate the spleen, lymph nodes, or central nervous system. Myelogenous or myelocytic leukemia involves the myeloid stem cells in the bone marrow and interferes with the maturation of all blood cell types (granulocytes, erythrocytes, and thrombocytes).

The exact cause of leukemia is unknown. There is a higher incidence in people who have been exposed to high levels of radiation, who have had exposure to benzene, or who have a history of aggressive chemotherapy for a different type of cancer. There may be a genetic predisposition to develop acute leukemia. Patients with Down's syndrome, Fanconi's anemia, or a family history of leukemia also have a higher-than-average incidence of this disease.

Prognosis

Patients with acute leukemia typically have a more aggressive disease process, which may have a shorter course from the time of diagnosis. Patients have increased incidence of anemia, bleeding, and infections. Patients with chronic leukemia are more likely to have a less aggressive disease process that runs over a longer course. The chronic patients typically have an insidious onset and a better prognosis. Adults typically develop Acute Myeloid Leukemia (AML) or Chronic Lymphocytic Leukemia (CLL).

Hallmark Signs and Symptoms

Acute patients:

- Fatigue and weakness due to anemia.
- Night sweats.
- Frequent infections.
- Fever due to increased susceptibility to infection.
- Bleeding, petechiae, ecchymosis (bruising), epistaxis (nosebleed), and gingival (gum) bleeding owing to decreased platelet count.

- Bone pain because of bone infiltration and marrow expansion.
- Lymph nodes (lymphadenopathy) enlarged as leukemic cells invade nodes.
- Liver (hepatomegaly) and spleen (splenomegaly) enlarged as leukemic cells invade. Enlarged spleen may cause swollen, tender abdomen (typically left upper quadrant).
- Headache, nausea, anorexia, vomiting, and weight loss.
- Papilledema, cranial nerve palsies, seizure if there is central nervous system involvement.

Chronic patients:

- Fatigue due to anemia.
- Weight loss because of chronic disease process and poor or loss of appetite.
- Enlarged lymph nodes (lymphadenopathy) due to infiltration of lymph nodes.
- Enlarged spleen (splenomegaly) owing to involvement of the spleen.

Common Test Results

- Low RBC count, low hemoglobin—anemia
- Low platelet count—thrombocytopenia
- Elevated WBC count—leukocytosis
- Abnormal amount of immature WBC shown in bone marrow biopsy

Treatment

Actual treatment protocols will vary depending on evidence-based guidelines for the specific type of leukemia and patient comorbidities.

- Chemotherapy, biologic therapy, or targeted therapy
  - Commonly used medications can include imatinib, idarubicin, daunorubicin, fludarabine, etoposide, asparaginase, dasatinib, and vincristine, azacitidine.
- Radiation therapy
  - Administer platelet transfusions.
  - Administer filgrastim for neutropenia.
  - Administer antibiotics for infections.

- Bone marrow or stem cell transplant
  - Administer immunosuppressives to avoid transplant rejection.
- Transfusion if hemolytic anemia or bleeding
  - Packed RBCs.
  - Whole blood.
  - Platelets.
- Dietary modification to ensure adequate nutritional intake

Nursing Diagnoses

- Risk for infection
- Chronic pain
- Imbalanced nutrition, less than what body requires

NURSING INTERVENTION

- Monitor for bleeding—platelet count may be decreased.
- Monitor for infection—patients have increased susceptibility to infection.
- Monitor pain control.
- Small, frequent meals.
- Teach patients about infection control.
  - Avoid others with infection.
  - Report signs of infection, sore throat, fever, etc.
- **Explain to the patient:**
  - Use an electric razor.
  - Use a soft toothbrush.
  - Watch for bleeding or bruising.
  - Maintain a healthy diet.
  - Balance rest and exercise, avoid overexertion.

11. Multiple Myeloma

What Went Wrong

A malignancy of the plasma cells causes an excessive amount of plasma cells in the bone marrow. Plasma cells grow out of control within the marrow. Platelets and blood cells have difficulty forming within the crowded marrow. Masses within the bone marrow cause destructive lesions in the bone. Normal bone marrow function is reduced as the abnormal plasma cells continue to grow. Immune function is diminished, and the patient develops anemia. The disease typically affects older adults and, it is twice as common in African-Americans. There is an increased risk for patients with a prior history of radiation exposure.

Prognosis

Patients are susceptible to infection and often have significant pain from bone involvement of the disease. The survival time from diagnosis averages about 3 years.

Hallmark Signs and Symptoms

- Severe bone pain most commonly in the back or hips or skull
- Anemia due to invasion of the bone marrow
- Fatigue because of anemia
- Bleeding due to decreased platelet count (thrombocytopenia)
- Fever
- Shortness of breath owing to anemia
- Broken bones because of loss of normal bone structure (osteoporosis) or plasmacytoma
- Broken bones due to minor injury
- Numbness and weakness of extremities if spine is affected
- Increased risk of infection because of bone marrow failure to produce adequate WBCs (leukopenia)
- Spinal cord compression as mass enlarges
- High serum calcium levels (hypercalcemia)
- Hyperviscosity (thickening) of the blood as myeloma protein increases
- Renal failure due to protein effect in renal tubules

Common Test Results

- Presence of the Bence Jones protein in urine.
- Protein in urine (proteinuria).
- Quantitative immunoglobulins to check levels of antibodies IgA, IgD, IgE, IgG, and IgM.

- Serum protein electrophoresis shows a monoclonal protein spike.
- Immunofixation (immunoelectrophoresis) determines the type of antibody present.
- CBC shows anemia.
- Rouleaux formation on peripheral smear, a group of RBCs clump together in a stack (like a stack of coins).
- Abnormal plasma cells in bone marrow biopsy.
- X-rays of bone show lytic lesions.
- Elevated level of calcium in blood (hypercalcemia).
- Elevated erythrocyte sedimentation rate.
- Decreased bone density.

Treatment

Treatment regimens undergo changes based on patient's response and current research findings. Combination therapy is common in treatment of multiple myeloma.

- Pain management.
- Chemotherapy.
  - Commonly used medications include melphalan, vincristine, cyclophosphamide, etoposide, doxorubicin, and bendamustine.
- Immunomodulating agents (often in combination with a blood thinner or aspirin).
  - thalidomide, lenalidomide, and pomalidomide
- Proteasome inhibitors to help control cell division time.
  - bortezomib, carfilzomib, and ixazomib
- Monoclonal antibodies have been developed to have a specific target on the surface of myeloma cells.
  - daratumumab and elotuzumab
- Diet high in protein, carbohydrates, vitamins, and minerals.
- Small frequent meals.
- Transfusion of packed RBCs if anemia is severe.
- Bone marrow or stem cell transplantation.
  - Autologous (patient's own cells—increased survival in younger patients) or allogeneic (donor cells—more risk)

- Radiation therapy for bone pain or bone tumors.
- Bisphosphonates to decrease bone pain and prevent fractures.

Nursing Diagnoses

- Pain
- Impaired mobility
- Risk for injury

NURSING INTERVENTION

- Protect the patient from falling.
- Monitor input and output due to renal function changes.
- Perform muscle-strengthening exercises.
- Increase fluids to enhance kidney clearance.
- **Explain to the patient:**
  - No lifting.
  - Be alert for fractures.

---

12. Polycythemia Vera

What Went Wrong

Polycythemia vera is a cancerous disorder of the bone marrow (myeloprolif-erative disorder) resulting in an overproduction of blood cells and a thickening of blood. Predominantly due to increased RBCs, but WBCs and platelets may also increase. The hallmarks of polycythemia vera include excessive produc-tion of RBCs, WBCs, and platelets. The excess of cells present in the blood causes problems with the flow of blood through vessels, especially the smaller ones. There will be an increase in peripheral vascular resistance causing increased pressure, and vascular stasis in the smaller vessels, potentially caus-ing thrombosis or tissue hypoxia. Blood clots may form. Organ damage may result because of these changes.

Prognosis

After diagnosis of polycythemia vera, the average survival time is 10 to 15 years with appropriate treatment and less than 2 years without treatment. Some patients may go on to develop acute leukemia. Complications usually arise from thrombosis or tissue hypoxia. It is associated with a gene mutation (JAK2V617F). It is more in men and those over the age of 40 years.

Hallmark Signs and Symptoms

- Facial skin and mucous membranes are dark and flushed (plethora).
- Hypertension due to increased peripheral vascular resistance and thickening of the blood.
- Difficulty breathing when lying flat (orthopnea).
- Itching worse after warm shower because of histamine release from increased basophils within dilated vessels.
- Excessive sweating.
- Unexplained weight loss.
- Fevers.
- Headache and difficulty concentrating.
- Vision blurred, tinnitus (ringing in ears), and hearing changes.
- Easy bruising, epistaxis (nosebleeds), and gingival (gum) bleeding.
- Thrombosis owing to vascular stasis.
- Spleen enlargement (splenomegaly).
- Sensation of fullness in the LUQ of the abdomen due to enlarged spleen.
- Tissue hypoxia and possible infarction of heart, spleen, kidneys, and brain as a result of thrombosis.

Common Test Results

- Increased RBC count.
- Increased hemoglobin.
- Increased hematocrit level.
- Increased WBC count.
- Increased basophils.
- Increased eosinophils.
- Increased platelet count.
- Low erythropoietin level
- Increased uric acid level.
- Increased potassium.
- Increased vitamin B12 level.
- Bone marrow panhyperplasia; iron stores absent.
- Genetic testing may show JAK2 or TET2 mutation.

Treatment

Treatment is aimed at maintaining blood flow to the smaller vessels and diminishing the amount of excess blood cells being made by the bone marrow.

- Periodic scheduled phlebotomy—the removal of up to 500 mL of blood—to reduce the hematocrit level to below 45 in male patients or 42 in female patients; may be done weekly.
- Adequate hydration.
- Administer anticoagulants such as aspirin.
- Administer myelosuppressive medication to reduce the number of RBCs being made.
  - hydroxyurea, anagrelide, and radioactive phosphorus-32
- Administer medication to lower uric acid level if necessary.
  - allopurinol
  - Alkylating agents.
  - melphalan
  - busulfan
- Radiation therapy.
  - Interferon-alpha or selective serotonin reuptake inhibitors for pruritus.
  - Aspirin to reduce the risk of clotting.

Nursing Diagnoses

- Ineffective tissue perfusion
- Disturbed sensory perception
- Risk for injury

NURSING INTERVENTION

- Monitor vital signs.
- Monitor for bleeding.
- Monitor for signs of infections.
- Keep the patient mobilized to decrease the chance of clot formation.
- Increase fluid intake.
- **Explain to the patient:**
  - Maintain activity.

> - Use an electric razor, a soft toothbrush, and avoid flossing to decrease chances of bleeding.
> - Avoid activities that could cause injury.

13. Von Willebrand Disease

What went wrong

Von Willebrand disease is most commonly a genetically transmitted disease, present at birth. In this case, there is a faulty gene that controls Von Willebrand factor which is necessary for hemostasis or clotting. Von Willebrand factor also binds factor VIII and platelets, which is integral in clotting. In some instances, the disease is acquired, typically in the setting of an autoimmune disease or following treatment with certain medications.

Prognosis

Von Willebrand disease is the most common bleeding disorder, and it affects both men and women. Since the symptoms can be mild, some patients are not diagnosed until adulthood. Most patients lead normal lives. Extra care should be taken prior to surgery, dental procedures, childbirth, or other situations that can be associated with blood loss.

Hallmark Signs and Symptoms

- Nosebleeds lasting longer than 10 minutes
- Easy bruising and excessive bleeding
- Extended bleeding after dental procedures
- Heavy and/or longer than average menstrual periods (menorrhagia)—changing pads and/or tampons more frequently than every 2 hours
- Hemorrhaging after childbirth

Common Test Results

- **Prothrombin time** typically within normal range.
- Activated **partial thromboplastin time** (aPTT) may be mildly prolonged.
- Factor VIII coagulant activity.
- Concentration of Von Willebrand factor antigen. This test may be a quantitative measure or an enzyme-linked immunosorbent assay (ELISA).

- Ristocetin cofactor activity to assess the functional ability of Von Willebrand factor to bind with platelets. This test should be performed at specialized centers familiar with the testing protocol.
- Von Willebrand factor activity assay to assess the binding ability of Von Willebrand factor. This test does not require the use of Ristocetin (an antibiotic) and is easier to perform and more reliable.

Treatment

- Administer desmopressin acetate (DDAVP) IV or nasal spray to stimulate the release of Von Willebrand factor.
- Fluid restriction due to the antidiuretic effect of desmopressin to avoid hyponatremia.
- Von Willebrand/factor VIII replacement.
- Recombinant Von Willebrand factor.
- Contraceptives for women of childbearing age to decrease the amount of menstrual bleeding.
- Antifibrinolytic medications (aminocaproic acid or tranexamic acid) to help stop active bleeding.
- Platelet transfusion for active bleeding that is not responding adequately to other therapy.
- Fibrin sealants applied topically for cuts.

Nursing Diagnoses

- Risk for bleeding
- Risk for powerlessness

NURSING INTERVENTION

- Avoid IM injections.
- No aspirin.
- To stop bleeding:
  - Elevate site.
  - Apply direct pressure to the site.
- **Explain to the patient:**
  - Inform your healthcare providers (including dentists) about your disease.

- Avoid aspirin and other NSAIDs.
- Appropriate prophylactic therapy should be considered.
- Contact physician, nurse practitioner or physician assistant for changes in bleeding.
- Avoid situations where injury might occur.

REVIEW QUESTIONS

1. **A patient is diagnosed with anemia and is often fatigued. He or she asks you why he or she feels this way. You tell him or her that it is because of:**
   A. Destruction (hemolysis) of the RBCs.
   B. Lack of oxygen getting to the cells in her body.
   C. Paleness (pallor) of the skin.
   D. Lack of nutritional intake of essential nutrients, such as iron or B12.

2. **A patient is diagnosed with iron deficiency anemia. She asks you if there is anything she should do to help correct this. Your best response is:**
   A. Sleep 7 to 8 hours each night.
   B. Decrease her salt intake and drink more water.
   C. Increase dietary iron intake with foods such as lean red meat, dark green leafy vegetables, and whole grains.
   D. Aerobic exercise for at least 30 minutes three times a week.

3. **A patient is showing signs of clotting and bleeding concurrently. You contact the physician immediately because you recognize this as signs of potential:**
   A. Disseminated intravascular coagulation.
   B. Hemophilia.
   C. Multiple myeloma.
   D. Polycythemia vera.

4. **Patients with ITP have an increased risk of bleeding. You would expect careful monitoring of:**
   A. Platelet count and RBC.
   B. WBC and bleeding time.
   C. PT and PTT.
   D. Iron and ferritin levels.

5. **A patient is diagnosed with DVT. A priority intervention is:**
   A. Monitoring of PT, PTT, and INR.
   B. Early ambulation and aerobic exercise

C. Application of ice packs to the affected area every 4 to 6 hours.

D. Increasing dietary intake of foods rich in vitamin K.

6. **A patient is recently diagnosed with hemophilia. What signs and symptoms should the nurse teach his/her patient to recognize?**

A. Clot formation, especially in the veins of the lower extremities.

B. Excessive bleeding after minor trauma.

C. Low blood counts and fatigue due to lack of adequate RBC production.

D. Anemia, bone pain, and infection.

7. **As part of a treatment plan for patients with leukemia, a bone marrow transplant may be performed. You know that as a result of the care needed after the bone marrow transplant, these patients will have an increased risk of:**

A. Bleeding.

B. Clot formation.

C. Infection.

D. Nausea and vomiting.

8. **You are reviewing a health history of a college-aged patient and discover that she experiences intermittent nose bleeds lasting 15 to 20 minutes and she also has heavy menstrual bleeding every month. You are concerned that these symptoms are consistent with:**

A. Von Willebrand disease.

B. Polycythemia vera.

C. Multiple myeloma.

D. Disseminated intravascular coagulation.

9. **You are caring for a patient with sickle cell anemia during a sickle cell crisis. You would expect the treatment plan for this patient to include:**

A. IV fluids to adequately hydrate.

B. Narcotic pain management when pain is severe.

C. Transfusion of RBCs to correct anemia.

D. All of the above.

10. **Patients with pernicious anemia are treated with:**

A. Oral iron.

B. Oral folic acid.

C. Parenteral vitamin B12.

D. Oral prednisone.

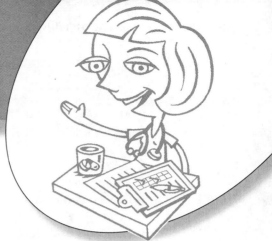

Chapter **5**

Nervous System

At the end of this chapter, the student will be able to:

- Identify normal anatomy and physiology related to the nervous system
- Discuss the disease-causing pathologic changes within the nervous system
- List four signs or symptoms of specific neurologic disease or injury
- Recognize expected nursing and medical treatment of neurologic injury or disease

KEY CONCEPTS

1. Abscess
2. Amyotrophic lateral sclerosis
3. Aneurysm
4. Bell's palsy
5. Encephalitis
6. Guillain-Barré syndrome
7. Head injury
8. Huntington's disease
9. Meningitis
10. Multiple sclerosis
11. Myasthenia gravis
12. Parkinson's disease
13. Spinal cord injury
14. Stroke
15. Seizure disorder
16. Tumor

KEY TERMS

Arachnoid mater
Astrocytoma
Battle's sign
Broca's area
Cerebral edema
Closed head injuries
Concussion
Dura mater
Electromyogram
Epidural
Glioma
Hematoma
Idiopathic facial paralysis

Intracerebral
Lou Gehrig's disease
Meningiomas
Occipital lobe
Open head injuries
Pia mater
Raccoon sign
Skull fractures
Subarachnoid
Subdural
Wernicke's area
Widened pulse pressure

How the Nervous System Works

The nervous system is divided into the central and peripheral nervous systems (see Fig. 5–1). The central nervous system is composed of the brain and spinal cord. The peripheral nervous system contains the spinal nerves and peripheral nerves.

The basic component of the nervous system is the nerve cell or neuron (see Fig. 5–2). A neuron is composed of the nucleus (within the cell body), a dendrite (which receives the signal), an axon (the extension of the cell that can

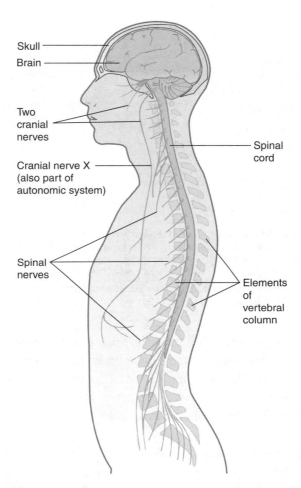

Skull
Brain
Two
cranial
nerves
Cranial nerve X
(also part of
autonomic system)
Spinal
nerves
Spinal
cord
Elements
of
vertebral
column

FIGURE 5−1 • Structure of the central nervous system and the peripheral nervous system.
Source: Reproduced with permission from: Waxman SG: *Clinical Neuroanatomy*, 26th ed. New York, NY: McGraw-Hill; 2010. Fig. 1–1.

pass on an impulse to the next nerve cell), and the axon terminals (which can transmit the signals to other cells). The messages are sent from one nerve cell to another, crossing a synapse (or gap) between cells. Neurotransmitters are chemicals released by the presynaptic neuron to enhance the communication between nerve cells. There are specific receptor sites for the different neurotransmitters on the postsynaptic neuron. Each neurotransmitter only fits into specific receptor sites. Electrically charged ions transmit signals along the cell membranes of the nerve cells. A myelin coating on the outer surface of the nerve cells helps to speed the transmission along the nerve cells. This myelin coating also gives a white color to the nerve cells.

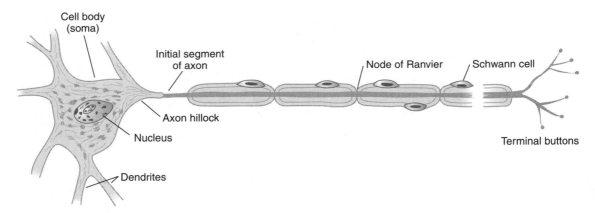

FIGURE 5–2 · Neuron with a myelinated axon. A motor neuron is composed of a cell body (soma) with a nucleus, several processes called dendrites, and a long fibrous axon that originates from the axon hillock. The first portion of the axon is called the initial segment. A myelin sheath forms from Schwann cells and surrounds the axon except at its ending and at the nodes of Ranvier. Terminal buttons (boutons) are located at the terminal endings.

Source: Reproduced with permission from: Barrett KE, Barman SM, Boitano S, Brooks HL: *Ganong's Review of Medical Physiology*, 24th ed. New York, NY: McGraw-Hill; 2012. Fig. 4–2.

Neurons transmit information from the body to the central nervous system and from the central nervous system to the body. Afferent neurons carry sensory information from the peripheral areas of the body to the central nervous system. These neurons do not have dendrites. Motor neurons that transmit information from the central nervous system to the muscles or glands are efferent neurons.

The brain is protected within the skull. The outermost layer of the brain is the cerebral cortex, made up primarily of neural cell bodies, giving a gray appearance. The cerebral cortex is divided into right and left hemispheres, and it is also divided into frontal, parietal, occipital, and temporal lobes (see Fig. 5–3A). The frontal lobe has motor and premotor areas, as well as **Broca's area**, which controls speech articulation, behavior, moral decision making, and emotional outburst. The parietal area interprets sensory stimuli, pain, and touch. The temporal lobe is involved in auditory processing, language interpretation (**Wernicke's area**), memory formation, and storage. The **occipital lobe** houses the visual cortex. The diencephalon includes the thalamus, hypothalamus, and the basal ganglia (see Fig. 5–3B). The thalamus is like a relay center. It relays the ascending sensory information from the body to the appropriate part of the cerebral cortex. Descending messages from the cerebral cortex are passed through the thalamus to the body. The hypothalamus controls neuroendocrine function and maintains homeostasis, or constancy, within the body. The basal ganglia control highly skilled movements that require

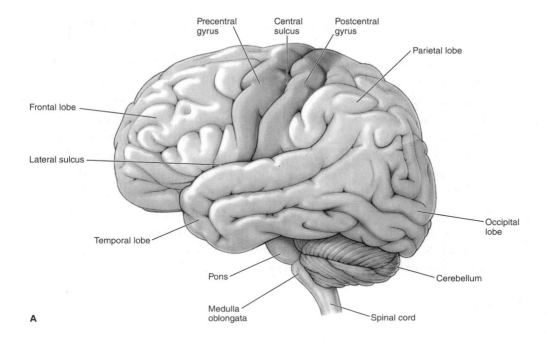

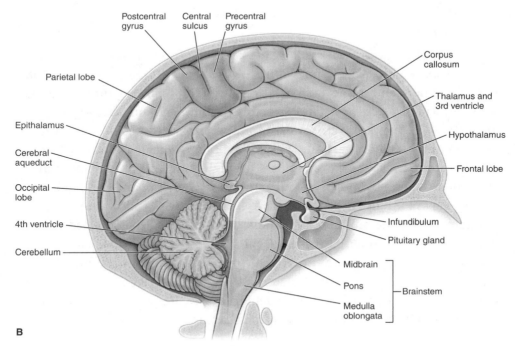

FIGURE 5–3 · Lateral view of the brain (A) and the medial view of the sagittal section of the brain (B).

Source: Reproduced with permission from: Morton DA, Foreman KB, Albertine KH: *The Big Picture: Gross Anatomy.* New York, NY: McGraw-Hill; 2011. Fig. 16–1.

precision without intentional thought. The brainstem is composed of the pons, medulla oblongata, and midbrain.

The spinal column is protected within the vertebral column. Both motor and sensory fibers are found within the spinal column. Motor nerves are located along the anterior horns, and sensory nerves are located along the posterior horns of the spinal column. The motor nerve fibers are more protected from traumatic injury this way. If a patient sustains an external injury to the back that damages the spinal column, the first area to be impacted will be the sensory nerves, hopefully maintaining motor function. If enough damage has occurred, then both sensory and motor functions will be lost. Peripheral nerve fibers leave the spinal column to travel to the rest of the body. Impulses travel from the central nervous system to muscle fibers to control voluntary motion and involuntary function of organs. Impulses are also sent from the body to the central nervous system for input.

Just the Facts

1. Abscess

What Went Wrong

Collection of pus within the skull creates a local increase in pressure. This can mimic a space-occupying lesion within the brain. Since the surrounding skull provides a hard and immovable covering, any additional structure within its confines will displace the normal structures within the skull (such as brain or blood vessels). Symptoms are similar to any other space-occupying lesion. The infection may be a primary site within the brain or may have traveled from nearby sites such as the ear or sinuses through bone erosion. Infection may also enter the brain via the systemic circulation from any infected site in the body, such as the lungs in bronchiectasis. The invading organism causes a local inflammatory reaction; there is pus and liquefication of the affected tissue. Edema of the surrounding tissue occurs. The area becomes encapsulated within 10 to 14 days from the onset of the infection. The most common infectious organisms are streptococci, staphylococci, anaerobes, or mixed-organism infections. Immunocompromised patients may have fungus or yeast present in the abscess. Up to 20% of the patients may have more than one abscess.

Prognosis

Identification of the organism and appropriate treatment is imperative to resolution of the infection. There is a significant mortality rate in these patients.

Hallmark Signs and Symptoms

- Headache owing to increased intracranial pressure
  - Drowsiness due to increased intracranial pressure
- Confusion or inattention
- Seizures because of irritation of brain tissue
- Increasing intracranial pressure
- **Widened pulse pressure** and bradycardia due to increased intracranial pressure
- Focal neurologic deficit, depending on the location of abscess
- Nystagmus with cerebral abscess
- Aphasia with frontal lobe abscess
- Loss of coordination (ataxia) with a cerebellar abscess

Common Test Results

- CBC shows elevated WBC count due to bacterial presence.
- CT scan shows the area of abscess site differentiated from surrounding tissue.
- MRI shows the area of abscess site possibly earlier than CT scan.
- Biopsy to positively identify the organism.

Treatment

- Surgically drain (aspiration or open) the abscess to relieve intracranial pressure.
- Administer antibiotic intravenously, depending on the organism.
  - nafcillin sodium (penicillinase-resistant penicillin)
  - penicillin G benzathine
  - chloramphenicol
  - metronidazole
  - vancomycin
- Administer corticosteroids in divided doses to decrease inflammation.
  - dexamethasone, prednisone—taper down dose of steroids before stopping
- Administer anticonvulsants to reduce seizure risk; watch for drug interactions.

- phenytoin
- phenobarbital
- Administer osmotic diuretics to decrease **cerebral edema**.
  - mannitol

Nursing Diagnoses

- Risk for disturbed thought process
- Risk for falls

NURSING INTERVENTION

- Assess the patient's ability to think, reason, and remember.
- Determine the level of orientation at regular intervals, compare findings to prior assessments.
- Assess the patient's speech capabilities.
- Assess the patient's movement and sensory function.
- Assess the patient's cranial nerve function.
- Supervise vital signs.
- Observe fluid intake and output.
- Monitor for signs of infection in postoperative patients.
- Examine for side effects of medications.
- **Explain to the patient:**
  - Need for continued antibiotic treatments.
  - How to administer IV antibiotics at home, how to monitor IV access, and when to call for problems.
  - Need for follow-up CT scan or MRI imaging for monitoring.

2. Amyotrophic Lateral Sclerosis

What Went Wrong

Amyotrophic lateral sclerosis (ALS) is commonly called **Lou Gehrig's disease,** and it is a progressive, degenerative disorder that involves both the upper and lower motor neurons. Coordination and muscle strength get progressively worse. Routine daily activities become difficult. There is usually no change in mental status or sensory function with the disease. There is an eventual paralysis of the motor system, except the eyes. As the disease is more progressed, families often can communicate with the patient through eye movements. Males are affected more commonly than females.

The disorder may present at any age, but the age at onset is usually between 40 and the late 60s. There is a familial form of the disease that has been linked to an abnormality in chromosome 21. This genetic disorder accounts for a small percentage of cases.

Prognosis

The disease is rapidly progressive and there is currently no known cure. As the muscles weaken and atrophy, paralysis develops. Over time, the respiratory muscles become involved. At first this results in poor air exchange, increasing the risk for respiratory infections, such as pneumonia. Eventually, the respiratory compromise leads to death from respiratory failure. Death is common within 3 to 5 years of diagnosis.

Hallmark Signs and Symptoms

- Fatigue, especially with exertion
- Atrophy of muscles due to weakness
- Dysphagia (trouble swallowing) owing to muscular weakness
- Weight loss
- Muscle weakness
- Muscle twitching (fasciculation) because of changes within the muscles
- Muscle cramps
- Paralysis
- Slurred speech as a result of muscle weakness
- Abnormal reflexes (deep tendon reflexes increased, gag reflex lost)

Common Test Results

- **Electromyogram** (EMG) shows fibrillation and fasciculation; motor conduction velocity is normal or slightly slowed.
  - Swallowing study to determine the loss of swallowing ability.
  - Elevated creatine kinase due to muscle changes.
  - Muscle biopsy shows lower neuron degeneration.
  - Pulmonary function testing shows decreased vital capacity.

Treatment

- Maintain adequate nutrition. Increase in calories needed due to illness and difficulty swallowing.

- Consult with a nutritionist or dietician to meet caloric needs.
- Consult with speech pathologist for potential swallowing difficulties.
- Administer spasmolytic agent specific for ALS, which reduces the transmission of glutamine across the neural synapse. Use of the following drug appears to slow the progression of the disease.
  - riluzole
- Administer medications to control symptoms.
  - baclofen or diazepam for muscle spasm
  - trihexyphenidyl for improvement in swallowing
- Bilevel positive airway pressure (BLPAP) to assist respiration either at nighttime, intermittently as needed, or all day.
- Mechanical ventilation necessary as the disease progresses.
- Physical therapy.
- Gastrostomy tube to decrease the chance of aspiration.
- Refer to hospice for end-of-life care.

Nursing Diagnoses

- Impaired physical mobility
- Ineffective airway clearance

NURSING INTERVENTION

- Develop a method of communication within the patient's capabilities—verbal communication may not be possible; the patient may not be able to use call bell system.
- Monitor vital signs—monitor respiratory function and cardiovascular status; as muscular function decreases the respiratory muscles may be affected.
- Supervise input and output.
- Assess gag reflex—as muscular changes occur, normal protective gag reflex will diminish.
- **Explain to the patient:**
  - How to suction oropharynx to remove secretions or food particles. As muscle function decreases, the cough reflex will not be sufficient to remove these.
  - How to tuck chin while drinking and eating to decrease the chance of aspiration.

3. Aneurysm

What Went Wrong

A cerebral aneurysm is a balloon-like outpouching caused by a congenital or developed weakness in a cerebral artery. Trauma, infection, or vessel wall lesions due to atherosclerosis can all lead to the development of an aneurysm. Increased pressure within the vessel lumen may cause the aneurysm to rupture, causing significant intracranial bleeding.

Prognosis

Patients are often asymptomatic with the aneurysm, until the time of the rupture. Some patients have the aneurysm identified on a radiologic study as an incidental finding. The decision can then be made to monitor or treat the aneurysm. If an arterial aneurysm ruptures without warning, the patient will have significant bleeding—a hemorrhagic stroke. The blood may need to be evacuated from the intracranial area to relieve pressure. The rupture of the aneurysm may be fatal, or the patient may have long-term disability following the event.

Hallmark Signs and Symptoms

- Asymptomatic until rupture
- Severe headache due to hemorrhage and increasing intracranial pressure
- Decreased level of consciousness owing to increased intracranial pressure from blood accumulating within the brain

Common Test Results

- Angiogram highlights the aneurysm due to structural abnormality.
- CT scan shows the aneurysm unless it is very small.
- Digital subtraction angiography shows the detail of the vasculature—abnormal structure.
- Diffusion/perfusion MRI or magnetic resonance angiography (MRA) shows vessel structure.
- Single-photon emission computed tomography (SPECT) shows the perfusion of blood flow to a specific area of the brain.

Treatment

- Surgical repair of the aneurysm.
- Monitor level of consciousness and neurologic status.
- Administer corticosteroid drugs to reduce inflammation.
  - dexamethasone
- Administer anticonvulsant drugs to reduce seizure risk due to irritation of brain.
  - phenytoin, phenobarbital
- Administer stool-softener drugs to decrease the need to strain (straining increases intracranial pressure).
  - docusate sodium
- Bed rest until otherwise ordered by the physician, nurse practitioner, or physician assistant.
- Elevate head of bed 30 degrees.

Nursing Diagnoses

- Ineffective tissue perfusion
- Decreased intracranial adaptive capacity

NURSING INTERVENTION

- Monitor the patient's neurologic function for changes—typically use Glasgow Coma Scale or a similar tool to grade response to stimuli (highest score 15):

• Eye-opening response	spontaneous	4
	to sound	3
	to pain	2
	none	1
• Motor responses	spontaneously obeys commands	6
	localizes pain	5
	withdrawal (normal)	4
	abnormal flexion	3
	extension	2
	none	1

• Verbal responses	oriented	5
	confused conversation	4
	inappropriate words	3
	incomprehensible sounds	2
	none	1

- Check vital signs for changes—widened pulse pressure with bradycardia indicative of increased intracranial pressure.
- **Explain to the patient:**
  - When to call the healthcare provider.
  - Needs for home care.

4. Bell's Palsy

What Went Wrong

This is an acute **idiopathic facial paralysis** or weakness of the muscles supplied by the seventh cranial nerve (facial nerve) that affects one side of the face. Often due to inflammation, the disorder is more common in diabetic patients. One side of the face is paralyzed, making the patient unable to close the eyelid, raise the eyebrow, or smile on the affected side of the face. Some patients will experience pain around the ear on the affected side. The patient may have an associated change in taste. Bell's palsy may be associated with herpes, HIV infection, sarcoidosis, Lyme disease, or other localized infection.

Prognosis

The more severe the symptoms at the time of presentation, the worse the prognosis. Some patients will have long-term persistence of symptoms, like facial disfigurement due to muscle weakness. The majority of patients will have complete resolution of symptoms.

Hallmark Signs and Symptoms

- Unilateral facial paralysis—inability to close eye, wrinkle forehead, puff out cheeks, or smile
- Pain near the ear and jaw
- Altered taste
- Dryness in eye

- Headache
- Hyperacusis (sound perceived as louder on the affected side)

Common Test Results

- EMG used to indicate recovery time; it can determine prognosis.
- Nerve conduction study.
- MRI or CT of the brain to rule out tumor.

Treatment

Treatment may not be needed.

- Administer corticosteroids to decrease inflammation (unclear if there is a definitive benefit).
  - prednisone in divided doses for first few days, then tapered down
- Administer artificial tears to maintain moisture within eyes.
- Eyepatch for nighttime to maintain moisture.

Nursing Diagnoses

- Disturbed sensory perception
- Disturbed body image

NURSING INTERVENTION

- Monitor for pain control.
- Observe visual changes—dryness of eye can lead to irritation of cornea.
- Examine the patient for reaction to medications.
- Provide meals in private—the patient may have difficulty keeping food in mouth and may not feel food or liquid that is drooling outside of the mouth.
- **Explain to the patient:**
  - How to properly instill artificial tear drops.
  - How to use eye patch.

---

5. Encephalitis

What Went Wrong

Encephalitis is the inflammation of the brain tissue, most often caused by a virus, although it can also be due to bacteria, fungus, or protozoa. In the case of viral encephalitis, the patient typically will have had viral symptoms prior to the current illness. The virus enters the central nervous system through the bloodstream and begins to reproduce. Inflammation in the area follows, causing damage to the neurons. Demyelination of the nerve fibers in the affected area and hemorrhage, edema, and necrosis occur, which create small cavities within the brain tissue. Herpes simplex virus 1, cytomegalovirus, echovirus, coxsackievirus, and herpes zoster can all cause encephalitis. Some forms of encephalitis can be transmitted by insects (such as mosquitoes or ticks) to humans, such as West Nile virus, St. Louis encephalitis virus, or equine encephalitis.

Prognosis

Identification of the organism is important in order to individualize the treatment for the patient. The earlier those symptoms are recognized and the earlier the patient enters the healthcare system, the better. Some patients will incur permanent disability from the irreversible damage that occurs to the brain. These patients may be in need of rehabilitation or long-term custodial care. The elderly and very young have the greatest incidence of severe cases.

Hallmark Signs and Symptoms

- Fever due to infection
- Nausea and vomiting owing to increased intracranial pressure
- Photophobia (light sensitivity)
- Stiff neck because of meningeal irritation
- Drowsiness, lethargy, or stupor due to increased intracranial pressure
- Altered mental status—irritability, confusion, disorientation, personality change
- Headache due to increased intracranial pressure
- Seizure activity possible owing to irritation of brain tissue
  - Abnormal reflexes
  - Skin rash

Common Test Results

- Lumbar puncture to examine cerebrospinal fluid (CSF)
- Electroencephalogram (EEG)
- Blood work to detect viral antibodies or viral DNA (polymerase chain reaction—PCR)
- Blood cultures used to help identify the organism when the patient is febrile
- MRI or CT of the head

Treatment

- Supportive care.
- Monitor respiratory status for compromise.
- Monitor vital signs for widened pulse pressure and bradycardia—signs of increased intracranial pressure.
- Monitor neurologic function for change.
- Antiviral medication to treat viral infection.
  - acyclovir
- Antibiotics to combat bacterial infection.
- Administer corticosteroid to decrease inflammation.
  - dexamethasone
- Administer antipyretics to reduce fever.
  - acetaminophen
- Administer anticonvulsants to decrease the chance of seizure activity.
  - phenytoin, phenobarbital
- Administer diuretics to decrease cerebral edema, if indicated.
  - furosemide
  - mannitol

Nursing Diagnoses

- Impaired physical mobility
- Disturbed thought processes

NURSING INTERVENTION

- Range of motion exercises—active or passive.
- Turn and position the patient to prevent skin breakdown.
- Monitor neurologic status for changes—typically use Glasgow Coma Scale or a similar tool to grade response to stimuli (highest score 15):
  - Eye-opening response

spontaneous		4
to sound		3
to pain		2
none		1

• Motor responses	spontaneously obeys commands	6
	localizes pain	5
	withdrawal (normal)	4
	abnormal flexion	3
	extension	2
	none	1
• Verbal responses	oriented	5
	confused conversation	4
	inappropriate words	3
	incomprehensible sounds	2
	none	1

- Provide a quiet environment to decrease unnecessary stimulation.
- Monitor fluid input and output.
- **Explain to the patient and family:**
  - Home care needs.
  - Necessity of turning and positioning.
  - Medication actions, side effects, and interactions.

6. Guillain-Barré Syndrome

What Went Wrong

This is an acute, progressive autoimmune condition that affects the peripheral nerves. Symptoms occur as the myelin surrounding the axon on the peripheral nerves is damaged by the autoimmune effect. The disease typically follows a viral infection, surgery, other acute illness or immunization by a couple of weeks. Ascending Guillain-Barré exhibits muscle weakness and/or paralysis that begins in the distal lower extremities and travels upwards. The patient may also experience altered sensory perception in the same areas, such as the sensation of crawling, tingling, burning, or pain. The progression of symptoms may take hours or days. Descending Guillain-Barré begins with muscles in the face, jaw, or throat and travels downward. Respiratory compromise is a concern as the paralysis reaches the level of the intercostal muscles and diaphragm. Breathing can become compromised more quickly in patients with descending disease. Level of consciousness, mental status, personality, and pupil size are not affected.

Prognosis

Patient support and monitoring are important during symptom progression. Involvement of respiratory muscles may result in respiratory compromise or failure. Involvement of ocular areas may cause blindness. If the nerve cell body is damaged during the acute phase, there may be permanent deficits for the patient in the involved area. Otherwise, the axons of the nerves may be able to repair the damage over several months.

Hallmark Signs and Symptoms

- Burning, numbness, or a tickling feeling due to demyelination of the nerve axons.
- Symmetrical weakness or flaccid paralysis, typically ascending in pattern.
- Absence of deep tendon reflexes owing to changes within the nerves—reflexes are a sensory-motor response that happens at the spinal level, not the brain.
- Recent infection or other acute illness.
- Facial weakness, dysphagia, visual changes in descending disease.
- Labile blood pressure and cardiac dysrhythmias due to autonomic nervous system response.
- Difficulty breathing as the intercostal and diaphragmatic areas become involved.

Common Test Results

- Lumbar puncture will show CSF with increased protein; may not be present initially.
- Nerve conduction studies show slowed velocity.
- Pulmonary function tests show diminished tidal volume and vital capacity.

Treatment

- Monitor respirations and support ventilation if necessary.
- Plasmapheresis for plasma exchange to remove the antibodies in the circulation.
- Administer immunoglobulin intravenously after drawing labs for serum IgA.
- NG tube feeding if swallowing is a problem.

Nursing Diagnoses

- Ineffective breathing pattern
- Impaired gas exchange
- Impaired physical mobility
- Powerlessness

NURSING INTERVENTION

- Monitor for progression of change of sensation.
- Examine respiratory status for change in effort or rate, use of accessory muscles, cyanosis, change in breath sounds, breathlessness when talking, irritability, and decreased cognitive awareness.
- Call healthcare provider (physician, nurse practitioner, or physician assistant) if there are respiratory changes or decrease in pulse oximeter reading.
- Monitor gag reflex.
- Check for visual changes.
- Observe communication ability; the patient may need a special method to communicate with staff if not able to use the call bell system.
- Turn and reposition.
- Consult with social worker or chaplain for support services available to the patient.
- **Explain to the patient:**
  - Importance of turning and positioning.
  - Care of the plasmapheresis access site.
  - Importance of planning for home care needs.

7. Head Injury

What Went Wrong

The patient experiences a trauma to the head. The resulting injury may be a minor scalp laceration or a major internal injury with or without a skull fracture. There may be internal hemorrhage or cerebral edema resulting in hypoxia and a decrease in cognitive and functional capabilities. There are a variety of injuries that may be sustained. **Open head injuries** are typical of projectile wounds from gunshots or knives. **Closed head injuries** are typical of trauma from falls, motor vehicle accidents, sports, or fights.

Concussion involves a blow to the head where there is a bruising-type injury as the brain is thrust against the inside of skull. The point of injury where the brain makes an impact against the skull is referred to as a coup injury.

There is also a contrecoup injury as the head recoils away from the point of impact and the brain is thrust against the inside of the skull at the opposite point of the head, resulting in injury there as well. Patients with concussion may experience a transient loss of consciousness associated with bradycardia, or slowing of the heart rate; low blood pressure; slow, shallow breathing; amnesia of the injury and the events immediately following the injury; headache; and temporary loss of mental focus. Cerebral contusion is a more serious injury than concussion. Greater damage is done to the brain; cerebral edema or hemorrhage may occur and lead to necrosis. Patients typically have longer loss of consciousness with a cerebral contusion.

Hemorrhages can occur at a variety of levels, between the skull and the outer coverings (dura) of the brain, within the layers covering the brain, or within the brain tissue. The bleeding may occur acutely, at the time of injury, or hours to weeks later. An **epidural** hematoma happens at the time of injury from an arterial site. The blood accumulates between the skull and the **dura mater**, or the outermost layer covering the brain. The site is often in the temporal area. The patient is typically awake and talking immediately after the blow to the head. Within a short time, the patient becomes unstable and then unconscious. Emergency neurosurgery is necessary to relieve the pressure and stop the bleeding. **Subdural** hematoma is typically bleeding from a venous source into the area below the dura mater and above the **arachnoid mater**. This may occur acutely in some patients, but can also occur as a slow, chronic bleed, especially in the elderly patient. The elderly patient with a chronic bleed may have a significant amount of blood accumulate before symptoms occur due to age-related changes in the volume of brain tissue. A **subarachnoid** hemorrhage causes blood to accumulate within the area below the arachnoid mater and above the **pia mater**. The CSF is found in this area. An **intracerebral** bleed is an accumulation of blood within the tissues of the brain. This may be owing to a shearing force on the brain tissue from a twisting motion between the upper part of the brain (cerebrum) and the brain stem or tearing of small vessels within the brain. There will be associated edema and elevation of intracranial pressure.

Simple **skull fractures** are displaced and do not require specific intervention. Depressed skull fractures have bone fragments that have been broken off from the skull and pressed down toward the brain tissue. These fractures need to be corrected surgically. A basilar skull fracture has classic signs that include periorbital bruising (**raccoon sign**), blood behind the eardrum (**Battle's sign**), and leaking of CSF from the nose or ear (check for glucose content to distinguish from a runny nose).

Prognosis

The prognosis following head injury varies greatly depending on the location of the injury, the severity of the damage that occurred, and the treatment that was received. Patients with loss of consciousness over 2 minutes have a more severe injury and therefore worse prognosis. Patients who have loss of memory, either about the incident or the events immediately following, also have a more severe injury and worse prognosis. Some patients develop hemorrhage as a late effect of head injury, occurring hours, or in some cases, days after the initial injury. Post-traumatic seizure disorder can also occur as a late effect of head injury.

Hallmark Signs and Symptoms

- Headache owing to direct trauma and/or increasing intracranial pressure
- Disorientation or cognitive changes
- Changes in speech
- Changes in motor movements
- Nausea and vomiting because of increased intracranial pressure
- Unequal pupil size—important to determine if due to neurologic change or if the patient has always had unequal pupil size (small percentage of population has unequal pupil size)
- Diminished or absent pupil reaction owing to neurologic compromise
- Decreased level of consciousness or loss of consciousness
- Amnesia

Common Test Results

- Skull x-ray shows fractures.
- MRI shows edema and hemorrhage.
- CT scan shows hemorrhage, cerebral edema, and displacement of midline structures.
- EEG indicates focal seizure activity.

Treatment

- Surgical interventions may be necessary (craniotomy).
  - Removal of **hematoma**
- Ligation of bleeding vessel
- Bur holes (drilling holes) for decompression

- Debridement of foreign material and dead cells
- Administer antibiotics for open head injuries to prevent infection.
- Ventilatory assist if needed—intubation and mechanical ventilation.
- Administer low-dose opioids for restlessness, agitation, and pain in ventilator-dependent patients.
  - morphine sulfate or fentanyl citrate
- Administer osmotic diuretics to reduce cerebral edema.
  - mannitol
- Administer loop diuretics to decrease edema and circulating blood volume.
  - furosemide
- Administer analgesics.
  - acetaminophen (Tylenol)
- High-protein, high-calorie, high-vitamin diet.
- Platelet and packed RBC transfusions—if blood counts warrant transfusion.

Nursing Diagnoses

- Risk for injury
- Ineffective tissue perfusion
- Decreased intracranial adaptive capacity
- Risk for disturbed thought processes

NURSING INTERVENTION

- Avoid discussing the patient's condition in the presence of the patient—remember the patient can still hear you even though he or she is not conscious, and may recall the conversations after he or she regain consciousness.
- Monitor vital signs for stability—increased blood pressure with widening pulse pressure and slow pulse, suggestive of increased intracranial pressure.
- Check neurologic status for changes—typically use Glasgow Coma Scale or a similar tool to grade response to stimuli (highest score 15):

• Eye-opening response	spontaneous	4
	to sound	3
	to pain	2
	none	1

• Motor responses	obeys commands	6
	localizes pain	5
	withdrawal (normal)	4
	abnormal flexion	3
	extension	2
	none	1
• Verbal responses	oriented	5
	confused conversation	4
	inappropriate words	3
	incomprehensible sounds	2
	none	1

- Monitor for signs of intracranial pressure—report changes.
- Check for signs of infection at the wound site in postoperative patients.
- Examine signs for diabetes insipidus—increased risk due to injury to the pituitary gland.
- Monitor intake and output.
- Observe urine specific gravity, serum, and urine osmolarity.
- Collaborate with a dietician for appropriate diet, if any swallowing or oral sensory concerns.
- Seizure precautions per institution policy.
- **Explain to the patient and family:**
  - Any dietary restrictions.
  - Any activity restrictions.
  - Medication actions, side effects, interactions.
  - What to do in case of a seizure, how to protect the patient from further injury, time the seizure, monitor for breathing, when to call the doctor or EMS.
  - Call your physician at any signs of change in the level of consciousness—drowsiness, lethargy, change in personality.

8. Huntington's Disease

What Went Wrong

Huntington's disease (chorea) is a degenerative disease that presents with a gradual onset of involuntary, jerking movements (chorea), and a progressive decline in mental ability, resulting in behavioral changes and dementia. The disease is transmitted genetically, as an autosomal dominant trait located on chromosome 4. Family members of patients can have genetic testing done to identify the presence of the gene. The symptoms typically appear between the ages of 30 and 50 years.

Prognosis

The patient may present with either abnormalities of movements or changes in intellectual function. In time, both will be present. The mental status changes will progress to dementia. The disease will prove to be fatal within 10 to 20 years from the time of onset.

Hallmark Signs and Symptoms

- Personality changes
- Irritability or moodiness
- Psychiatric disturbance
- Progressive dementia as disease causes further neurologic degeneration
- Restlessness or fidgeting due to dyskinesia
- Abnormal, jerking movements (chorea)
- Depression

Common Test Results

- Genetic testing can detect gene presence even prior to the onset of symptoms.
- CT scan shows cerebral atrophy later in disease.
- MRI shows atrophy later in disease.
- Positron emission tomography (PET) shows a decrease in glucose uptake in specific areas in a structurally normal brain.

Treatment

Huntington's disease is progressive and while there is no cure for it, medications can be used to control symptoms.

- Genetic counseling.
- Control dyskinesia and behavior with medication to block dopamine receptors.
- phenothiazines
- haloperidol
- reserpine

Nursing Diagnoses

- Risk for injury
- Impaired physical mobility
- Ineffective health maintenance

NURSING INTERVENTION

- Provide basic needs for the patient, assist with ADLs as needed.
- Protect the patient from suicide attempts due to depression.
- Assist the patient with positioning for safety and comfort.
- **Explain to the patient:**
  - Nature of disease.
  - Genetic counseling available for family members of patients.

---

9. Meningitis

What Went Wrong

Meningitis is the inflammation of the meningeal coverings of the brain and the spinal cord, most commonly due to bacteria or viral cause, although it can also be caused by fungus, protozoa, or toxic exposure. Bacterial meningitis is the second most common, and it is typically due to *Streptococcus pneumoniae* (pneumococcal) and *Neisseria meningitidis* (meningococcal). The incidence of *Haemophilus influenzae* meningitis infections has decreased since the vaccine against *H influenzae* began to be used routinely in infants in the early 1990s. Other organisms that can cause bacterial meningitis include *Staphylococcus aureus*, *Escherichia coli*, and *Pseudomonas*. Organisms typically travel either through the bloodstream to the central nervous system or enter by direct contamination (skull fracture or extension from sinus infections). Bacterial meningitis is more common in colder months when upper respiratory tract infections are more common. People in close living conditions, such as prisons, military barracks, or college dormitories, are at greater risk for outbreaks of bacterial meningitis due to the likelihood of transmission.

Viral meningitis may follow other viral infections, such as mumps, herpes simplex or zoster, enterovirus, measles, or West Nile virus. Viral meningitis is more common than bacterial meningitis, tends to be milder, and is often a self-limiting illness. Late summer and early fall is the most common time for viral meningitis.

Patients who are immunocompromised have an increased risk for contracting fungal meningitis. This may travel from the bloodstream to the central nervous system or by direct contamination. *Cryptococcus neoformans* may be the causative organism in these patients.

Prognosis

Identification of meningitis and the causative organism is important in order to adequately treat the patient. Bacterial meningitis still has a significant mortality rate (about 10% of cases are fatal) and these patients need to be managed in the hospital soon after the onset of symptoms. Some patients will have permanent neurologic effects following the acute episode. Viral meningitis is typically self-limiting. Fungal meningitis often occurs in patients who are immunocompromised. Patients who have comorbidities or are elderly have greater difficulty with the symptoms of meningitis.

Hallmark Signs and Symptoms

- Stiff neck due to meningeal irritation and irritation of the spinal nerves
- Nuchal rigidity (pain when flexing chin toward chest) owing to meningeal irritation and irritation of the spinal nerves
- Headache as a result of increased intracranial pressure
- Nausea and vomiting because of increased intracranial pressure
- Photophobia (sensitivity to light) due to irritation of the cranial nerves
- Fever owing to infection
- Malaise and fatigue due to infection
- Myalgia (muscle aches) because of viral infection
- Petechial rash on skin and mucous membranes with meningococcal infection
- Seizures due to irritation of the brain from increased intracranial pressure

Common Test Results

- Lumbar puncture for CSF analysis, glucose (bacterial low), protein (bacterial elevated), cell counts (bacterial elevated neutrophils), and culture.
- Increased CSF pressure noted.
- PCR test of CSF to test for organisms—results within a couple of hours.
- Culture and sensitivity—final results may take up to 72 hours.

- Blood cultures.
- CT scan of the brain to rule out space-occupying lesion as a cause of symptoms.

Treatment

There is no specific treatment for viral meningitis. Bed rest, fluids, antipyretics, and analgesics are commonly given.

- Administer antibiotics as soon as possible to improve the outcome of bacterial meningitis.
  - penicillin G
  - ampicillin
  - ceftriaxone
  - cefotaxime
  - vancomycin plus ceftriaxone or cefotaxime
  - ceftazidime
  - rifampin
- Fungal infections are typically treated with:
  - fluconazole
  - acyclovir
- Administer corticosteroid to decrease inflammation in pneumococcal infection.
  - dexamethasone
- Administer osmotic diuretics for cerebral edema.
  - mannitol
- Administer analgesics for headache if needed.
  - acetaminophen
- Administer anticonvulsant if necessary.
  - phenytoin, phenobarbital
- Bed rest until neurologic irritation improves.

Nursing Diagnoses

- Risk for injury
- Powerlessness

NURSING INTERVENTION

- Monitor fluid intake and output to check balance.
- Keep room darkened due to photophobia.
- Monitor neurologic function at least every 2 to 4 hours: look for changes in mental status, level of consciousness, pupil reactions, speech, facial movement symmetry, and signs of increased intracranial pressure.
- Seizure precautions per institution policy.
- Isolation per policy depending on the organism.
- **Explain to the patient:**
  - Why restrictions (bed rest) are necessary.
  - Vaccine available for meningococcal meningitis—the two different types are meningococcal polysaccharide vaccine (MPSV4) and conjugate vaccine (MCV4).

---

10. Multiple Sclerosis

What Went Wrong

Multiple sclerosis (MS) is an autoimmune disease that results in demyelination of the white matter of the nervous system. Nerve impulses travel along the myelin coating on the outside of the nerve cells. With the disruption in the myelin on the outside of the nerve cells, the transmission of information from cell to cell within the nervous system is altered. The patient's sensations, movements, or mental function may be affected. A patient with relapsing-remitting disease will have episodes of exacerbation when symptoms occur and then months or years of symptom-free episodes (see Fig. 5–4). A portion of these patients will progress to enter a disease state that has a steady pattern of deterioration without relation to the periodic exacerbations; this is referred to as a secondary progressive multiple sclerosis (SPMS). Other patients have a primary progressive multiple sclerosis (PPMS) and develop the steady deterioration from the onset of the disease.

Prognosis

The actual cause of the disease is unknown, although it is thought to be auto-immune. The disease is progressive. Stress may be noted to aggravate symptoms. When damage is done to the nerve cells, it is not repairable, even when symptoms resolve in between periods of exacerbation. The pattern of symptoms will vary from one patient to the next. The time frame between exacerbations will also vary. As the disease progresses, the patient will lose more

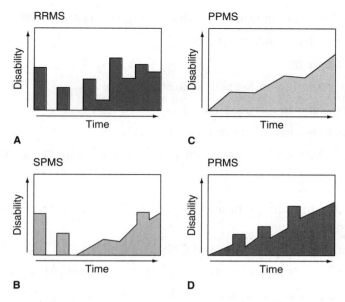

FIGURE 5–4 · Clinical course of multiple sclerosis (MS). A. Relapsing/remitting MS (RRMS). B. Secondary progressive MS (SPMS). C. Primary progressive MS (PPMS). D. Progressive/relapsing MS (PRMS).

Source: Reproduced with permission from: Longo DL, Fauci AS, Kasper DL, Hauser SL, Jameson JL, Loscalzo J: *Harrison's Principles of Internal Medicine*, 18th ed. New York, NY: McGraw-Hill; 2012. Fig. 380–2.

functional ability and will ultimately need assistance with basic self-care needs. The disease is more common in women and most often diagnosed between the ages of 20 and 40.

Hallmark Signs and Symptoms
Symptoms have periods of exacerbation and remission. Symptoms typically resolve completely in between exacerbations early in the disease process. Symptoms will vary depending on the actual location of the demyelination.

- Double vision (diplopia)
- Blurred vision
- Fatigue
- Muscle weakness or unsteadiness
- Unsteady gait due to muscle weakness and general unsteadiness
- Intolerance of temperature changes

- Ataxia (decrease in motor coordination, gross motor movements)
- Increased deep tendon reflexes
- Slurred speech
- Burning tingling on the skin (paresthesia)
- Paralysis later in disease state
- Memory loss; loss of attention or mental focus
- Urinary urgency or hesitancy due to changes in sphincter control

Common Test Results

- Increased immunoglobulin G (IgG) in CSF. CSF tested for oligoclonal banding.
- MRI shows demyelination and CNS plaques.
- CT scan shows increased density of white matter or plaque formation.
  - Nerve conduction studies will show alteration in affected areas.

Treatment

- Use one of the following biologic response modifiers on a continuous basis, not just during periods of exacerbation.
  - interferons
  - natalizumab
  - glatiramer acetate
- Administer immunosuppressants—may be helpful for SPMS.
  - cyclophosphamide
  - azathioprine
  - methotrexate
  - cladribine
  - mitoxantrone
- Administer corticosteroids.
  - methylprednisolone intravenously
  - prednisone 60 to 80 mg daily the first week, then tapered over the next couple of weeks
  - dexamethasone
- Administer one of the following for muscle relaxation.
  - dantrolene

- baclofen
- carisoprodol
- metaxalone
- tizanidine
- diazepam
- Use of the following medications may help with fatigue symptoms.
    - modafinil
    - methylphenidate
    - amantadine
- Administer antidepressants if indicated.
    - fluoxetine (selective serotonin reuptake inhibitor—SSRI)
    - sertraline (SSRI)
    - paroxetine (SSRI)
    - citalopram (SSRI)
    - escitalopram (SSRI)
    - venlafaxine (inhibits norepinephrine, serotonin, and dopamine reuptake)
    - bupropion (inhibits norepinephrine and dopamine reuptake)
    - duloxetine (inhibits norepinephrine and serotonin reuptake)
    - amitriptyline (tricyclic) may help with discomfort associated with paresthesia
- Administer medications to help with altered bladder function.
    - oxybutynin
    - hyoscyamine sulfate
    - darifenacin
    - solifenacin
    - tolterodine
- Remove antibodies by removing plasma (plasmapheresis).
- Administer medication that reduces the rates of immune system attacks on myelinated neurons by targeting B-lymphocytes that express a protein called CD20 that is related to the autoimmune response. Used for relapsing-remitting MS (RRMS) and primary-progress MS (PPMS).
    - ocrelizumab (Ocrevus)

Nursing Diagnoses

- Impaired physical mobility
- Fatigue
- Self-care deficit

NURSING INTERVENTION

- Monitor motor movements for interference with ADLs.
- Encourage activity balanced with rest periods.
- Assess cognitive function for changes or deterioration.
- **Explain to the patient:**
  - Bladder training.
  - Teach self-catheterization if necessary (for patients with flexi bladder).
  - Increase fluid intake unless other medical problems contraindicate.
  - Importance of positioning.
  - Avoid temperature extremes.
  - Medication compliance.

---

11. Myasthenia Gravis

What Went Wrong

This is an autoimmune disorder of the peripheral nervous system involving antibodies that have been produced by the body; they bind to receptor sites that normally bind acetylcholine. This prevents the acetylcholine from binding to the receptor sites on the skeletal muscle, inhibiting normal muscle contraction in the affected area. The areas of the body most commonly affected by the autoimmune disease include the muscles in the eyes, face, lips, tongue, throat, and neck, resulting in weakness and fatigue of these areas. The disease does not seem to be hereditary but does have a family tendency toward autoimmune disorders. The majority of the patients have a hyperplasia (excessive growth of normal cells) of the thymus gland. Myasthenia gravis is more likely to develop in young women or older men.

Prognosis

The disease can take a variety of forms from mild weakness of voluntary muscles and drooping of the eye muscles to generalized, progressive weakness that ultimately affects respiratory function. Progression of symptoms will vary from patient to patient. There are typically episodes of exacerbations and remissions. The aggressive form of the disease progresses more rapidly, resulting in death from respiratory failure.

Hallmark Signs and Symptoms

- Ptosis (drooping of the upper eyelid) due to muscular weakness
- Diplopia (double vision) owing to inability to keep both eyes focused on the same object
- Trouble closing eyes completely; dry eyes because of muscle weakness
- Difficulty swallowing (dysphagia) as a result of muscle weakness
- Muscle weakness later in the day or with activity due to fatigue
- Proximal muscle weakness
- Fatigue
- Normal deep tendon reflexes
- In advanced disease—loss of bowel and bladder control; difficulty with respiratory function
- Myasthenic crisis is an exacerbation of symptoms owing to insufficient medication.
  - Tachycardia
  - Tachypnea
  - Elevated blood pressure
  - Cyanosis
  - Decrease in urinary output
  - Incontinence of bowel and bladder
  - Loss of gag reflex
- Cholinergic crisis is an exacerbation of weakness due to too much cholinergic medication.
  - Blurred vision
  - Nausea, vomiting, diarrhea
  - Abdominal cramping
  - Paleness
  - Twitching of facial muscles

- Small pupils (miosis)
- Low blood pressure

Common Test Results

Symptoms are relieved temporarily after administering edrophonium (Tensilon) or neostigmine bromide (Prostigmin) because the drug will allow the acetylcholine to bind at the postsynaptic receptor site on the muscle at which it should normally bind.

- Acetylcholine receptor antibodies are present in more than 80% of patients with myasthenia gravis.
- EMG shows reduced muscle response to repeated stimulations.
- CT scan to rule out thymoma.

Treatment

There is no specific cure for myasthenia gravis.

- Administer immunosuppressants to induce remission and help control symptoms.
  - prednisone or dexamethasone initially to improve symptoms
  - azathioprine and cyclophosphamide in the long term to help control symptoms
- Administer cholinesterase inhibitors for long-term control of symptoms. These drugs have short duration of action; therefore, they have to be dosed several times during the day.
  - neostigmine
  - pyridostigmine
  - ambenonium
- Administer natural tears or other lubricants to keep eyes moist.
  - patch eyes if unable to close
- High-calorie diet of appropriate food type—patient may have difficulty swallowing.
- Removing antibodies from plasma (plasmapheresis) may be beneficial.
- BiPAP or CPAP for enhanced air movement and oxygenation.
- Thymectomy (surgical removal of thymus gland) for patients with thymoma.
- Avoid aminoglycoside antibiotics that may exacerbate symptoms.

Nursing Diagnoses

- Impaired physical mobility
- Impaired verbal communication
- Ineffective air exchange
- Self-care deficit

NURSING INTERVENTION

- Encourage frequent rest periods.
- Monitor vital signs.
- Monitor nutritional intake.
- Monitor weight.
- Monitor neurologic status for changes in pupil reaction, extraocular movements, eyelid movement, facial symmetry, hand grip strength, coordination, fine motor skills, and gait.
- Monitor respiratory status for changes in rate, effort, skin color, use of accessory muscles, or change in mental status.
- Monitor gag reflex.
- Arrange for appropriate communication with staff if the patient is unable to use the call bell system or unable to be heard over intercom from the room.
- **Explain to the patient:**
  - Home care needs.
  - Medication use; need to maintain time schedule for medications.
  - Time meals an hour after medications to decrease the chance of aspiration.
  - Teach use of oral-pharyngeal suctioning catheter to clear secretions.
  - Avoid heat extremes (hot tubs, saunas).
  - Alcohol may exacerbate symptoms.

12. Parkinson's Disease

What Went Wrong

There is a gradual degeneration of the midbrain area known as the substantia nigra. The neurons use the neurotransmitter dopamine to send their signals from cell to cell. The loss of neurons within the substantia nigra continues and results in diminished voluntary fine motor skills due to dopamine loss. There is also development of sympathetic noradrenergic lesions, causing norepinephrine loss within the sympathetic nervous system. There is excess effect of the excitatory neurotransmitter acetylcholine on the neurons; this causes increased muscle tone, leading to rigidity and tremors. There seems to be a genetic tendency toward the development of Parkinson's disease. Environmental factors such as exposure to airborne contaminants, occupational chemicals, toxins, or a virus have been implicated in the development of the disease. Typical age of onset is after the fifth decade of life.

Prognosis

Parkinson's disease is a progressive disorder, and it does not have a cure. The symptoms can be managed with medicines, but will return as the medications wear off. The dosages will need to be adjusted periodically, and additional medications may be needed to address the side effects of the medicines used. Some patients develop mental status changes or dementia in conjunction with Parkinson's disease.

Hallmark Signs and Symptoms

- Mask-like facial expressions
- Slow, shuffling gait
- Pill-rolling movements of hands
- Stooping posture
- Tremor at rest
- Change in handwriting—gets progressively smaller over time
- Bradykinesia (slow movement)
- Trouble chewing or swallowing
- Drooling
- Inability to control voluntary movement (dyskinesia) and fine-skilled movement, or to initiate movement—due to loss of dopamine which has an inhibitory effect and helps refine movements while acetylcholine retains the excitatory effect on the neurons
- Rigidity of limbs
  - Cogwheeling—there is a rhythmic stopping or interruption of the movement of the extremity.
  - Lead pipe—no bending; resists movement completely.
- Orthostatic hypotension due to lack of norepinephrine within the sympathetic nervous system, affecting the cardiovascular system.

Common Test Results

- CSF levels may show low levels of dopamine.

Treatment

- Administer antiparkinsonian agents that are able to cross the blood-brain barrier. These drugs absorb better on an empty stomach.
  - levodopa
  - carbidopa-levodopa
- Administer dopamine receptor agonists to act directly on the dopamine receptor sites.
  - pergolide
  - bromocriptine
  - pramipexole
  - ropinirole
- Administer selegiline, a selective monoamine oxidase B inhibitor that slows the breakdown of dopamine and allows lower doses of levodopa to be used because it prolongs its effect.
- Administer catechol O-methyltransferase (COMT) inhibitors that help block the breakdown of levodopa.
  - entacapone
  - tolcapone
- Administer acetylcholine blocking drugs to decrease tremor and rigidity in patients.
  - biperiden
  - benztropine mesylate
  - procyclidine
  - orphenadrine
  - trihexyphenidyl
- Diet high in protein and calories.
- Soft food diet.
- Physical therapy.

Nursing Diagnoses

- Activity intolerance
- Impaired mobility
- Risk for injury

NURSING INTERVENTION

- Monitor neurologic status for changes.
- Examine respiratory status for changes.
- Encourage self-care, allow patient extra time.
- Encourage exercise; assist with passive ROM if necessary.
- Weigh patient.
- Record food intake.
- **Explain to the patient:**
  - Importance of following medication time schedule as well as effects of medication wearing off.
  - Reduce risk of falls at home.

13. Spinal Cord Injury

What Went Wrong

Injury to the spinal cord results in compression, twisting, severing, or pulling on the spinal cord. The damage to the cord may involve the entire thickness of the cord (complete), or only a partial area of the spinal cord (limited). The most common cause of spinal cord injury is trauma. Any level of the spinal cord may have been affected by the injury. Loss of sensation, motor control, or reflexes may occur below the level of injury or within 1 to 2 vertebrae or spinal nerves above the level of injury. The loss may be unilateral or bilateral. Motor neurons are located on the anterior surface of the spinal cord, with sensory neurons located on the posterior aspect. Damage to the vertebrae may have occurred at the same time as the spinal cord injury. Swelling due to the initial trauma may make the injury seem more severe than it actually is. When the initial swelling resolves, the actual degree of permanent injury can be more accurately assessed.

Prognosis

The level of injury will determine the degree of disability the patient is likely to sustain. A high-level injury, such as a cervical injury, will more likely result in quadriplegia (paralysis of all four extremities) and compromise of the respiratory drive. A complete spinal cord injury will result in greater disability than an incomplete injury. Spinal cord tissue does not regenerate after an injury. Swelling that occurs immediately following an injury may be controlled with medications and some clinical improvement may occur, but the damage to the cord cannot be undone.

Hallmark Signs and Symptoms

- Loss of motor control due to damage to the anterior horn of the spinal cord
- Loss of reflexes because of damage of the spinal cord, the point of synaptic transmission of sensory impulse to motor response
- Flaccid paralysis
- Lack of bowel and bladder control
- Altered sensation (tingling—paresthesia; diminished—hypoesthesia; increased—hyperesthesia)
- Bradycardia, hypotension, hypothermia due to problems with the autonomic nervous system

Common Test Results

- MRI shows vertebral or spinal cord injury and edema.
- CT scan shows vertebral or spinal cord injury and edema.
- Spinal x-ray may show damage to the vertebrae.
- Somatosensory-evoked potentials will show the ability of nerve signals to pass through the tissue.

Treatment

Immediate treatment needs to be initiated as soon as possible after the injury.

- Immobilize the affected area of the spinal cord to decrease the chance of further irritation.
- Place the patient on bed rest in a flat position to avoid flexion or misalignment of the spine.
- Moderate systemic hypothermia to reduce damage and improve chances for maximal recovery of function.
- Monitor traction or collar to prevent skin irritation.
- Administer corticosteroid to decrease inflammation at the point of injury.
  - methylprednisolone
  - prednisone
  - dexamethasone
- Administer dextran, a plasma expander, which increases blood flow in the spinal cord, increasing oxygenation to the tissue.
- Assist respirations if indicated.

- Administer H2 receptor antagonists to protect the stomach from stress ulcer formation.
  - cimetidine, ranitidine, famotidine, nizatidine
- Administer gastric mucosal protective agent to coat stomach lining.
  - sucralfate
- Place patient in a rotation bed for repositioning to prevent pressure on the skin.
- Surgical repair of vertebral fracture or decompression may be necessary.
- Physical therapy.

Nursing Diagnoses

- Impaired physical mobility
- Powerlessness

NURSING INTERVENTION

- Monitor respiratory status—assess for changes in rate, effort, use of accessory muscles, cyanosis, altered mental status, and pulse oximetry reading.
- Examine neurologic status for changes—assess sensation, temperature, touch, position sense, comparing right to left.
- Check for spinal shock.
  - Flaccid paralysis, loss of reflexes below the level of injury, hypotension, brady-cardia, possible paralytic ileus.
- Monitor pulse and blood pressure for changes—change in heart rate, hypoten-sion, or hypertension.
- Assess skin for signs of pressure (redness) or breakdown.
- Assess abdomen and listen for bowel sounds.
- **Explain to the patient:**
  - Importance of regular bowel and bladder function to avoid autonomic dys-reflexia due to distension: severe headache, hypertension, bradycardia, flush-ing, nasal congestion, sweating, and nausea.
  - Use of an incentive spirometer.
  - Need for turning and positioning or a special rotating bed to decrease pressure.
  - Monitor fluid intake and output.
  - Home care needs—accessibility, equipment needs.
  - Proper way to transfer from a bed to a wheelchair.
  - Care of pin sites for cervical traction devices (eg, halo traction).

14. Stroke

What Went Wrong

A stroke is also known as a cerebrovascular accident (CVA) or a brain attack. Blood supply is interrupted to part of the brain, causing brain cells to die, resulting in the loss of brain function in the affected area. Interruption is usually caused by an obstruction of arterial blood flow, referred to as *ischemic* stroke (see Fig. 5–5), such as formation of a blood clot, but can also be caused by a leaking or ruptured blood vessel, referred to as *hemorrhagic* stroke. A blood clot may develop from a piece of unstable plaque lining a vessel wall that breaks free, or an embolus that travels from

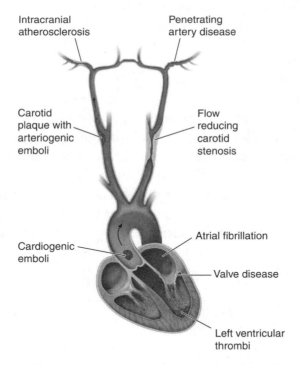

Intracranial atherosclerosis

Penetrating artery disease

Carotid plaque with arteriogenic emboli

Flow reducing carotid stenosis

Cardiogenic emboli

Atrial fibrillation

Valve disease

Left ventricular thrombi

FIGURE 5–5 · The three major mechanisms that underlie ischemic stroke: (1) occlusion of an intracranial vessel by an embolus that arises at a distant site (eg, cardiogenic sources such as atrial fibrillation or artery-to-artery emboli from carotid atherosclerotic plaque), often affecting the large intracranial vessels; (2) in situ thrombosis of an intracranial vessel, typically affecting the small penetrating arteries that arise from the major intracranial arteries; (3) hypoperfusion caused by flow-limiting stenosis of a major extracranial (eg, internal carotid) or intracranial vessel, often producing "watershed" ischemia.

Source: Reproduced with permission from: Longo DL, Fauci AS, Kasper DL, Hauser SL, Jameson JL, Loscalzo J: *Harrison's Principles of Internal Medicine*, 18th ed. New York, NY: McGraw-Hill; 2012. Fig. 370–3A.

elsewhere in the body and lodges within the vessel. The bleeding may occur as a result of trauma or it may occur spontaneously, as in the setting of uncontrolled hypertension. Ischemia occurs when insufficient blood is getting to the brain tissue. This leads to lack of available oxygen (hypoxia) and glucose (hypoglycemia) for the brain. When these nutrients are not available for a sustained period, the brain cells die, causing an area of infarction. Permanent deficits result from infarction. There is increased risk of stroke in patients with a history of hypertension, diabetes mellitus, high cholesterol, atrial fibrillation, obesity, smoking, or oral contraceptive use.

Patients may also experience a transient ischemic attack (TIA) in which the symptoms result from a temporary problem with blood flow to a specific area of the brain. The symptoms have duration between a few minutes and 24 hours. Patients who have had a TIA have a significantly increased risk of subsequent stroke.

Prognosis

The degree of damage and location of the stroke will determine the outcome for the patient. Strokes occur suddenly and patients should seek immediate treatment for the best possible outcome. The majority of strokes are ischemic. Rapid entry into the healthcare system and treatment with thrombolytic agents (unless there are contraindications to this treatment) to break up a clot that has caused the ischemia give the patient the best chance for recovery without permanent disability. Patients with hemorrhagic stroke may need surgery to relieve intracranial pressure or stop the bleeding. A large area of damage may lead to significant permanent disability or death.

Hallmark Signs and Symptoms

- Mental impairment
- Disorientation, confusion
- Emotional changes, personality changes
- Aphasia (difficulty with speech; may be receptive, expressive)
- Slurring of words
- Sensory changes (paresthesia, visual changes, hearing changes)
- Unilateral numbness or weakness in face or limbs
- Seizure

- Severe headache due to increased intracranial pressure from hemorrhage
- TIA symptoms are similar but have a shorter duration (< 24 hours) and resolve completely.

Stroke scales (such as the NIH Stroke Scale) are often used to evaluate the severity of patient's symptoms. These scales typically grade the current level of consciousness, assess the patient's gaze, visual perception, motor and sensory function of the face, upper and lower extremities, language ability and clarity of speech and whether there is any neglect (inattention to the affected side of the body). A normal score on the NIH Stroke Scale is 0 (zero) with increasing scores reflecting increasing deficits.

Common Test Results

- CT scan identifies the area of bleeding (usually for emergency use).
- MRI identifies the location of ischemic areas (slower than CT scan).
- MRA can identify abnormal vasculature or vasospasm.
- Diffusion/perfusion MRI or MRA will show areas that are not getting adequate blood supply but have not yet suffered an infarction.
- SPECT will show an area that is not perfusing adequately.
- Carotid duplex ultrasound to determine if the arteries are narrowed (due to plaque buildup).
- Echocardiogram to determine if a blood clot within the heart may have caused the stroke.
- EKG to determine if an underlying rhythm abnormality (such as atrial fibrillation) caused the stroke.

Treatment

It is most important to determine whether the patient has suffered an ischemic or hemorrhagic stroke as the treatment is different. Giving a thrombolytic agent to the patient who has had a hemorrhagic stroke will only cause further bleeding into the brain. Caution is also recommended in patients with head trauma, uncontrolled hypertension, hemorrhagic retinopathy, gastrointestinal bleeding, recent surgery, recent MI, or pregnancy.

- Administer thrombolytic agent (TPA) within 3 hours of onset of symptoms, unless contraindicated.

- Contraindications typically include:
  - Evidence of intracranial bleeding
  - Suspected subarachnoid bleed
  - Head trauma within the past 90 days
  - History of previous intracranial bleeding, neoplasm, arteriovenous malformation (AVM), or aneurysm
  - Major surgery within the past 2 weeks
  - Recent use of heparin products with prolonged thromboplastin time (PTT) and low platelet count
  - Lumbar puncture within the past week
  - International normalized ratio (INR) more than 1.7
  - Uncontrolled blood pressure (>185/110 mmHg after medication)
  - Unknown or prolonged time since symptom onset
  - Terminal illness with short (<6 months) life expectancy
- Administer anticoagulants to patients with ischemic stroke after use of TPA.
  - heparin, warfarin, low–molecular-weight heparin, aspirin
- Administer antiplatelet medications to decrease platelet adhesiveness; used to prevent recurrent stroke.
  - clopidogrel, ticlopidine hydrochloride, dipyridamole
- Administer corticosteroid to decrease swelling.
  - dexamethasone (Decadron)
- Physical therapy to help maintain muscle tone or return function.
- Speech therapy to help with speech and swallowing.
- Occupational therapy to help regain function.
- Bed rest to reduce the chance of injury.
- Adequate nutrition in an appropriate food type for the patient.
- Carotid artery endarterectomy to remove plaque from within the carotid artery if stenosis is present.
- Stenting of carotid artery to maintain blood flow.
- Surgical correction of arteriovenous malformation, aneurysm, intracranial bleeding.

Nursing Diagnoses

- Risk for injury
- Ineffective tissue perfusion

NURSING INTERVENTION

- Monitor vital signs for changes.
- Assess neurologic status for signs of deterioration—perform neurologic checks at least every 4 hours—typically use Glasgow Coma Scale or a similar tool to grade response to stimuli (highest score 15):

  - Eye-opening response
spontaneous	4
to sound	3
to pain	2
none	1

  - Motor responses
obeys commands	6
localizes pain	5
withdrawal (normal)	4
abnormal flexion	3
extension	2
none	1

  - Verbal responses
oriented	5
confused conversation	4
inappropriate words	3
incomprehensible sounds	2
none	1

- Monitor for signs of increased intracranial pressure—diminished level of consciousness, headaches, restlessness, confusion, nausea and vomiting, speech changes, or seizures.
- Notify healthcare provider of changes in neurologic status.
- Develop means of communication with the patient—aphasia may compromise the use of the call bell system or intercom.
- Assess for neglect syndrome—patient may act as if unaware of the side affected by paralysis due to the stroke.
- Need for rehabilitation to return to prior functional ability.
- **Explain to the patient:**
  - Home care needs.
  - Proper technique to transfer from the bed to the chair.

- Use of ambulatory assist devices: cane, crutch, walker.
- Special dietary needs: use of Thick-It for liquids.
- Medication schedule, use, side effects, and interactions.

15. Seizure Disorder

What Went Wrong

This is a disorder that involves a sudden episode of abnormal, uncontrolled discharge of the electrical activity of the neurons within the brain. The patient may experience a variety of symptoms depending on the type of seizure and the cause. Seizures may be a symptom of another condition—such as a tumor or stroke which has increased the intracranial pressure, a metabolic disorder, withdrawal from alcohol or drugs—or may be due to a chronic seizure disorder such as epilepsy. Prior to the seizure, the patient may experience an aura, a sensory alteration involving sight, sound, or smell. After the seizure, the patient enters a postictal stage where there may be confusion, and the patient is often fatigued. The patient may not recall any of the seizure or the time immediately surrounding the seizure.

Generalized seizures	
Tonic clonic	Begins with stiffening or rigidity of muscles in the limbs (tonic), loss of consciousness, and then rhythmic jerking (clonic)
Tonic	Stiffening or rigidity of muscles; loss of consciousness
Clonic	Rhythmic jerking due to muscle contraction and relaxation
Absence	Brief loss of conscious awareness and staring into space; appears to be daydreaming
Myoclonic	Brief stiffening or jerking of extremity, either singly or in groups
Atonic	Loss of muscle tone
Partial seizures	
Simple partial	Begins with aura; may have unilateral unusual sensation or movement of extremity, autonomic (heart rate, flushing), or psychic changes; no loss of consciousness
Complex partial	Loss of consciousness; automatisms (lip smacking, picking, patting)

Common Test Results

- EEG to identify areas of abnormal electrical activity within the brain. This may be a scheduled one-time test or an ambulatory study with a 24-hour recording of electrical activity during normal activity.

- Implanted EEG electrodes provide monitoring of electrical activity and can pinpoint the area of involvement more accurately than electrodes placed on the scalp. This is an invasive procedure (electrodes are inserted in the operating room). The patients are monitored in the hospital for several days or longer. Risk of infection is a concern in these patients.
- CT scan of the brain to identify causes of increased intracranial pressure (rule out tumor or bleed).
- MRI to identify causes of increased intracranial pressure (rule out tumor or bleed).
- PET or SPECT to determine areas in the brain that are not adequately perfused.

Treatment

If there is an underlying condition causing the disorder, removal of this condition will often result in resolution of the disorder. The patient with a primary seizure disorder will typically be managed with anticonvulsant medications. Some patients will need multidrug regimens to adequately control the seizure disorder. Patients who do not respond to multiple antiepileptic drugs may be candidates for surgical intervention.

- Administer antiepileptic medications.
  - carbamazepine
  - phenytoin
  - phenobarbital
  - clonazepam
  - valproic acid
  - lamotrigine
  - gabapentin
  - levetiracetam
  - oxcarbazepine
  - primidone
  - tiagabine
  - topiramate
- Seizure precautions—these may vary slightly by the institution.
- Maintain IV access with saline lock if no intravenous fluids needed for hospitalized patients.

- Surgery to remove seizure focal area or sever the connection between the cerebral hemispheres (corpus callosotomy) to limit the amount of seizure activity for patients who do not have adequate control of seizures with medications.
- Vagal nerve stimulation where there is implantation of an electrical device that provides a predetermined pattern of vagal stimulation. This is used to decrease the frequency of seizures.

Nursing Diagnoses

- Risk for ineffective breathing pattern or airway clearance
- Risk for fall
- Anxiety

NURSING INTERVENTION

- Monitor patient during the seizure for breathing, skin color (cyanosis)—patient may have diminished oxygenation during seizure.
- May need supplemental oxygen post-seizure.
- Keep oxygen equipment, suction equipment, and emergency airway management equipment at the bedside (intubation may be performed by anesthesiologist, nurse anesthetist, or respiratory therapist).
- Monitor duration of seizure and progression of symptoms.
- Monitor for incontinence of bladder or bowel.
- Monitor for status epilepticus—prolonged seizures or repeated seizures, considered a medical emergency.
- Position patient to decrease the risk of injury:
  - Remove objects that may injure patient.
  - Turn patient on side to reduce risk of aspiration.
  - Do not insert anything in patient's mouth during seizure.
- Assess the patient post-seizure.
- **Explain to the patient:**
  - Medication use, side effects, and interactions.
  - Importance of taking medications on time, not skipping doses.
  - Importance of checking with prescriber before taking any new medications or over-the-counter (OTC) medications or supplements.
  - Have lab tests for drug level of antiepileptic drugs checked as directed.

16. Tumor

What Went Wrong

A brain tumor is a growth of abnormal cells within the brain tissue. The tumor may be a primary site that originated in the brain or a secondary site that has metastasized from a cancer site elsewhere in the body. Because the tumor is growing within the confined space of the skull, the patient will eventually develop signs of increased intracranial pressure. Some cell types grow faster than others; the patients with the more aggressive, fast-growing cancers will develop symptoms more quickly.

Prognosis

Meningiomas are typically benign tumors that begin from the meninges (covering the brain). They are more common in women and in people as they age. Treatment is surgical removal, but the growth tends to recur.

Gliomas are malignant brain tumors of the neuroglia cells that tend to be fast-growing. Patients have nonspecific symptoms of increased intracranial pressure. Treatment typically includes surgical debulking of the tumor; complete removal is often not possible at the time of diagnosis. Surgery is followed by radiation and chemotherapy. **Astrocytoma** is the most common glioma and has a variable prognosis.

Oligodendroglioma is more slow-growing and may be calcified. Glioblastoma is a poorly differentiated glioma with a poor prognosis.

Hallmark Signs and Symptoms

- Cerebellum or brain stem:
  - Lack of coordination—cerebellum helps coordinate gross movements
  - Hypotonia of limbs
  - Ataxia
- Frontal lobe:
  - Inability to speak (expressive aphasia)
  - Slowing of mental activity
  - Personality changes
  - Anosmia (loss of sense of smell)

- Occipital lobe:
  - Impaired vision—defect in visual fields; patient may deny or be unaware of defect
  - Prosopagnosia (patient is unable to recognize familiar faces)
  - Change in color perception
- Parietal lobe:
  - Seizures
  - Sight disturbances result in visual field defect
  - Sensory loss—unable to identify object placed in hand without looking
- Temporal lobe:
  - Seizures
  - Taste or smell hallucinations
  - Auditory hallucinations
  - Depersonalization
  - Emotional changes
  - Visual field defects
  - Receptive aphasia
  - Altered perception of music

Common Test Results

- MRI with gadolinium (contrast) defines tumor location and size.
- CT scan shows a characteristic appearance of meningioma.
- Angiography will show blood flow to the area; some tumors will displace vessels as they grow.

Treatment

- Chemotherapeutic agents alone or in combination with radiation and surgery—may be given orally, intravenously, or through an Ommaya reservoir. Drugs are chosen based on cell type.
  - carmustine, lomustine, procarbazine, vincristine, temozolomide, erlotinib, gefitinib
- Irradiation of the area to decrease tumor size.

- Craniotomy to remove the tumor if appropriate; this depends on location, size, primary site of cancer, and number of tumors. Some patients may have several small, scattered tumors, making surgery impractical.

- Administer glucocorticoid to reduce swelling or inflammatory response within confined space inside the skull (no room to expand, bone does not give).

  - dexamethasone

- Administer osmotic diuretic to reduce cerebral edema.

  - mannitol

- Administer anticonvulsant to reduce the chance of seizure activity.

  - phenytoin, phenobarbital, carbamazepine, divalproex sodium, valproic acid, levetiracetam, lamotrigine, clonazepam, topiramate, ethosuximide

- Administer mucosal barrier fortifier to reduce the risk of gastric irritation.

  - sucralfate

- Administer H2 receptor antagonists to reduce the risk of gastric irritation.

  - ranitidine, famotidine, nizatidine, cimetidine

- Administer proton pump inhibitors (PPIs) to reduce the risk of gastric irritation.

  - lansoprazole, omeprazole, esomeprazole, rabeprazole, pantoprazole

Nursing Diagnoses

- Disturbed sensory perception
- Risk for injury

NURSING INTERVENTION

- Monitor neurologic function.
- Check for side effects to medications.
- Seizure precautions per institution protocol.
- Assess for pain control.
- **Explain to the patient:**
  - Home care needs.
  - Possible need for hospice.

REVIEW QUESTIONS

1. **A patient is admitted to a unit diagnosed with advanced ALS. Which is the priority intervention?**

    A. Provide six small meals high in protein and assist with feeding.

    B. Do not involve the patient in decisions about his healthcare because he does not have the mental status to respond.

    C. Develop a method of communication.

    D. Provide six normal meals high in protein and assist with feeding.

2. **A patient who was in an automobile accident 30 minutes ago reports that he or she is unable to move his or her legs. What is the best response?**

    A. Swelling due to the initial trauma may make the injury seem more severe than it actually is. A more accurate assessment will be made once the swelling goes down.

    B. Swelling owing to the initial trauma prevents you from moving your legs.

    C. There are good rehabilitation centers that will help restore sensation to your legs.

    D. You should have been wearing your seatbelt.

3. **The wife of a patient who has a ruptured aneurysm asks how this could have happened considering that he passed a physical 3 months ago. What is the best response?**

    A. Aneurysms are often asymptomatic.

    B. The physician must have misread the x-ray.

    C. The aneurysm must have developed since his physical.

    D. Do not be too concerned because this happens all the time.

4. **A patient has unilateral facial paralysis and is unable to close his or her right eye. He or she is diagnosed with Bell's palsy. He or she asks the physician if there is any special care required for his or her eye. What is the best response?**

    A. No, since the symptoms will go away in a few weeks.

    B. Wear sunglasses.

    C. Increase fluid intake to prevent dryness of the eye.

    D. Yes, you will need to instill artificial teardrops and use an eye patch.

5. **A patient arrives in the ER with blurred and double vision, muscle weakness, and intolerance of temperature changes. The physician suspects multiple sclerosis. What test would you expect the physician to do in order to confirm his or her suspicions?**

    A. CBC with a very low WBC count.

    B. MRI with gadolinium showing demyelination of nerve fibers.

    C. Endocrine function study with a low growth hormone and high T3 and T4.

    D. Fasting glucose test with a result over 300 mg/dL.

6. **A patient diagnosed with Guillain-Barré syndrome has a burning, tickling feeling and asks what causes that feeling. What is the best response?**

    A. The myelin cover of the nerve endings is absent.

    B. You are lying too long on the affected side.

    C. This is in response to the medication.

    D. This is secondary to dysphagia.

7. **A patient arrived in the ER with a head injury. She is unconscious. The physician and a fellow nurse are the only staff members near the patient. Her husband begins to criticize the attending physician and suggest that a different physician should care for this patient. What is the best response?**

    A. Report the nurse to the attending physician.

    B. Call the nurse away from the patient and remind him that the patient can still hear even if unconscious.

    C. Ask the nurse why he has such feelings.

    D. Simply nod your head in agreement.

8. **A husband visiting his wife in the hospital suddenly becomes confused and has difficulty with speech and starts slurring his words. The physician caring for his wife recognizes this as a cerebrovascular accident. What would you expect the physician to do?**

    A. Administer TPA since this is within 3 hours of the CVS.

    B. Assess if the husband had an ischemic or hemorrhagic CVS.

    C. Tell the husband to go home, get rest, and to call the physician in the morning if the symptoms continue.

    D. Admit the husband and place him on bed rest.

9. **A new patient arrived in a physician's unit. He or she has been diagnosed with a brain tumor. The physician is told that the patient is unable to speak. Based on this sign, where is the tumor located?**

    A. Frontal lobe.

    B. Occipital lobe.

    C. Cerebellum.

    D. Parietal lobe.

10. **A 49-year-old patient is diagnosed with Huntington's disease. He thought he saw symptoms of the disease in his 15-year-old son. What is the best response?**

    A. Your son probably has the early symptoms of the disease.

    B. Huntington's disease is genetically transmitted.

C. Symptoms usually appear between the ages of 30 and 50 years; however, the patient may want to ask his physician about genetic testing that can detect if his son has the gene that is associated with Huntington's disease.

D. Symptoms usually appear before the age of 30 years; however, the patient may want to ask his physician about genetic testing that can detect if his son has the gene that is associated with Huntington's disease.

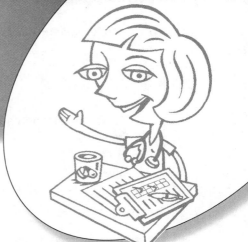

Chapter **6**

Musculoskeletal System

KEY CONCEPTS

1. Carpal tunnel syndrome
2. Fractures
3. Gout
4. Ligament sprain
5. Muscle/tendon strain

6. Osteoarthritis
7. Osteomyelitis
8. Osteoporosis
9. Tendonitis

KEY TERMS

Abduction
Adduction
Bursa
Cartilage
Circumduction
Connective tissues
Crepitus
Eversion
Extension
Flexion

Inversion
Osteoblasts
Osteoclasts
Phalanges
Pronation
Rotation
Supination
Synovial joints
Synovium
Tendons

How the Musculoskeletal System Works

The musculoskeletal system provides both structure and function for the body. The bones protect and support the vital organs (see Fig. 6–1). The skeleton is divided into the axial and appendicular areas. The axial skeleton protects the vital organs, surrounding the central nervous system and thoracic cavity. The appendicular skeleton attaches to the axial skeleton and consists primarily of the limbs. Bones are classified by both their shape and composition. Short bones (like the **phalanges**) are found in the fingers and toes. Long bones (like the humerus or femur) are found in the limbs. Irregular bones are named for their shapes and are found in the joints of the ankle or wrist and in the middle ear. Flat bones (ribs or scapula) protect inner organs. The outer layer of bone tissue is a dense compact-bone tissue called the cortex. Blood supply for the bone travels through small blood vessels within haversian canals located longitudinally within the cortical bone area. The inner layer is a spongier, cancellous tissue that has spaces filled with marrow. Production of blood cells occurs within the red bone marrow.

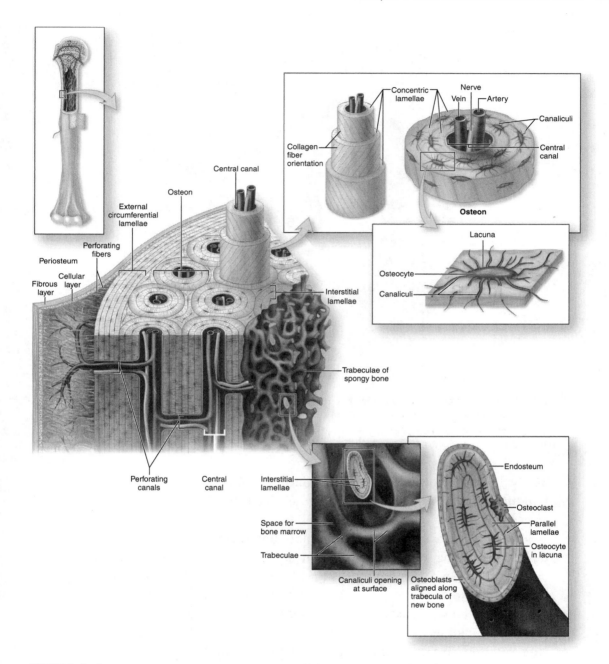

FIGURE 6–1 · Overview of the basic features of bone, including the three key cell types (osteocytes, osteoblasts, and osteoclasts), their usual locations, and the typical lamellar organizations of bone.

Source: Reproduced with permission from: Mescher AL: *Junqueira's Basic Histology: Text and Atlas,* 12th ed. New York, NY: McGraw-Hill; 2010. Fig. 8–1.

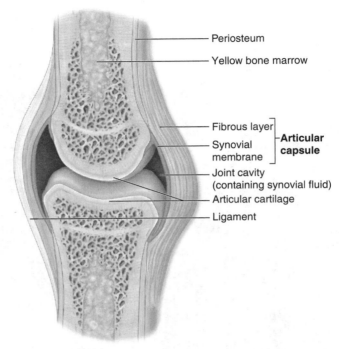

Typical synovial joint

FIGURE 6–2 · A typical synovial joint, also referred to as diarthroses, which are joints that allow free movement of the attached bones, such as knuckles, knees, and elbows.

Source: Reproduced with permission from: Mescher AL: *Junqueira's Basic Histology: Text and Atlas,* 12th ed. New York, NY: McGraw-Hill; 2010. Fig. 8–19A.

Yellow bone marrow is composed primarily of fat cells. **Osteoblasts** (bone-building cells) and **osteoclasts** (bone-resorbing cells) are found in the outer layer of the bone.

Joints are the areas where two or more bones come together. Joints are described as being freely movable (synovial joints like the hip), partially movable (pelvic bones), or immovable (suture lines in the skull). Synovial joints are lined with **synovium** (see Fig. 6–2). This membrane secretes synovial fluid to lubricate the joint and act as a shock absorber during motion or weight bearing. **Synovial joints** have a variety of range of motion including **flexion, extension, rotation, circumduction, supination, pronation, abduction, adduction, inversion**, and **eversion**. Partially movable joints have specific small amounts of motion that are typical of the joint space. Pelvic bones and individual joints between the vertebral bones are partially movable. Immovable joints are areas where bones come together, but no movement is allowed.

Muscles work in groups, with one set of muscles relaxing as other set contracts, to create motion (see Fig. 6–3). A small amount of muscle contraction

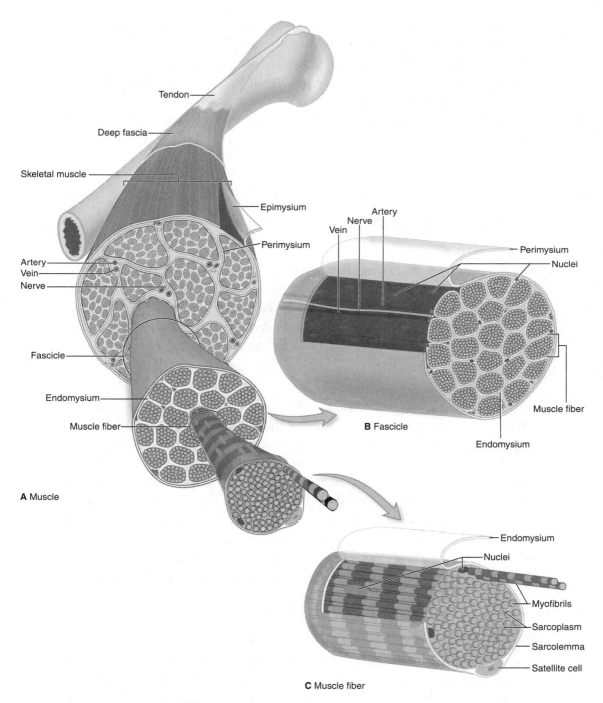

FIGURE 6–3 • Organization of skeletal muscle.

Source: Reproduced with permission from: Mescher AL: *Junqueira's Basic Histology: Text and Atlas*, 12th ed. New York, NY: McGraw-Hill; 2010. Fig. 10–3.

is typical to maintain muscle tone within the muscles. Skeletal muscle is striated and voluntary. **Connective tissues** are the pieces that hold other parts together. **Tendons** attach muscles to bones; ligaments attach bones to bones. **Cartilage** provides a smooth surface within joints to ease movement and provide cushioning to weight-bearing joints. **Bursa** are small fluid-filled sacs, within joint areas or adjacent to bone, which provide cushioning at points of friction.

Just the Facts

1. Carpal Tunnel Syndrome

What Went Wrong

The median nerve that passes through the carpal tunnel in the anterior wrist is compressed, resulting in pain and a numb sensation in the thumb, index finger, middle finger, and lateral aspect of the fourth finger in the hand. This is often the result of repetitive hand motions and may be work or hobby related. Carpal tunnel syndrome tends to be more common in women.

Prognosis

Some patients respond to conservative treatments including nonsteroidal anti-inflammatory drugs (NSAID) and rest of the affected area. A wrist brace may help to keep the wrist in a neutral position during this time. If this conservative treatment fails, the patient may need surgery to decompress the carpal tunnel area to relieve pressure on the nerve as it passes through the wrist into the hand. The long-term presence of carpal tunnel syndrome can lead to atrophy of muscles in the palm of the hand. The thenar eminence (area on the anterior palm between the proximal interphalangeal joint of the thumb and the mid-palm just distal to the wrist area) is the area of atrophy in carpal tunnel. Hand grip strength may be affected. After treatment, carpal tunnel syndrome may recur in the future.

Hallmark Signs and Symptoms

- Tingling, numbness, or burning sensation (paresthesia) in the hand (more specifically—the anterior surface of the palm, the thumb, index, middle finger, and the lateral portion of the ring finger) due to nerve compression

- Weakness in the hand owing to nerve compression and, eventually, muscle wasting
- Pain in the hand because of nerve compression
- Tapping over the carpal tunnel area will cause tingling, numbness, or pain through the palm and affected fingers (Tinel's sign)
- Pain, tingling, and burning sensation in the wrist and hand as a result of the blood pressure cuff being inflated on the upper arm to the level of the patient's systolic blood pressure

Common Test Results

- Electromyography (EMG) or nerve conduction studies will show nerve dysfunction.
- Magnetic resonance imaging (MRI) will show swelling of the median nerve within the carpal tunnel.

Treatment

- Splint the wrist for 2 weeks to keep it in a neutral position or slightly extended and decrease compression on the carpal tunnel area.
- Administer NSAID to decrease inflammation.
  - aspirin, diclofenac, diflunisal, etodolac, fenoprofen, flurbiprofen, ibuprofen, indomethacin, ketoprofen, ketorolac, meloxicam, nabumetone, naproxen, oxaprozin, piroxicam, sulindac, tolmetin
- Administer corticosteroids to decrease inflammation.
  - hydrocortisone, dexamethasone, methylprednisolone, prednisolone, prednisone.
- Some are given orally.
- Some may be injected into the carpal tunnel area.
- Surgery when decompression of the carpal tunnel is necessary to relieve pressure on the median nerve.

Nursing Diagnoses

- Pain
- Impaired mobility
- Disturbed sensory perception: tactile

NURSING INTERVENTION

- Assist the patient with hygiene if necessary before surgical correction and with postoperative dressings after surgery.
- Patients wearing wrist splints may need assistance with certain activities of daily living (ADLs).
- Assist the patient in exercising the hand; encourage performance of activities through physical therapy.
- Monitor the motion and sensation in the hand following surgery—check capillary refill, color, and sensation of fingers.
- Encourage movement of fingers after surgery.
- Monitor postoperative dressing for drainage.
- Keep the patient's hand elevated above the level of the heart to decrease the chance of postoperative swelling.
- **Explain to the patient:**
  - Use, interactions, and side effects of anti-inflammatory medications.
  - Proper use of wrist splints.
  - Encourage appropriate exercises.
  - Use of ergonomic devices, such as wrist rests or keyboard trays, for computer work.

2. Fractures

What Went Wrong

Excess stress or direct trauma is placed on a bone, causing a break. This results in damage to surrounding muscles and tissue, leading to hemorrhage, edema, and local tissue damage. Initially after the fracture, bleeding in the area leads to hematoma formation at the site. Inflammatory cells enter the area. Granulation tissue replaces the hematoma. Cellular changes continue, and a non-bony union known as a callus develops. Osteoblasts continue to enter the area. Fibrous tissue in the fractured area changes to bone.

The fracture site may be just a crack in the bone, without displacing any of the bone itself. A fracture that does not go all the way through the bone is considered an incomplete fracture. The fracture may also go all the way through a bone, breaking it into two (or more) pieces, which is referred to as a complete fracture. The surrounding muscle tissue that attaches above and below the fracture area in a limb will continue to create tension on their attachment points to the bone and pull the pieces further out of alignment.

Some fractured bone pieces may penetrate through the skin; this is known as an open or compound fracture. Those that do not penetrate the skin are considered closed or simple fractures.

Prognosis

The area of fracture needs to be identified (via an x-ray) and properly treated in order to heal. The fractured area typically needs to be realigned and then immobilized to allow for proper healing. During this time of immobilization, the bone cells come into the area to rebuild new bone to repair the damaged area. The period of immobilization typically lasts for 6 to 8 weeks, depending on the site and degree of damage. The full structural strength is not typically restored until months after the break, depending on the size and location of the fracture. Time for full healing varies from 6 weeks in young healthy adults with simple fractures to a couple of months in older patients with other health problems. Older patients have a significant increase in both morbidity and mortality following a hip fracture.

Complications following fractures include compartment syndrome, fat embolism, deep vein thrombosis (DVT), delayed union, nonunion, or misalignment. Compartment syndrome occurs when excess pressure builds up within a muscle compartment sheath. The pressure may be coming from internal or external sources of pressure. This is most common with fractures involving the lower leg or the lower arm. Fat globules may be released from the yellow bone marrow into the bloodstream and embolize to other areas of the body. The risk for this is highest in the elderly and in men between 18 and 40 years. A decrease in mobility following fracture will increase the risk for DVT. Smoking, obesity, heart disease, and lower extremity surgery all increase this risk. Delayed union is when a fracture has not joined within 6 months, despite appropriate treatments. Nonunion is a fracture site that fails to completely heal. Misalignment is when the fracture site heals, but the anatomic alignment is not as it should be.

Muscle wasting may occur in the area that has been immobilized. Physical therapy can be very helpful for the patient to regain full functional strength of the area.

Hallmark Signs and Symptoms

- Local bleeding—may or may not see skin level discoloration; it depends on the amount of blood loss and distance between fracture and skin.
- Edema at site due to inflammatory reaction to tissue damage

- Abnormal range of motion—need intact bone in order for muscle to pull and create movement; if fracture occurs near joint, swelling may limit ROM.
- Shortening of the leg and external rotation are common following hip fracture.

Common Test Results

- X-ray shows fracture—may be displaced or not.
- Computed tomography (CT) scan shows fracture—useful when patient's body part cannot be turned or positioned for imaging (eg, the neck).
- Bone scan will show increased cellular activity in the area of fracture as the body is attempting to heal the fracture—useful for sites where fracture is not easily seen or for hairline fractures not previously diagnosed.

Treatment

- Immobilize broken bone—to stabilize area, initially may be done with splint until fracture reduced (replaced into proper position) and cast applied or a fixation device applied surgically.
- Open reduction is the surgical repair and direct visual realignment of fracture.
- Pain management as needed.

Nursing Diagnoses

- Risk for impaired skin integrity
- Risk for activity intolerance
- Impaired physical mobility

NURSING INTERVENTION

- Monitor circulation: check peripheral pulses, capillary refill, and skin temperature distal to the break. Compromise of blood flow will diminish pulses, slow capillary refill, and cause cool skin temperature. Compare bilateral areas for symmetry.
- Monitor vital signs: check for elevated pulse, low BP, and elevated respiratory rate. The broken bone ends can lacerate a vessel causing internal bleeding; monitor for signs of shock. May see elevated temperature with infection from open fracture.

> • **Explain to the patient:**
>   • How to provide self-care—depending on the fracture area, the patient's ability to care for himself or herself may be compromised.
>   • The importance of performing range-of-motion exercise to maintain muscle tone in the areas not immobilized.
>   • Not to insert anything into the cast. The padding may become dislodged, causing pressure points under the hard cast, which would lead to skin breakdown. The skin integrity may also be broken when scratching under the cast, leading to an infection.

3. Gout

What Went Wrong

This is a metabolic disorder in which the body does not properly metabolize purine-based proteins. As a result, there is an increase in the amount of uric acid, which is the end product of purine metabolism. As a result of hyperuricemia, uric acid crystals accumulate in joints, most commonly the big toe (podagra), causing pain when the joint moves. Uric acid is cleared from the body through the kidneys. These patients may also develop kidney stones as the uric acid crystallizes in the kidney.

A person may also develop secondary gout. This is due to another disease process or use of medication, such as thiazide diuretics or some chemotherapeutic agents.

Prognosis

Gout is typically a chronic disorder. Patients need to understand the disease and its treatment so that medications can be initiated at the earliest point during a painful flare. Repeated flares in the same joint will ultimately cause joint damage. Chronic elevation of serum uric acid is associated with progression of atherosclerosis.

Hallmark Signs and Symptoms

- Acute onset of excruciating pain in joint due to the accumulation of uric acid within the joint
- Redness owing to inflammation around the joint
- Nephrolithiasis (kidney stones) because of uric acid deposits in the kidney

Common Test Results

- Elevated erythrocyte sedimentation rate (ESR) or C-reactive protein—tests that identify inflammation.
- Elevated serum uric acid level—not seen in all patients with gout. Typical of primary gout patients prior to the episode of acute joint pain.
- Elevated urinary uric acid levels.
- Arthrocentesis shows uric acid crystals within the joint fluid.

Treatment

Acute treatment is managed with colchicine and NSAIDs. These medications are continued until the pain is controlled. Chronic gout is treated with febuxostat, allopurinol, or a uricosuric agent to reduce the amount of uric acid in the system. These medications are used in the long term to reduce the amount of painful flares that occur.

- Administer colchicine during an acute episode to decrease the inflammatory response resulting from uric acid deposits. This will help reduce pain.
- Administer NSAID to decrease inflammation to aid in pain relief.
  - indomethacin, ibuprofen, naproxen
- Not aspirin; regular dosing causes retention of uric acid.
- Administer xanthine oxidase inhibitor medication to reduce the total body uric acid. Given as long-term treatment to patients with recurrent episodes of gout.
  - allopurinol
  - febuxostat
- Administer uricosuric medications when the total body amount of urate needs to be decreased. Not used in patients who are already excreting a large amount of uric acid. Given to patients with chronic gout or recurrent episodes.
  - probenecid, sulfinpyrazone
- Low-fat, low-cholesterol diet—elevated uric acid levels accelerate atherosclerosis.
- Immobilize the joint for comfort.

Nursing Diagnoses

- Impaired mobility
- Acute pain

> ### NURSING INTERVENTION
>
> - Have the patient drink 3 L of fluid every day to avoid crystallization of uric acid in the kidneys. Increased fluids help flush the uric acid through the kidneys.
> - Monitor uric acid levels in serum.
> - Assist with positioning for comfort.
> - Avoid touching inflamed joint unnecessarily. May need to keep clothing or bed linen away from area.
> - **Explain to the patient:**
>   - Which foods are high-purine proteins—turkey, organ meats, sardines, smelts, mackerel, anchovies, herring, bacon.
>   - Avoid alcohol, which inhibits renal excretion of uric acid.

4. Osteoarthritis

What Went Wrong

Osteoarthritis is a degenerative joint disease caused by the wear and tear of the articular cartilage. As the protective joint cartilage is worn away, the underlying bone becomes exposed, causing the exposed bones to rub. Degenerative changes within the bone tissue produce small areas of regrowth, causing jagged joint spaces and bone spurs. These rough areas project out into soft tissue or joint spaces, causing pain.

Prognosis

Pain associated with osteoarthritis typically is related to activity and is relieved with rest. The major weight-bearing joints are more affected in overweight patients due to the excess wear and tear on the joints, especially affecting hips and knees. Initially, patients respond well to rest periods and over-the-counter medications for pain control. As joints become more damaged over time, a joint replacement may be necessary to correct pain and to improve quality of life and mobility.

Hallmark Signs and Symptoms

- Stiff joints for short time in the morning, usually 15 minutes or less due to changes within joints.
- Joint pain with movement or weight bearing because of joint remodeling.
- **Crepitus** (grating feeling on palpation over joint during range of motion) owing to loss of articular cartilage and bony overgrowth in joint.
- Pain relief when joints are rested because lack of movements will relieve irritation in joint space.

- Enlargement of joint as a result of bony overgrowth or remodeling.
- Heberden's nodes—swelling of the distal interphalangeal joints.

Common Test Results

- X-ray shows narrowed joint spaces, bone spurs, or osteophytes around joints.
- Tests for inflammation will be normal—ESR, C-reactive protein.

Treatment

Initial treatment is usually with over-the-counter medications. The patients respond well to these medications. There is no underlying inflammatory disorder, so the medications can be used on an as-needed basis. Many of the patients are older and will be on other medications, so it is important that you check for medication interactions.

- Administer NSAID—for any local inflammation from irritation at the joint area due to osteophytes or bone spur formation.
  - aspirin, ibuprofen, naproxen
  - diclofenac, diflunisal, etodolac, fenoprofen, flurbiprofen, indomethacin, ketoprofen, ketorolac, meloxicam, nabumetone, oxaprozin, piroxicam, sulindac, tolmetin
- Administer acetaminophen for pain relief.
- Glucosamine and chondroitin sulfate for relief of pain and stiffness.
- Capsaicin cream topically.
- Intra-articular injections of corticosteroid up to 3 or 4 times in a year.
- Intra-articular injections of
  - hyaluronate sodium; series of 3 to 5 injections
  - **hyaluronan;** series of 3 injections
  - hylan GF 20; series of 3 injections
- Exercise to maintain joint mobility and muscle tone.
- Walking aid for stability.

Nursing Diagnoses

- Pain
- Activity intolerance
- Impaired mobility

NURSING INTERVENTION

- Monitor pain to adequately treat pain, as needs may change.
- Diet modification for weight loss for overweight patients to decrease excess stress on weight-bearing joints.
- **Explain to the patient:**
  - When and how to take medications.
  - Importance of maintaining activity.
  - Disease process.

5. Osteomyelitis

What Went Wrong

Osteomyelitis is an infection of the bone. In an adult, it is most commonly due to direct contamination of the site during trauma, such as an open fracture. Bacteria that cause infections elsewhere in the body may also enter the bloodstream and become deposited into the bone, starting a secondary infection site there. This is more common in children and adolescents. Some of the patients have been treated with antibiotics previously for the initial infection.

The causative organism is not always identified. More than three-quarters of the identified organisms are *Staphylococcus aureus*. Acute infection is associated with inflammatory changes in the bone and may lead to necrosis. Some patients will develop chronic osteomyelitis.

Prognosis

The sooner the infected area can be made infection-free, the better the prognosis for the patient. There is a risk of developing chronic osteomyelitis. This risk is greater in patients with a compromised immune system or poor blood supply to the area (such as diabetics).

Hallmark Signs and Symptoms

- Pain
- Fever, chills
- Malaise

Common Test Results

- Elevated white blood count (WBC).
- X-ray osteolytic lesions (localized loss of bone density).

- Bone scan shows the area of increased cellular activity—detects the site of infection.
- Culture and sensitivity tests to determine the infecting organism and antibiotic—may be difficult to determine the infecting organism.
- Bone biopsy to identify the organism.

Treatment

Removal of necrotic bone tissue and local pus or drainage is often necessary to speed healing. Typically, patients need antibiotics for several weeks to properly treat the infection.

- Debridement of the area to remove necrotic tissue.
- Drain the infected site.
- Immobilize or stabilize the bone if necessary.
- Administer antibiotics parenterally for 4 to 6 weeks or orally for 6 to 8 weeks.
  - nafcillin, vancomycin, penicillin G, piperacillin, ticarcillin/clavulanate, ampicillin/sulbactam, piperacillin/tazobactam, clindamycin, cefazolin, linezolid, ceftazidime, ciprofloxacin
- Administer analgesic to relieve discomfort as needed.
  - ibuprofen, naproxen, acetaminophen
  - oxycodone, hydrocodone
  - If there is vascular insufficiency or gangrene, amputation may be needed.

Nursing Diagnoses

- Impaired mobility
- Activity intolerance

NURSING INTERVENTION

- Monitor vital signs, changes in blood pressure, elevated pulse, elevated temperature, and respiratory rate.
- Monitor wound site for redness, drainage, and odor.
- Monitor IV access site for patency.

- **Explain to the patient:**
  - When and how to take medications.
  - Importance of completing antibiotic medication.
  - How to flush venous access device.
  - Signs of infection, infiltration, clotting of venous access device.
  - When to call for assistance with venous access.

6. Osteoporosis

What Went Wrong

There is a decrease in bone density, making bones more brittle and increasing the risk of fracture. The body continuously replaces older bone with new bone through a balance between the osteoblastic and osteoclastic activity. When bone-building activity does not keep up with bone-resorption activity, the structural integrity of the bone is compromised (see Fig. 6–4).

Increased age, lack of physical activity, poor nutrition, having a small frame, being Caucasian, Asian, or female all increase the risk of osteoporosis. Osteoporosis can also occur as a secondary disease due to another condition. These causes include the use of medications such as corticosteroids or some anticonvulsants, hormonal disorders (Cushing's or thyroid), and prolonged immobilization.

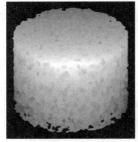 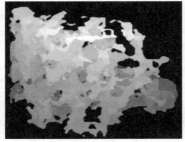 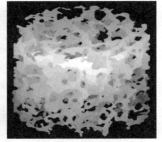

Young female	76-year-old woman	80-year-old woman

FIGURE 6–4 · High-resolution Micro-MRI images of a radial trabecular bone in a young woman at peak bone mass and in 76-year-old and 80-year-old women demonstrating loss of trabecular connectivity (trabecular horizontal struts) with age.

Source: Reproduced with permission from: Gardner DG, Shoback D: *Greenspan's Basic & Clinical Endocrinology*, 9th ed. New York, NY: McGraw-Hill; 2011. Fig. 23–12.

Prognosis

The risk of fracture is significantly increased in patients with osteoporosis. The most common fracture sites in patients with osteoporosis are hip, vertebrae, pelvis, and distal radius. Some fractures such as vertebral compression fractures affect the quality of life. There is increased morbidity and mortality in patients who sustain a hip fracture. The cost of healthcare for these patients is significant and includes the immediate care of the fracture as well as the necessary rehabilitation.

Hallmark Signs and Symptoms

- Asymptomatic
- Back pain due to compression fractures in vertebral bodies
- Loss of height
- Excessive forward curvature of the thoracic spine (kyphosis) owing to pathologic vertebral fractures; collapsing of the anterior portion of the vertebral bodies in the thoracic area
- Fracture with minor trauma

Common Test Results

- X-ray shows demineralization of the bone—not an early sign.
- Dual-energy x-ray absorptiometry (DEXA) shows a decrease in bone mineral density in the hip and spine compared to young patients with normal bone density, and compared to age-matched, race-matched, and gender-matched patients.

Treatment

It is much more cost-effective to focus on prevention of osteoporosis. Encourage adequate exercise and nutrition. Calcium supplementation may be necessary for patients who are not getting the recommended daily requirement of calcium in the diet. The body stores calcium in the bones. If there is insufficient dietary intake, the body will remove the calcium from the bone, further weakening the structural integrity. Once osteoporosis occurs, proper medical management is important to prevent fractures and increase bone density.

- Administer bisphosphonate drugs to inhibit osteoclastic bone resorption and increase bone density.
  - alendronate, risedronate, ibandronate sodium orally

- • Parenteral preparations, zoledronic acid, pamidronate
- Administer biologic medication via injection.
  - • denosumab
- Administer calcitonin nasal spray to increase bone density and also has an analgesic effect on bone pain after 2 to 4 weeks.
- Administer a selective estrogen receptor modulator for postmenopausal women for prevention of osteoporosis.
  - • raloxifene
- Administer teriparatide to stimulate the production of collagenous bone to increase bone density.
- Administer vitamin D, which enhances the absorption of calcium; many patients with osteoporosis are also deficient in vitamin D.
- Administer calcium, 1000 to 1500 mg per day in divided doses to enhance absorption.
- Encourage weight-bearing activity.
- Perform range-of-motion activities.
- Increase vitamins and calcium in the diet.

Nursing Diagnoses

- Impaired mobility
- Pain
- Risk for injury

NURSING INTERVENTION

- Pain control if fracture occurs.
- **Explain to the patient:**
  - How to properly take medications.
  - Bisphosphonates must be taken first thing in the morning on an empty stomach with a full glass of water. The patient cannot lie down for 30 to 60 minutes after taking the medication; this is to reduce the risk of esophageal irritation.
  - Monitor for side effects of medications—GI effects with bisphosphonates.
  - Encourage weight-bearing activity.
  - Encourage appropriate nutrition.

7. Tendonitis

What Went Wrong

A tendon connects muscle to bone. Over repetitive motion of the tendon causes irritation and inflammation of the tendon. Inflammation can also be caused by impact injury to the tendon. Tendonitis can be a secondary condition to arthritis, poor posture, thyroid disorder, and an adverse reaction to medication. The most common places where tendonitis occurs are elbow, fingers, hips, knees, and shoulders.

Prognosis

Depending on the severity of the inflammation, tendonitis usually resolves within a few weeks of treatment. However, more severe inflammation can take months to resolve, especially if surgical treatment is required. Tendinitis may return if the underlying cause of tendinitis such as repetitive motion continues once the inflammation has subsided.

Hallmark Signs and Symptoms

- Gradual or sudden severe pain at the location of the tendon.
- Loss of motion in the area (adhesive capsulitis). This is also known as frozen shoulder when the inflammation occurs in the shoulder.
- Swelling in the tendon area.
- Redness and warmth in the tendon area.

Common Test Results

- X-ray may be ordered to rule out other causes for the symptoms.
- No other test is used to diagnose tendonitis.

Treatment

A combination of physical and medication therapies is used to treat tendonitis. In rare cases, surgical intervention may be required.

- Administer NSAIDs medication.
  - ibuprofen (Advil, Motrin)
  - naproxen (Aleve)

- Administer corticosteroid medication via injection. (Not for chronic tendonitis. Frequent injections may weaken the tendon.)
- Dry needling stimulation. A needle is inserted into the tendon making small holes in the tendon to stimulate the body's immune response to increase the inflammatory response.
- Surgery if the tendon is torn from the bone.
- Physical therapy stretches and strengthens the tendon and muscle at the site of the tendonitis.

Nursing Diagnoses

- Impaired mobility
- Pain
- Risk for injury

NURSING INTERVENTION

- Pain control.
- **Explain to the patient:**
  - How to properly take medications.
  - The importance of finding alternatives to repetitive motions that caused the tendonitis.
  - Monitor for side effects of medications.
  - Encourage weight-bearing activity.
  - Encourage the performance of exercise suggested by physical therapy.

---

8. Ligament Sprain

What Went Wrong

A ligament contacts bones to bones at a joint. A sprain is a stretch or tear in a ligament during a fall, or when a joint is twisted. A sprain can also occur during an accident that places force causing the joint to twist unnaturally. Ligament sprains are common in ankles, knees, wrists, and thumbs. A sprain differs from a strain. A strain happens in muscles or tendons.

A sprain is graded based on the damage to the ligament.

Grade I: A mild tear or stretching with little or no instability of the joint.

Grade II: An incomplete tear with some looseness in the joint.

Grade III: Complete tear or rupture of the ligament. Impossible to bear weight on the joint. The joint is unstable.

Prognosis

Healing may take a few days to months for a Grade I sprain, and for a Grade III sprain that may require surgery to reattach the ligaments. A typical recovery for a Grade II sprain is from 3 to 8 weeks.

Hallmark Signs and Symptoms

- Pain at the site.
- Difficulty using the joint. In Grade III sprain the joint may not be mobile.
- Swelling at the site.

Common Test Results

- X-ray may be ordered to rule out fractures.
- MRI to assess the joint.
- CT scan to assess the ligament.

Treatment

A combination of non-medication and medication therapy is used to treat a ligament sprain. In rare cases, surgical intervention may be required.

- Administer NSAIDs medication.
  - ibuprofen (Advil, Motrin)
  - naproxen (Aleve)
- Administer analgesic medication.
  - acetaminophen (Tylenol)
- Rest for 2 days without using the affected joint.
- Ice the affected area on and off for 10 minutes for a 30-minute period for 3 days following the injury to reduce swelling.
- Compression on the site with a compression sleeve to reduce swelling.
- Elevate the affected area above the heart to prevent fluid from collecting at the site to reduce swelling.
- Rehabilitation to gradually restore motion.
- Surgery in severe cases to attach the ligament.

Nursing Diagnoses

- Impaired mobility
- Pain
- Risk for injury

NURSING INTERVENTION

- Pain control.
- **Explain to the patient:**
  - How to properly take medications.
  - The importance of rehabilitation to regain motion.
  - Monitor for side effects of medications.
  - Encourage not to rush to return to activity to prevent reinjury.
  - Encourage performance of exercise suggested by physical therapy.

---

9. Muscle/Tendon Strain

What Went Wrong

A strain is a stretch or tear of a muscle or tendon sometimes referred to as a pulled muscle that occurs during a fall, or when muscles and tendons are twisted. A strain can also occur during an accident that places force to muscle or tendon. Sometimes small blood vessels rupture leading to bruising. Exposed nerve endings cause pain.

Prognosis

Healing may take a few days or months depending on the severity of the strain.

Hallmark Signs and Symptoms

- Pain at the site when at rest and with movement.
- Weaken sensation at the site or inability to move the muscle.
- Swelling at the site.

Common Test Results

- X-ray may be ordered to rule out fractures.
- MRI to rule out fractures.

- CT scan to assess the muscles and tendons.
- Range-of-motion assessment to identify pain in the affected muscles and tendons:
  - Sit-up: abdominal muscle
  - Walking: calf muscle
  - Bending: lumbar back muscle
  - Rowing motion: rhomboid muscle
  - Head movement: neck muscle
  - Pulling down from an overhead position: trapezius muscle
  - Squeezing knees together: adductor muscle
  - Extending the knee from a flexed position: quadriceps muscle
  - Flexing the thigh into the body at the hip: hip flexor muscles
  - Walking up stairs: gluteal muscle
  - Accelerating during sprinting: hamstring muscle
  - Lifting against resistance at the elbow: bicep muscle
  - Throwing or chopping motion: intercostal muscle

Treatment

A combination of non-medication and medication therapy is used to treat a muscle/tendon strain. In rare cases, surgical intervention may be required.

- Administer NSAIDs medication.
  - ibuprofen (Advil, Motrin)
  - naproxen (Aleve)
- Administer analgesic medication.
  - acetaminophen (Tylenol)
- Rest for 2 days without using the affected joint.
- Ice the affected area on and off for 10 minute for a 30-minute period for 3 days following the injury to reduce swelling.
- Compression on the site with a compression sleeve to reduce swelling.
- Elevate the affected area above the heart to prevent fluid from collecting at the site to reduce swelling.
- Rehabilitation to gradually restore motion.
- Surgery in severe cases to attach the tendon.

Nursing Diagnoses

- Impaired mobility
- Pain
- Risk for injury

NURSING INTERVENTION

- Pain control.
- **Explain to the patient:**
  - How to properly take medications.
  - The importance of rehabilitation to regain motion.
  - Monitor for side effects of medications.
  - Encourage not to rush to return to activity to prevent reinjury.
  - Encourage performance of exercise suggested by physical therapy.

REVIEW QUESTIONS

1. **Teaching patients about proper use of bisphosphonate medications for treatment of osteoporosis should include taking medication:**
   A. On a full stomach.
   B. First thing in the morning on an empty stomach with a full glass of water, 30 to 60 minutes before eating, without lying down.
   C. Just before getting into bed.
   D. With an acidic liquid, like orange juice.

2. **The patient with gout will have periodic exacerbations of painful joint inflammation. Acute episodes are treated with:**
   A. Nonsteroidal anti-inflammatory medications and colchicine.
   B. Allopurinol and aspirin.
   C. Antibiotics and acetaminophen.
   D. Bisphosphonates and calcium.

3. **In order to allow for proper healing, patients with osteomyelitis may need to have:**
   A. Debridement and drainage of the area.
   B. Immobilization of the area.
   C. Ice packs alternating with moist heat applied externally.
   D. Internal fixation device inserted.

4. **Initial treatment of the patient with a fracture should include:**

    A. Surgical reduction of the fracture.

    B. Insertion of internal fixation device.

    C. Reduction of the fracture.

    D. Immobilization of the area.

5. **You have been caring for a patient with osteomyelitis. In preparing the patient for discharge, you include teaching about:**

    A. The importance of completing the multiple-week treatment with antibiotics.

    B. The side effects and interactions of the medications.

    C. Symptoms that necessitate a call to the physician, nurse practitioner, or physician assistant.

    D. All of the above.

6. **You are caring for a patient who has just had open carpal tunnel release surgery. The surgeon has requested that the patient's hand and arm remain elevated above the level of the heart after the surgery. This is to:**

    A. Reduce lymphatic drainage.

    B. Reduce postoperative swelling.

    C. Restrict hand movements.

    D. Decrease possibility of nosocomial infection.

7. **The first priority of care of the patient with a new fracture includes assessing:**

    A. Respiratory rate and effort, pulse.

    B. The fracture site for bleeding.

    C. For signs of infection at the wound site of an open fracture.

    D. For circulation and sensation distal to the fracture site.

8. **Patients who work in settings that require repetition of the same hand movements over a long period of time have an increased risk for which of the following disorders?**

    A. Osteomyelitis.

    B. Osteoporosis.

    C. Carpal tunnel syndrome.

    D. Fracture of the overused area.

9. **Patients with a history of osteoporosis have an increased risk for:**

    A. Infection in the bone.

    B. Peripheral blood clot formation.

    C. Painful joint inflammation.

    D. Fracture formation.

10. **In obtaining the history for the patient with carpal tunnel syndrome, you would expect to note a history of:**

   A. Pain and numbness or tingling sensation in the hand (over the palmar surface of the thumb, index finger, middle finger, and lateral aspect of the ring finger) that is worse at night.

   B. Crepitus (grating feeling on palpation over joint during range of motion) due to loss of articular cartilage and bony overgrowth in joint.

   C. Excessive forward curvature of the thoracic spine (kyphosis) owing to pathologic vertebral fractures, and collapsing of the anterior portion of the vertebral bodies in the thoracic area.

   D. Acute onset of excruciating pain in joint because of accumulation of uric acid within the joint.

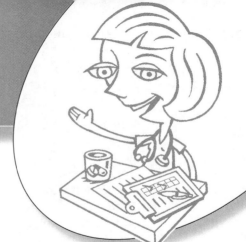

Chapter **7**

Gastrointestinal System

LEARNING OBJECTIVES

At the end of this chapter, the student will be able to:

- Identify normal anatomy and physiology related to the gastrointestinal (GI) system
- Discuss the disease-causing pathologic changes within the GI system
- List four signs or symptoms of specific GI disease or injury
- Recognize expected nursing and medical management of GI injury disease

KEY CONCEPTS

1. Appendicitis
2. Cholecystitis
3. Cirrhosis
4. Crohn's disease
5. Diverticulitis disease
6. Gastroenteritis
7. Gastroesophageal reflux disease
8. Gastrointestinal bleed
9. Gastritis
10. Hepatitis
11. Hiatal hernia
12. Intestinal obstruction and paralytic ileus
13. Pancreatitis
14. Peritonitis
15. Peptic ulcer disease
16. Ulcerative colitis

KEY TERMS

Accessory organs
Alimentary canal
Fatty acids
Gastrin
Glucagon
Hydrochloric acid
Ileocecal valve
Insulin
Islets of Langerhans
Lipase
Lower esophageal sphincter (LES)
Oropharynx
Pepsin
Pepsinogen
Plasma
Proteins
Secretin
Sphincter of Oddi
Triglycerides
Trypsin
Upper esophageal sphincter (UES)

How the Gastrointestinal System Works

The gastrointestinal (GI) system includes the **alimentary canal** (mouth, esophagus, stomach, small intestine, large intestine, rectum), **accessory organs** (salivary glands, liver, pancreas, gallbladder), and ducts (see Fig. 7–1). The alimentary canal is a hollow tube lined with a mucous membrane. The GI tract functions to digest food, absorb nutrients, propel the contents through the lumen, and eliminate the waste products.

Digestion of food has both mechanical and chemical components. Both processes begin in the mouth. Chewing, movement through the GI tract, and churning within the stomach are parts of the mechanical process.

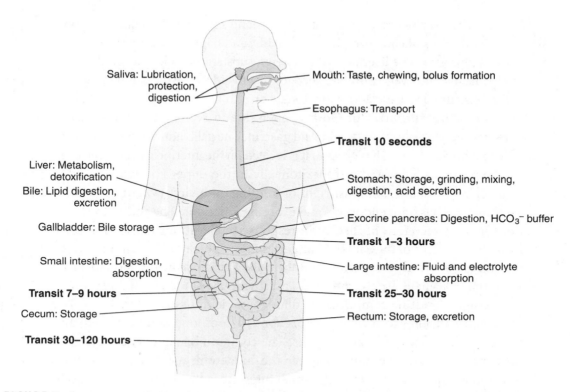

Saliva: Lubrication, protection, digestion

Mouth: Taste, chewing, bolus formation

Esophagus: Transport

Transit 10 seconds

Liver: Metabolism, detoxification

Bile: Lipid digestion, excretion

Gallbladder: Bile storage

Stomach: Storage, grinding, mixing, digestion, acid secretion

Exocrine pancreas: Digestion, HCO_3^- buffer

Transit 1–3 hours

Small intestine: Digestion, absorption

Large intestine: Fluid and electrolyte absorption

Transit 7–9 hours

Transit 25–30 hours

Cecum: Storage

Rectum: Storage, excretion

Transit 30–120 hours

FIGURE 7–1 · Overview of the gastrointestinal system. Components of digestion and transport of food from the mouth to the rectum/anus are shown, including a summary of their contributions and the average amount of time for food to reach their location after ingestion.

Source: Reproduced with permission from: Janson LW, Tischler ME: *The Big Picture: Medical Biochemistry.* New York, NY: McGraw-Hill; 2012. Fig. 11–1.

Saliva, **hydrochloric acid**, bile, and other digestive enzymes all contribute to the chemical process of digestion.

The esophagus extends from the **oropharynx** to the stomach. At the top of the esophagus is the **upper esophageal sphincter (UES)** to prevent the influx of air into the esophagus during respiration. At the bottom of the esophagus is the **lower esophageal sphincter (LES)** to prevent the reflux of acid from the stomach into the esophagus.

The contents of the esophagus empty into the stomach through the cardiac sphincter. The stomach secretes gastrin, which promotes secretion of **pepsinogen** and hydrochloric acid, **pepsin**, and lipase, all of which aid digestion and mucous that helps protect the stomach lining.

The liver is a very vascular organ located in the right upper quadrant (RUQ) of the abdomen under the diaphragm. It has two main lobes that comprise smaller lobules. The liver stores a variety of vitamins and minerals. It metabolizes proteins; synthesizes **plasma proteins**, **fatty acids**, and **triglycerides**; and stores and releases glycogen. The liver detoxifies foreign substances such as alcohol, drugs, or chemicals. The liver forms and secretes bile to aid in the digestion of fat. Bile will release into the gallbladder for storage or into the duodenum if needed for digestion if the **sphincter of Oddi** is open due to secretion of the digestive enzymes **secretin**, cholecystokinin, and **gastrin**. The gallbladder is a small receptacle that holds bile until it is needed. It is located on the inferior aspect of the liver.

The pancreas is located retroperitoneally in the upper abdomen near the stomach and extends from just right of midline to the left toward the spleen. The pancreas has both endocrine and exocrine functions. The endocrine functions include secretion of **insulin** in response to elevations in blood glucose from the beta cells of the **islets of Langerhans** and **glucagon** in response to the decrease in blood glucose from the alpha cells. The exocrine function includes secretion of **trypsin**, **lipase**, amylase, and chymotrypsin to aid in digestion.

The small intestine comprises the duodenum, jejunum, and the ileum. The duodenum attaches to the stomach, is about 1-foot long and C-shaped, and curves to the left around the pancreas. The common bile duct and pancreatic duct enter here. The jejunum is between the duodenum and ileum and is about 8-feet long. The last portion of the small intestine is the ileum, which is up to 12-feet long, depending on the size of the patient. The **ileocecal valve** separates the ileum from the large intestine. The appendix is found at this juncture. The large intestine can be broken down into the ascending colon, transverse colon, descending colon, and sigmoid colon. The sigmoid colon joins the rectum and ultimately the anal canal.

Just the Facts

1. Appendicitis

What Went Wrong

Inflammation of the vermiform appendix (a blind pouch located near the ileocecal valve in the right lower quadrant of the abdomen) is known as appendicitis. It may be due to obstruction from stool, a foreign body or, in rare cases, a tumor. The mucosal lining of the appendix continues to secrete fluid, which will increase the pressure within the lumen of appendix, causing a restriction of the blood supply to the appendix. This decrease in blood supply may result in gangrene or perforation as the pressure continues to build. Pain localizes at McBurney's point, located midway between the umbilicus and right anterior iliac crest.

Appendicitis may occur at any age, but the peak occurrence is from the teenage years to 30. Appendicitis is a common reason for emergency surgery.

Prognosis

Rupture of the appendix is more likely to occur in acute appendicitis within the first 36 to 48 hours. Symptoms of peritonitis (inflammation of the peritoneum—the membrane lining the abdominal cavity) may occur as a complication of appendicitis. Rapid diagnosis and surgical intervention are necessary to avoid rupture of the appendix. Most patients heal fairly quickly after surgery. If the appendix has ruptured prior to the surgery, healing may be prolonged, and the potential for complications such as peritonitis increases.

Hallmark Signs and Symptoms

- Abdominal pain begins periumbilical and travels to right lower quadrant.
- Rebound pain (pain when pressure on the abdomen is quickly removed) occurs with peritoneal inflammation.
- Guarding (protecting the abdomen from painful exam).
- Rigidity of the abdomen (abdomen feels more firm when palpating).
- Fever, chills due to infection.
- Nausea, vomiting, loss of appetite.
- Diarrhea or constipation owing to inflammation of an area of the bowel.
- Right lower quadrant pain that improves with flexing the right hip suggests perforation.

Common Test Results

- Elevated white blood cell (WBC) count.
- CT scan shows enlarged appendix or fecalith.
- Ultrasound may show enlarged appendix.

Treatment

- Surgical removal of the appendix—appendectomy (may be done via laparoscopy or open laparotomy).
- Nothing by mouth (NPO) to avoid further irritation of the intestinal area, and preparation for surgery.
- Intravenous fluids until diet resumed.

- Pain medications after surgery as needed; pain medication is used cautiously preoperatively to maintain awareness of the increase in pain due to possible rupture of appendix.
- Antibiotics postoperatively if needed.
- Treatment for peritonitis may be necessary if appendix has ruptured.

Nursing Diagnoses

- Acute pain
- Hyperthermia (HT)
- Nausea

NURSING INTERVENTION

- Monitor vital signs for fever, increased heart rate, respiratory rate, and decrease in blood pressure.
- Assess pain level for changes.
- Monitor surgical site for appearance of wound, drainage.
- Monitor abdomen for distention, presence of bowel sounds.
- Monitor intake and output.
- Monitor bowel function.

---

2. Cholecystitis

What Went Wrong

An inflammation of the gallbladder, often accompanied by the formation of gallstones (cholelithiasis), is cholecystitis. The inflammation may be either acute or chronic in nature. In an acute cholecystitis, the blood flow to the gallbladder may become compromised which in turn will cause problems with the normal filling and emptying of the gallbladder. A stone may block the cystic duct which will result in bile becoming trapped within the gallbladder due to inflammation around the stone within the duct. The majority of patients (9 out of 10) will have gallstones development; the remaining patients will have inflammation without stone formation, or an acalculous cholecystitis. Blood flow to the inflamed area will be minimized, localized edema develops, the gallbladder distends due to retained bile, and ischemic changes will occur within the wall of the gallbladder. This buildup of bile causes further irritation and pressure within the organ causing pain. Chronic cholecystitis occurs when there have been recurrent episodes of blockage of the cystic duct, usually because of stones. There is chronic inflammation. The gallbladder is often contracted, which leads to problems with storing and moving the bile. Patients may develop jaundice due to backup of bile or obstructive jaundice. They will exhibit a yellowish tone to skin and mucous membranes. If patients have a naturally dark pigmentation to their skin, check palms and soles. Icterus is the yellow color change seen in the sclera (white) of the eye.

There is increased risk for gallbladder inflammation and development of gallstones with increasing age, being female or overweight, having a family history of gallbladder disease, people on rapid weight loss diets, and during pregnancy. Acalculous cholecystitis is more common in older men. In some cases, gallstones are an incidental finding when radiology studies are performed for an unrelated reason.

Prognosis

The ischemic changes of the gallbladder wall increase the risk of perforation of the organ or development of gangrene. Cholangitis (inflammation of the common bile duct) may develop secondary to cholecystitis. Peritonitis is a potential risk in patients if a significant area of gallbladder perforates, or there is associated infection or abscess that spreads. A small percentage of patients will develop cancer of the gallbladder. There is increased surgical risk for older patients or patients with comorbidities. Some patients may develop pancreatitis secondary to the development of gallstones.

Hallmark Signs and Symptoms

- Upper abdominal, epigastric, or right upper quadrant abdominal pain which may radiate to the right shoulder or to the upper-midline area of the back
- Pain often follows eating and may be intermittent or constant
- RUQ pain increases with palpation of right upper abdomen during inspiration (Murphy's sign) causing the patient to stop taking the deep breath (an inspiratory pause)
- Nausea and vomiting, especially following fatty foods
- Loss of appetite
- Fever
- Increased air in intestinal tract (eructation, flatulence)
- Pruritus (itching) of skin due to the buildup of bile salts

- Clay-colored stools because of lack of urobilinogen in the gut (normally converted from bilirubin which was blocked with bile flow)
- Jaundice—yellowish skin, sclera (eyes), and mucous membrane discoloration
- Icterus—yellowish discoloration of sclera (white of the eye)
- Dark, foamy urine as kidneys attempt to clear out bilirubin

Common Test Results
- Ultrasound of gallbladder shows cholelithiasis, inflammation.
- Hepatobiliary iminodiacetic acid (HIDA scan) may be more sensitive than ultrasound in showing obstructed duct.
- CT scan shows inflammation or cholelithiasis.
- Magnetic resonance cholangiopancreatography (MRCP).
- Endoscopic retrograde cholangiopancreatography (ERCP).
- Bilirubin direct (conjugated) and indirect (unconjugated) will be elevated if there is obstruction.
- WBC count elevation with inflammation.
- Alkaline phosphatase, aspartate aminotransferase (AST), and lactate dehydrogenase (LDH) will be elevated with abnormal liver function.
- Amylase and lipase may be mildly elevated.

Treatment
- Low-fat diet.
- Wait-and-see approach if the patient is asymptomatic.
- Intravenous fluid replacement for vomiting.
- Administer antiemetics for control of nausea and vomiting.
  - prochlorperazine
  - trimethobenzamide
- Nasogastric (NG) tube connected to suction for emesis.
- Replace fat-soluble vitamins (A, D, E, K) as needed.
- Administer analgesics for adequate pain control.
  - meperidine
  - morphine
  - ketorolac (not if surgery is planned)

- Administer antibiotics for acute symptoms.
  - piperacillin/tazobactam IV
  - ampicillin/sulbactam
  - third-generation cephalosporin plus metronidazole
  - meropenem or imipenem/cilastatin for more severe infections
- Placement of stent into the gallbladder if the patient is not a candidate for surgery.
- Ultrasound-guided aspiration of gallbladder.
- Surgical removal of gallbladder.
  - Laparoscopic cholecystectomy
  - Open cholecystectomy
  - Lithotripsy (breaks down stone) if single stone measuring less than 2 cm

Nursing Diagnoses

- Acute pain
- Chronic pain
- Risk for imbalanced nutrition: less than what body requires
- Nausea

NURSING INTERVENTION

- Monitor vital signs for changes in temperature, pulse rate, respiratory rate, and blood pressure.
- Assess abdomen for bowel sounds, distention, and tenderness.
- Assess pain level for adequate pain control.
- Assess postoperative wound for drainage, signs of infection.
- Monitor T-tube drainage in postoperative open cholecystectomy patients; empty and record at least every 8 hours.
- Advance diet to low-fat diet postoperatively as tolerated.

---

3. Cirrhosis

What Went Wrong

Injury to the cellular structure of the liver causes fibrosis due to chronic inflammation and necrotic changes, resulting in cirrhosis. There are nodular changes to the liver. The bile ducts and blood vessels through the liver may become blocked owing to both the nodular changes and fibrosis. These changes to the liver cause enlargement of the organ and change in texture. There is increased pressure within the portal vein. This causes resistance to blood flow throughout the venous system in the liver and also backs up venous blood to the spleen, causing enlargement of this organ. Damage to the liver may be reversible if the cause is identified early and removed. The most common causes of cirrhosis include chronic alcohol use and hepatitis C. Liver damage secondary to exposure to drugs or toxins, viral hepatitis (especially hepatitis B, and hepatitis D in those already infected with hepatitis B), fatty liver, steatohepatitis, autoimmune hepatitis, cystic fibrosis, metabolic disorders (excess iron storage—hemochromatosis or excess copper in Wilson's disease), or genetic causes.

Prognosis

As cirrhosis progresses, the patient may develop encephalopathy and coma. Early signs and symptoms of encephalopathy include altered level of consciousness, neuromuscular changes, and elevated serum ammonia levels.

Hallmark Signs and Symptoms

- Initially asymptomatic
- Weakness, fatigue due to chronic disease
- Muscle cramps
- Weight loss
- Anorexia
- Indigestion
- Nausea with possible vomiting
- Ascites—the accumulation of fluid within the abdominal cavity due to portal hypertension
- Pale, clay-colored stool
- Abdominal pain
- Portal hypertension
- Pruritus (itching)
- Ecchymosis (bruises) or petechiae (small, pinpoint, round, reddish purple marks)
- Coagulation defects because of problems with vitamin K absorption, causing problems with production of clotting factors
- Nosebleeds, bleeding gums

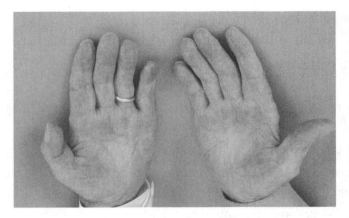

FIGURE 7−2 · Palmar erythema in a patient with alcoholic cirrhosis. The erythema is peripheral over the palm with central pallor.

Source: Reproduced with permission from: Longo DL, Fauci AS, Kasper DL, Hauser SL, Jameson JL, Loscalzo J: *Harrison's Principles of Internal Medicine*, 18th ed. New York, NY: McGraw-Hill; 2012. Fig. 308–1.

- Amenorrhea
- Impotence due to inactivity of hormones
- Gynecomastia
- Jaundice owing to problems with excretion of bilirubin
- Hepatomegaly (enlarged liver) in over one-half of the patients
- Spider veins—spider angiomas or telangiectasias on cheeks, nose, shoulders, or upper chest
- Dilated venous pattern over abdomen
- Redness of palms—palmar erythema (see Fig. 7–2)
- Glossitis due to vitamin deficiency
- Peripheral edema
- Dyspnea as a result of pressure on diaphragm from ascites
- Encephalopathy (asterixis, tremors, delirium, drowsiness, dysarthria, coma)

Common Test Results

- AST elevated.
- Alanine aminotransferase (ALT) elevated.
- Lactate dehydrogenase elevated.
- Bilirubin direct (conjugated) and indirect (unconjugated) elevated.

- Urinary bilirubin elevated.
- Fecal urobilinogen decreased with biliary tract obstruction.
- Serum protein decreased.
- Serum albumin decreased.
- Anemia with elevated mean corpuscular volume (MCV) and mean corpuscular hemoglobin (MCH).
- WBC count is low.
- Prothrombin time is prolonged due to changes in hepatic production of clotting factors.
- Platelet count low (thrombocytopenia).
- Ammonia level elevated as the disease advances.
- Abdominal x-rays show hepatomegaly.
- Abdominal CT scan shows hepatomegaly and ascites.
- Ultrasound shows hepatomegaly, ascites, and portal vein blood flow.
- Liver biopsy shows fibrosis and regenerative nodules.
- Esophagogastroduodenoscopy (EGD) detects esophageal varices.

Treatment

- Low-sodium diet; adequate calorie intake.
- Restrict fluid intake if hyponatremic (low serum sodium) or fluid overloaded.
- Stop alcohol intake to prevent further damage.
- Administer vitamin supplements—folate, thiamine, and multivitamin.
- Administer diuretics to reduce excess fluids.
  - furosemide
  - spironolactone
- Paracentesis to remove ascitic fluid.
- Monitor electrolytes for imbalance.
- Monitor coagulation profile (PT, PTT, INR).
- Administer lactulose to promote removal of ammonia in the gut.
- Administer antibiotics to destroy the normal GI flora, which decreases protein breakdown and the rate of ammonia production.
  - neomycin sulfate
  - metronidazole

- Shunt placement.
  - Peritoneovenous—moves ascitic fluid from abdomen to superior vena cava.
  - Portocaval—diverts venous blood flow from liver to decrease portal and esophageal pressures.
  - Transjugular intrahepatic portal systemic—nonsurgical procedure performed in interventional radiology—sheath placed into jugular and hepatic vein; needle threaded through sheath and pushed into portal vein through the liver; balloon enlarges the tract and stent maintains.
- Gastric lavage.
- Esophagogastric balloon tamponade for control of bleeding from esophageal varices.
- Administer blood products as needed for patients with bleeding esophageal varices.
- Sclerotherapy for esophageal variceal bleeding.
- Vaccine for influenza, hepatitis A, and hepatitis B recommended.

Nursing Diagnoses

- Ineffective breathing pattern
- Excess fluid volume
- Risk for infection

NURSING INTERVENTION

- Monitor intake and output.
- Monitor vital signs.
- Weigh patient daily.
- Measure abdominal girth—making sure to measure at level of umbilicus for consistency; marks are typically made at sides of abdomen to align tape measure on subsequent days.
- Assess peripheral edema.
- Assess heart and lung sounds for excess fluid.
- Elevate head of bed 30 degrees or greater to ease breathing.
- Elevate feet to decrease peripheral edema.
- Monitor for signs of bleeding or bruising.
- Monitor level of consciousness, orientation, recent and remote memory, behavior, mood, and effect.

4. Crohn's Disease

What Went Wrong

Crohn's disease is an autoimmune disorder that can affect any point within the GI tract from the mouth to the anus. The damage to the GI tract is non-continuous with diseased patches interspersed among healthy tissue. The majority of cases involve the small intestine and large intestine, often in the right lower quadrant at the point where the terminal ileum and the ascending colon meet. Patients typically have an insidious onset of intermittent symptoms. The disease causes transmural inflammation, going deeper than the superficial mucosal layer of the tissue to affect all layers. Over time the inflammatory changes within the GI tract can lead to strictures or the formation of fistulas. The affected tissue develops granulomas and takes on a mottled appearance interspersed with normal tissue. There are a genetic predisposition and a bimodal peak of onset at 16 to 30 years and again at 50 to 70 years. The average age for onset of symptoms is in the late 20s. There is an increased risk with a family history, smoking, and living in an urban area or industrialized country.

Prognosis

Crohn's disease is a chronic disorder with periods of exacerbation and remission. Many patients will ultimately need surgery to deal with bowel obstruction, development of strictures, or fistula formation. There is no cure, but medications can help to manage the disease.

Hallmark Signs and Symptoms

- Fever.
- Crampy abdominal pain, frequently occurring in the right lower quadrant.
- Diarrhea (non-bloody).
- Abdominal mass.
- Weight loss (unintentional) due to anorexia.
- Fatigue.
- Bloating after meals (postprandial).
- Tenesmus (feeling the need to pass stool, even though bowel is already empty; painful bowel movements or difficult bowel movements).

- Borborygmi (loud, frequent bowel sounds).
- Fistula formation (bowel-bowel, bowel-stomach, bowel-bladder, bowel-skin, bowel-vagina).
- Aphthous ulcers (oral ulcerations).
- Non-GI symptoms may include joint pain, skin lesions, eye inflammation, or nephrolithiasis.

Common Test Results

- Erythrocyte sedimentation rate (ESR) or C-reactive protein will be elevated during exacerbations.
- Anemia—due to both vitamin B_{12} and folic acid deficiency.
- Albumin level will be low.
- Electrolytes may be abnormal owing to loss from diarrhea and malabsorption.
- Barium studies will show an "apple core" appearance in areas of stricture formation, narrowing because of inflammation, and fistula formation. The test is not performed if bowel perforation is a concern.
- CT scan shows abscess formation and thickening of bowel wall due to inflammation.
- Sigmoidoscopy, colonoscopy, or endoscopy for direct visualization of the GI tract or for biopsy.

Treatment

- Dietary restriction.
- Nutritional supplementation.
- Administer vitamin B_{12} and folic acid as indicated.
- Administer aminosalicylates to induce or maintain remission.
  - mesalamine
  - sulfasalazine
  - olsalazine
  - balsalazide
- Administer glucocorticoids to reduce inflammation.
  - hydrocortisone
  - budesonide

- Administer purine analogs to induce or maintain remission.
  - azathioprine
  - 6-mercaptopurine
- Administer biologic agents to induce or maintain remission.
  - infliximab
  - adalimumab
  - certolizumab
  - natalizumab
- Administer methotrexate to induce or maintain remission.
- Administer antidiarrheal medications to decrease fluid loss; use with caution.
  - diphenoxylate hydrochloride and atropine sulfate
  - loperamide
- Intravenous fluids to maintain hydration.
- Surgical correction (bowel resection) of intestinal obstruction, strictures, fistula, perforation.

Nursing Diagnoses

- Acute pain
- Risk for imbalanced nutrition: less than what body requires
- Altered bowel elimination

NURSING INTERVENTION

- Monitor vital signs for temperature increase, pulse increase, and change in blood pressure.
- No single diet has been developed. Patients must identify which foods induce symptoms. Keeping a food diary is the easiest way to identify the foods to avoid. Common symptom-inducing foods include fatty or greasy foods, dairy products, gas-producing foods, and high-fiber foods.
- Monitor intake and output.
- Assess abdomen for bowel sounds, tenderness, and masses.
- Assess postoperative wound for signs of infection and drainage.
- Wound care postoperatively.

- Proper skin care if bowel-skin fistula.
  - Use of drainable pouch with skin wafer.
  - Cleaning skin promptly if drainage comes in contact with skin.
- Nutritional supplementation with Ensure, Sustacal, Vivonex.
- Teach patient about home care needs.

5. Diverticulitis Disease

What Went Wrong

Small outpouchings called diverticula develop along the intestinal tract. More than half of the Americans over the age of 60 years have developed diverticula. Diverticulosis is the condition of having these diverticula. Any part of the large or small intestine may be involved. The area of the intestinal tract that most commonly develops diverticula is the lower portion of the large intestine. Certain types of undigested foods can become trapped in the pouches of the intestine. Bacteria multiply in the area, causing further inflammation. Diverticulitis is an inflammation of at least one of the diverticula. Diets that have a low fiber content, seeds, or nuts have been implicated in the development of diverticulitis. Perforation of the diverticula is possible when they are inflamed.

Prognosis

Inflammation in diverticulitis increases the risk of perforation of the intestine. Peritonitis will develop from bacterial contamination after perforation of diverticula. Bleeding from the intestinal mucosa in the area of inflammation can also occur. The presence of diverticula and repeated periods of inflammation may allow development of fistula formation from the diverticula to other areas within the abdomen, such as the intestine or the bladder. Patients needing surgery may have a colostomy postoperatively. Depending on the location of the diverticulitis and the reason for the surgery, the colostomy may be reversible after healing has occurred.

Hallmark Signs and Symptoms

- Asymptomatic in diverticulosis
- Change in bowel habits
- Bloating, increased gas
- Loss of appetite, anorexia

- Abdominal pain most often in the left lower quadrant with diverticulitis
- Rectal bleeding due to inflammation with diverticulitis
- Fever with diverticulitis
- Nausea, vomiting
- Tachycardia because of fever
- Peritonitis if diverticula rupture

Common Test Results

- Barium enema will show diverticula—not done if there is increased risk of perforation.
- Colonoscopy will show diverticula—not done during acute inflammation.
- CT scan will show thickening of bowel wall due to inflammation or abscess in diverticulitis.
- Elevated WBC during diverticulitis.

Treatment

- Administer antibiotics.
  - ciprofloxacin
  - metronidazole
  - trimethoprim-sulfamethoxazole
- Administer adequate intravenous hydration.
- Manage pain as needed.
- NPO or clear liquids during acute inflammation to rest the intestinal tract.
- Surgical intervention to correct perforation of diverticula, abscess formation, bowel obstruction, fistula formation.
- NG tube postoperatively.

Nursing Diagnoses

- Acute pain
- Altered bowel elimination
- Disturbed body image

NURSING INTERVENTION

- Monitor vital signs for fever, increased heart rate, and decreased blood pressure.
- Assess abdomen for distention, presence of bowel sounds.
- Monitor intake and output.
- Postoperatively check:
  - Stoma at colostomy site.
  - Wound site for drainage or signs of infection.
  - Peripheral circulation, swelling due to increased risk of clot formation.
- **Explain to the patient:**
  - Eat low-residue foods during flare-ups.
  - Eat high-fiber diet—fresh fruits and vegetables, whole wheat breads, bran cereals—when asymptomatic.
  - Avoid laxatives and enemas due to increased irritation and intra-abdominal pressure.
  - Avoid lifting during exacerbation.
  - Avoid eating dried fruits, skins of fruits or vegetables, nuts and seeds, or drinking coffee, tea, or alcohol as these may exacerbate symptoms.

6. Gastroenteritis

What Went Wrong
Gastroenteritis is an acute inflammation of the gastric and intestinal mucosa which is most commonly due to bacterial, viral, protozoal, or parasitic infection. It may also be caused by irritation as a result of chemical or toxin exposure or allergic response. Viral exposure is more likely in winter; bacterial exposure is more common in summer when food-borne illness exposure is likely. Many people refer to these symptoms as "stomach flu."

Prognosis
Symptoms may be self-limiting or may need prescription medication to resolve the illness. Older or debilitated patients may have more severe symptoms or require hospitalization due to dehydration. The best prevention is thorough hand-washing. Dehydration is the most common complication.

Hallmark Signs and Symptoms
- Nausea and vomiting due to gastric irritation
- Diarrhea—watery, soft, may be mixed with mucous or blood

- Abdominal pain owing to intestinal irritation
- Abdominal distention
- Fever because of infection
- Anorexia due to gastric irritation
- Malaise owing to infection
- Headache as a result of viral illness
- Signs of dehydration—dry, flushed skin and mucous membranes, decreased urine output, tachycardia, poor skin turgor, and orthostatic blood pressure changes

Common Test Results

- CBC may show leukocytosis or eosinophilia (parasites).
- Electrolytes show imbalance due to GI loss.
- Blood urea nitrogen (BUN) and creatinine elevated because of dehydration.
- Stool for ova and parasites show positive with parasitic infection.

Treatment

- Monitor intake and output.
- Stop oral intake and resume initially with clear liquids and progress diet as tolerated.
- Replace fluids lost.
- Administer antiemetic medication for symptom relief.
  - prochlorperazine
  - trimethobenzamide
- Administer antidiarrheal medications for symptom relief.
  - loperamide
  - diphenoxylate
  - kaolin-pectin
  - bismuth subsalicylate
- Need to allow organism one way out of the GI system (either antiemetic or antidiarrheal, not both).

- Administer antimicrobials for infectious cause as indicated.
  - ciprofloxacin
  - metronidazole
  - Intravenous fluids to correct dehydration.

Nursing Diagnoses

- Risk for imbalanced nutrition: less than what body requires
- Deficient fluid volume
- Altered bowel elimination
- Diarrhea
- Fatigue

NURSING INTERVENTION

- Monitor vital signs for changes.
- Monitor intake and output.
- Replace fluids lost either orally (if tolerated) or IV.
- Assess skin and mucous membranes for signs of dehydration.
- Assess abdomen for bowel sounds, tenderness

7. Gastroesophageal Reflux Disease

What Went Wrong

Stomach acid and contents leak or reflux into the esophagus. This typically causes symptoms because the lining of the esophagus is not protected against the acid that is normally found only in the stomach. The pain that is produced is often referred to as heartburn or may be mistaken for cardiac pain. The pain may also be referred to the back. The pain occurs more frequently in men, people who are obese, smokers, and those who use alcohol or medications that decrease the muscle tone of the LES. The LES normally keeps the acid and other stomach contents within the stomach. The pain due to acid refluxing into the esophagus is worse after eating, when bending over or when lying down. Patients with a hiatal hernia may also experience reflux because of the increased pressure that exists from a portion of the stomach protruding upward through the diaphragm. Medications known to increase acid reflux include progesterone, anticholinergics, calcium channel blockers, nitrates, tricyclics, benzodiazepines, or opioids.

Prognosis

Control of symptoms is possible through lifestyle modification and use of medications to reduce acid production within the stomach. There has been no correlation shown between the severity of patient symptoms and the degree of damage being done to the tissue of the esophagus. Patients with ongoing symptoms should have an upper endoscopy to allow for visualization and biopsy of the area to monitor for the possibility of cancer of the esophagus developing because of long-term reflux. Barrett's esophagus is a premalignant condition of the esophagus that occurs due to reflux, where cellular changes have occurred, and the patient needs to be monitored for progression to a malignant cell type. Some patients may develop trouble with swallowing owing to the development of scarring from long-term exposure to acid. These patients may develop strictures over time. Procedures can be performed to help stretch the lumen of the esophagus to aid in swallowing.

Hallmark Signs and Symptoms

- Epigastric burning, worse after eating
- Heartburn
- Burping (eructation) or flatulence
- Sour taste in mouth, often worse in the morning
- Nausea
- Bloating
- Cough due to reflux high in the esophagus
- Sore throat
- Hoarseness or change in voice

Common Test Results

- Twenty-four-hour pH monitoring of lower esophageal area will show elevations.
- Barium swallow test or upper GI study may show reflux.
- Endoscopy or EGD shows irritation from cellular changes of chronic reflux which is also used to monitor patients with Barrett's esophagus.
- Esophageal manometry to measure lower esophageal sphincter tone.

Treatment

- Weight loss.
- Administer antacids to neutralize acid; these medications act quickly.
  - Maalox, Mylanta, Tums, Gaviscon
- Administer histamine type 2 (H2) blockers to decrease the production of acid.
  - ranitidine, famotidine, nizatidine, cimetidine
- Administer proton pump inhibitors (PPIs) to reduce the production of acid.
  - omeprazole, esomeprazole, pantoprazole, rabeprazole, lansoprazole
- Administer promotility agents.
  - metoclopramide
- Have patient eat six small meals rather than three large ones to reduce intra-abdominal pressure.
- Surgery or endoscopic procedures may be performed to prevent the reflux from occurring.

Nursing Diagnoses

- Risk for imbalanced nutrition: less than what body requires.
- Risk for imbalanced nutrition: more than what body requires.
- Acute pain.
- Chronic pain.

NURSING INTERVENTION

- Monitor vital signs.
- Assess abdomen for distention, bowel sounds.
- Teach about medication management.
- Teach patient about lifestyle modifications.
  - Not to lie down after eating.
  - Avoid exercise or bending over after meals.
- Elevate head of bed.
- Avoid wearing clothing that is tight at waist.
- Avoid acidic foods (citrus, vinegar, tomato), peppermint, caffeine, alcohol, carbonated beverages.
- Stop smoking.
- Lose weight if overweight.

8. Gastrointestinal Bleed

What Went Wrong

Bleeding from the GI tract may cause significant blood loss. The bleeding may be from either the upper or the lower GI tract. Upper GI bleeds are commonly from ulcers, esophageal varices, neoplasms, arteriovenous malformations, Mallory-Weiss tears secondary to vomiting, or anticoagulant use. Lower GI bleeds are commonly due to fissure formation, rectal trauma, colitis, polyps, colon cancer, diverticulitis, vasculitis, or ulcerations.

Prognosis

The amount and speed of blood loss coupled with the patient's age and comorbidities account for the prognosis. The greater the loss of blood, the harder it is for the system to overcome the stress. Multiple transfusions to replace the lost blood increase the patient's risk for a reaction. Patients with blood-clotting disorders have a greater risk of a significant bleed. Patients may go into shock if the amount of blood loss is great, as they become hemodynamically unstable.

Hallmark Signs and Symptoms

- Hematemesis—vomiting of blood (red, maroon, coffee ground)
- Melena—black, tarry stool
- Hematochezia—red or maroon blood rectally
- Orthostatic changes—drop in BP of at least 10 mmHg with position changes
- Tachycardia as body attempts to circulate lesser blood volume
- Pallor due to the decrease in circulating blood volume
- Light-headedness
- Diaphoresis (sweating)
- Nausea

Common Test Results

- Positive fecal occult blood.
- Hemoglobin drops.
- Hematocrit drops.
- Anemia (iron deficiency) with chronic slow bleed.

- Nasogastric aspirate positive with upper GI bleed.
- Anoscopy, sigmoidoscopy, or colonoscopy may show the site of lower GI bleed.
- Arteriography may show the site of bleed.
- Bleeding scan may show the site of bleed with radioisotope-tagged RBCs.

Treatment

- Maintain IV access.
- Administer isotonic fluids like normal saline.
- Monitor serial hemoglobin and hematocrit levels.
- Type and cross match for 3 to 6 units depending on the amount of blood loss.
- Transfuse packed RBCs, type-specific when possible (type O negative when type-specific unavailable—no time to get results back from laboratory yet).
- May need to administer albumin or fresh frozen **plasma**, depending on the amount of units transfused and comorbidities such as cirrhosis or clotting disorders.
- Endoscopic procedures to treat ulcer topically, with injectable or laser treatment.
- Esophageal varices may be treated by tamponade with Blakemore-Sengstaken tube.
- Surgery indicated when bleeding uncontrolled.

Nursing Diagnoses

- Deficient fluid volume
- Decreased cardiac output
- Anxiety

NURSING INTERVENTION

- Monitor vital signs for changes—drop in BP, increase in pulse, or respiration.
- Monitor intake and output.

- Replace volume lost.
- Monitor abdomen for bowel sounds, tenderness, or distention.
- Maintain large bore IV (14- to 18-gauge) access. Smaller size angiocatheters will not allow blood cells to pass through unharmed.
- Assess IV site for signs of redness or swelling.
- Monitor laboratory results—drop in laboratory values may lag behind blood loss.
- Monitor during blood transfusion as per institution protocol for checking blood unit, patient identity, frequency of vital signs, and documentation.

9. Gastritis

What Went Wrong

Gastritis is an inflammation of the stomach lining due to either erosion or atrophy. Erosive causes include stresses such as physical illness or medications such as nonsteroidal anti-inflammatory drugs (NSAIDs). Atrophic causes include a history of prior surgery (such as gastrectomy), pernicious anemia, alcohol use, or *Helicobacter pylori* infection.

Prognosis

Gastritis may cause changes within the cells of the stomach lining leading to malnutrition, lymphoma, or gastric cancer. Hospitalized patients, especially in critical care settings, should have preventive medications to avoid the development of gastritis.

Hallmark Signs and Symptoms

- Nausea and vomiting
- Anorexia
- Epigastric area discomfort
- Epigastric tenderness on palpation due to gastric irritation
- Bleeding from irritation of the gastric mucosa
- Hematemesis—red, maroon, bloody, or possible coffee ground emesis because of partial digestion of blood
- Melena—black, tarry stool

Common Test Results

- Hemoglobin and hematocrit decrease.
- Anemia (iron deficiency) due to chronic, slow blood loss.
- Fecal occult blood test positive.
- *H pylori* may be positive.
- Upper endoscopy shows inflammation, allows biopsy.

Treatment

- Administer antacids.
  - Maalox, Mylanta, Tums, Gaviscon
- Administer sucralfate to protect gastric lining.
- Administer H2 blockers.
  - ranitidine, famotidine, nizatidine, cimetidine
- Administer PPI.
  - omeprazole, esomeprazole, pantoprazole, rabeprazole, lansoprazole
- Eradicate *H pylori* infection if present.
- Diet modification.
- Monitor hemoglobin and hematocrit.

Nursing Diagnoses

- Risk for imbalanced nutrition: less than what body requires.
- Risk for imbalanced fluid volume.
- Nausea.

NURSING INTERVENTION

- Monitor vital signs.
- Monitor intake and output.
- Monitor stool for occult blood.
- Assess abdomen for bowel sounds, tenderness.

- **Explain to the patient:**
  - Diet restrictions: avoid alcohol, caffeine, and acidic foods.
  - Medications.
  - The need to avoid smoking.
  - The need to avoid NSAIDs.

10. Hepatitis

What Went Wrong

Hepatitis is an inflammation of the liver cells. This is most commonly due to a viral cause which may be either an acute illness or become chronic. The disease may also be as a result of exposure to drugs or toxins.

Hepatitis A is transmitted by an oral route, often due to contaminated water or poor sanitation when traveling; it is also transmitted in daycare settings and residential institutions. It can be prevented by vaccine.

Hepatitis B is transmitted through a percutaneous route, often due to sexual contact, IV drug use, mother-to-neonate transmission, or possibly blood transfusion. It can be prevented by vaccine. Infection may be acute or chronic.

Hepatitis C is transmitted via a percutaneous route, often due to IV drug use or, less commonly, sexual contact or history of blood transfusion. Transmission through sexual contact is more common among those with HIV infection. There is currently no vaccine available. Infection may be acute or chronic.

Hepatitis D is transmitted via a percutaneous route and needs hepatitis B to spread cell to cell. There is no vaccine available for hepatitis D.

Hepatitis E is transmitted by an oral route and it is associated with water contamination. There is no known chronic state of hepatitis E and no current vaccine available.

Hepatitis G is transmitted through a percutaneous route and it is associated with chronic infection but not significant liver disease.

Exposure to medications (even at therapeutic doses), drugs, or chemicals can also cause hepatitis. Onset is usually within the first couple of days of use and may be within the first couple of doses. Hepatotoxic substances include acetaminophen, carbon tetrachloride, benzenes, and valproic acid.

Prognosis

Hepatitis may occur as an acute infection (viral type A, E) or become a chronic state. The patient with chronic disease may be unaware of the illness until testing of liver function shows abnormalities and further testing reveals the presence of hepatitis. The chronic (viral type B, C) disease state creates the potential development of progressive liver disease. Some patients with chronic disease will need liver transplant. Recurrence rate posttransplant is high. Liver cancer may develop in those with chronic disease states.

Hallmark Signs and Symptoms

- Acute hepatitis:
  - Malaise
  - Nausea and vomiting
  - Diarrhea or constipation
  - Low-grade fever
  - Dark urine due to change in liver function
  - Jaundice owing to liver compromise
  - Tenderness in right upper quadrant of abdomen
  - Hepatomegaly
  - Arthritis, glomerulonephritis, and polyarteritis nodosa due to hepatitis B
- Chronic hepatitis:
  - Asymptomatic with elevated liver enzymes
  - Symptoms as acute hepatitis
  - Cirrhosis due to altered liver function
  - Ascites owing to the decrease in liver function, increased portal hypertension
  - Bleeding from esophageal varices
  - Encephalopathy as a result of diminished liver function
  - Bleeding due to clotting disorders
  - Enlargement of spleen

Common Test Results

- AST elevated.
- ALT elevated.
- IgM anti-HAV in acute or early convalescent stage of hepatitis A.

- IgG anti-HAV in the later convalescent stage of hepatitis A.
- HBeAg indicates current viral replication of hepatitis B and infectivity.
- HBsAg shows the presence of the hepatitis B surface antigen which is indicative of either current or past infection with hepatitis B.
- IgM anti-HBc shows acute or recent infection with hepatitis B.
- IgG anti-HBc shows convalescent or past infection with hepatitis B.
- HBV DNA shows the presence of hepatitis B DNA, most sensitive.
- Anti-HCV presents with hepatitis C infection.
- HCV RNA presents with hepatitis C infection (reverse transcriptase polymerase chain reaction or RT-PCR).
- Anti-HDV presents with hepatitis D infection.
- WBC count is normal to low.
- Liver biopsy shows hepatocellular necrosis.
- Urinalysis shows protein and bilirubin.

Treatment

- Avoid medications metabolized in the liver.
- Avoid alcohol.
- Remove or discontinue causative agents if drug-induced or toxic hepatitis.
- Intravenous hydration if vomiting during acute hepatitis.
- Activity as tolerated.
- High-calorie diet; breakfast is usually the best tolerated meal.
- Administer interferon or lamivudine for chronic hepatitis B.
- Administer interferon and ribavirin for hepatitis C.
- Administer prednisone in autoimmune hepatitis.
- Liver transplantation.

Nursing Diagnoses

- Fatigue
- Risk for injury
- Impaired tissue integrity

NURSING INTERVENTION

- Monitor vital signs.
- Assess abdomen for bowel sounds, tenderness, or ascites.
- Plan appropriate rest for the patient in acute phase.
- Monitor intake and output.
- Assess mental status for changes due to encephalopathy.
- **Explain to the patient:**
  - Plan palatable meals; remember that breakfast is generally the best tolerated meal.
  - Avoid smoking areas—intolerance to smoking.

11. Hiatal Hernia

What Went Wrong

This is also known as a diaphragmatic hernia. A part of the stomach protrudes up through the diaphragm near the esophagus into the chest (see Fig. 7–3). Patients may be asymptomatic or have daily symptoms of gastroesophageal reflux disease (GERD). The hernia may be a sliding hiatal hernia which allows movement of the upper portion of the stomach including the lower esophageal sphincter up and down through the diaphragm. These patients typically have symptoms of GERD. Another type of hiatal hernia is a rolling hernia in which a portion of the stomach protrudes up through the diaphragm, but the lower esophageal sphincter area remains below the level of the diaphragm. These patients do not generally suffer from reflux.

Prognosis

Lifestyle modifications may help control the symptoms of hiatal hernia. Some patients who do not get adequate control of symptoms or are refractory to treatment may need surgery to correct the movement through the diaphragm.

Hallmark Signs and Symptoms

- Sliding hernia:
  - Heartburn
  - Difficulty swallowing (dysphagia)

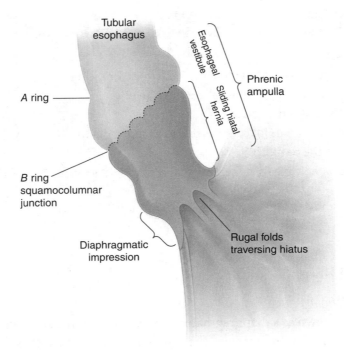

FIGURE 7–3 · Anatomy of the gastroesophageal junction where a sliding hiatal hernia occurs.
Source: Reproduced with permission from: Longo DL, Fauci AS, Kasper DL, Hauser SL, Jameson JL, Loscalzo J: *Harrison's Principles of Internal Medicine*, 18th ed. New York, NY: McGraw-Hill; 2012. Fig. 292–2.

- Burping (eructation)
- Chest pain
- Rolling hernia:
  - Chest pain
  - Shortness of breath after eating
  - Feeling of fullness after eating

Common Test Results

- Barium swallow test or upper GI study shows hiatal hernia
- EGD

Treatment

- Administer antacids for patients with reflux symptoms.
  - Maalox, Mylanta, Tums, Gaviscon

- Administer H2 blockers to reduce stomach acid.
  - ranitidine, nizatidine, famotidine, cimetidine
- Administer PPI to reduce the production of acid.
  - omeprazole, esomeprazole, pantoprazole, rabeprazole, lansoprazole
- Avoid lying down after eating.
- Modify eating schedule; small, frequent meals.
- Elevate head of bed.
- Avoid clothing that is tight around the waist.

Nursing Diagnoses

- Acute pain
- Chronic pain

NURSING INTERVENTION

- Monitor vital signs.
- Assess abdomen for distention, bowel sounds.
- **Explain to the patient:**
  - Lifestyle modifications.
  - Medication management.
  - Not to lie down after eating.
  - Elevate head of bed.
  - Avoid wearing clothing that is tight at waist.
  - Avoid acidic foods (citrus, vinegar, tomato), peppermint, caffeine, and alcohol.
  - Stop smoking.
  - Lose weight if overweight.

---

12. Intestinal Obstruction and Paralytic Ileus

What Went Wrong

An intestinal obstruction occurs when motility through the intestine is blocked. This may be caused by a mechanical obstruction due to the presence of a tumor, presence of adhesions from prior surgery, infection, or fecal impaction. A paralytic ileus results when motility through the intestine is blocked without any obstructing mass. This may occur during the postoperative period following intra-abdominal surgery, during a severe systemic illness (sepsis), electrolyte imbalance, or because of a metabolic disorder (diabetic ketoacidosis).

Prognosis

Disruption of intestinal function needs to be reestablished for return to homeostasis. In most cases, the underlying cause must also be corrected in order for the intestinal function to be restored. Nutritional needs must be met during the treatment period.

Hallmark Signs and Symptoms

- Obstruction:
  - Abdominal pain (cramping, intermittent, or constant)
  - Abdominal distention
  - Vomiting of GI contents (may eventually include stool as GI tract backs up)
  - Bowel sounds high-pitched
  - Constipation
  - Abdominal tenderness on palpation
- Paralytic ileus:
  - Abdominal pain (constant)
  - Abdominal distention
  - Vomiting of GI contents
  - Bowel sounds diminished or absent

Common Test Results

- Abdominal x-ray shows the dilation of small bowel with air-fluid levels in obstruction; diffuse distention in ileus.
- CT scan can identify the area of obstruction.

Treatment

- NPO to rest the intestinal tract.
- Nasogastric tube attached to suction the contents from the stomach.
- Intravenous fluid replacement with isotonic solution.

- Correction of electrolyte imbalances.
- Parenteral nutrition replacement and vitamin supplementation.
- Administer antiemetics if nausea continues after NG tube in place.
- Monitor electrolytes.

Nursing Diagnoses

- Risk for imbalanced nutrition: less than what body requires.
- Risk for imbalanced fluid volume.
- Altered bowel elimination.

NURSING INTERVENTION

- Monitor vital signs for changes.
- Assess abdomen for bowel sounds, tenderness.
- Monitor intravenous access site for irritation, redness, and swelling.
- Keep patient NPO.
- Monitor intake and output.
- Replace fluids lost from all sources.

---

13. Pancreatitis

What Went Wrong

Pancreatitis is an inflammation of the pancreas which causes destructive cellular changes. It may be an acute or a chronic process. Acute pancreatitis involves autodigestion of the pancreas by pancreatic enzymes and development of fibrosis. Blood glucose control may be affected by the changes in the pancreas. Chronic pancreatitis results from recurrent episodes of exacerbation, leading to fibrosis and a decrease in pancreatic function. Presence of gallstones blocking a pancreatic duct, chronic use of alcohol, postabdominal trauma or surgery, or elevated cholesterol are all associated with an increased risk of pancreatitis.

Prognosis

Acute pancreatitis may be life-threatening. Pleural effusion may develop as a complication of acute pancreatitis; older patients also have a greater risk of developing pneumonia. Disseminated intravascular coagulation is another complication that may occur, affecting the body's ability to clot due to depleted clotting factors in the development of small thrombi.

Hallmark Signs and Symptoms

- Epigastric pain due to inflammation and stretching of pancreatic duct
- Boring abdominal pain may radiate to back or left shoulder in acute pancreatitis
- Gnawing continuous abdominal pain with acute exacerbations in chronic pancreatitis
- Patient in knee-chest position for comfort—reduces tension on abdomen
- Nausea and vomiting
- Bluish-gray discoloration of periumbilical area of the abdomen (Cullen's sign)
- Bluish-gray discoloration of flank areas (Turner's sign)
- Ascites
- Weight loss
- Blood glucose elevation or fluctuation
- Fatigue

Common Test Results

- Elevated serum amylase and urine amylase levels.
- Elevated serum lipase.
- Elevated WBC due to inflammation.
- Elevated cholesterol.
- Elevated glucose because of labile effect on glucose control.
- Elevated bilirubin.
- CT scan shows inflammation.
- Chest x-ray may show pleural effusion.

Treatment

- NPO during acute stage to reduce release of pancreatic enzymes.
- Intravenous fluids for hydration.

- Total parenteral nutrition.
- Administer vitamin supplementation.
- Pain management with narcotics during acute stage.
- Avoid morphine that may increase pain due to spasm of the sphincter of Oddi at the opening to the small intestine from the common bile duct.
- Intravenous, patient-controlled analgesia, or transdermal delivery preferable to intramuscular.
- Acute:
  - NG tube connected to suction if vomiting.
  - Surgical intervention for abscess or pseudocyst.
- Chronic:
  - Blood glucose control with insulin.
  - Administer pancreatic enzymes with meals.
  - Surgical intervention for pain control, abscess.

Nursing Diagnoses

- Acute pain
- Imbalanced nutrition: less than what body requires

NURSING INTERVENTION

- Assess vital signs for elevated temperature, elevated pulse, and changes in blood pressure.
- Assess pain level.
- Monitor intake and output.
- Assess abdomen for bowel sounds, tenderness, masses, and ascites.
- Monitor fingerstick blood glucose.
- Assess lung sounds for bilateral equality.
- Frequent oral care for NPO patients.
- **Explain to the patient:**
  - Avoid alcohol and caffeine.
  - Bland, low-fat, high-protein, high-calorie, small, frequent meals.

- Use of blood glucose meter.
- Medication management, schedule, side effects.
- Plan rest periods until strength returns.

14. Peritonitis

What Went Wrong

Peritonitis is an acute inflammation of the peritoneum, which is the lining of the abdominal cavity. Peritonitis may be primary or secondary to another disease process. It typically occurs due to bacterial presence within the peritoneal space. The bacteria may have passed from the GI tract or the rupture of an organ within the abdomen or pelvis. After the introduction of the bacteria into the abdominal area, an inflammatory reaction occurs.

Prognosis

It is a life-threatening disease process. Patients may develop septicemia from the bacteria within the abdomen that enter the bloodstream.

Hallmark Signs and Symptoms

- Fever
- Tachycardia
- Abdominal distention
- Abdominal pain—may be localized or generalized
- Rebound pain (pain when quickly removing pressure during palpation of abdomen)
- Rigid abdomen
- Nausea, vomiting, and loss of appetite
- Decreased bowel sounds
- Decreased urine output

Common Test Results

- Elevated WBC.
- Blood cultures to identify infecting organisms.

- Abdominal x-rays to show free air from perforation.
- Ultrasound to identify causative problem (appendicitis, etc.).
- Peritoneal lavage to analyze fluid for WBC count, bacteria, and bile.
- CT scan to identify causative problem (appendicitis, salpingitis, etc.).

Treatment

- Intravenous fluids.
- Administer broad-spectrum antibiotics.
- Surgical intervention may be necessary to correct the cause of peritonitis.
- Pain management postoperatively.

Nursing Diagnoses

- Acute pain
- Impaired tissue integrity
- Impaired skin integrity

NURSING INTERVENTION

- Weigh daily.
- Monitor vital signs.
- Monitor intake and output.
- NPO to avoid irritation of intestinal tract, further stress on abdominal organs.
- Position for comfort, head of bed elevated.
- Assess for return of bowel sounds postoperatively.
- **Explain to the patient:**
  - Pain management.
  - Wound care, drains, etc.
  - Monitor for signs of infection.

---

15. Peptic Ulcer Disease

What Went Wrong

An ulcer develops when there is erosion of a portion of the mucosal layer of either the stomach or the duodenum. The ulcer may occur within the stomach (gastric ulcer) or the duodenum (duodenal ulcer). A break in the protective mucosal lining allows the acid within the stomach to make contact with the epithelial tissues. Gastric ulcers favor the lesser curvature of the stomach. Duodenal ulcers tend to be deeper, penetrating through the mucosa to the muscular layer. *H pylori* infection has been associated with duodenal ulcers. Stress ulcers are secondary to another acute medical condition or traumatic injury. As the body attempts to heal from the other physical condition (eg, major surgery), small areas of ischemia develop within the stomach or the duodenum. The ischemic areas then ulcerate.

Prognosis

The ulcerated areas may develop bleeding or may perforate. Depending on the location of the ulceration, a vessel may become exposed to the effects of the stomach acids. Damage to these vessels may result in significant bleeding. Perforation of the ulcer can occur as the ulcer continues to erode more deeply into the tissue. Perforation permits the contents of the stomach or the duodenum to enter the peritoneum, leading to peritonitis, paralytic ileus, septicemia, and shock. In this case, the patient will need emergency surgery due to a life-threatening condition.

Hallmark Signs and Symptoms

- Epigastric area pain
  - Worse just after eating as acid increases with gastric ulcer
  - Worse when the stomach is empty (with duodenal ulcer); may awaken during the night due to pain
- Weight changes
- Loss with gastric ulcer
- Gain with duodenal ulcer
- Bleeding from ulcer causes
  - Hematemesis (vomiting bloody fluid—red, maroon); more likely with gastric ulcer
  - Coffee ground emesis (partially digested blood)
  - Melena (tarry stool) more likely with duodenal ulcer
- Perforation of ulcer causes
  - Sudden, sharp pain
  - Tender, rigid, board-like abdomen

- Knee-chest position reduces pain
- Hypovolemic shock

Common Test Results

- Anemia due to bleeding.
- Stool for occult blood positive owing to bleeding.
- *H pylori* may test positive.
- Upper GI or barium swallow shows areas of ulceration—not done if perforation suspected.
- Upper endoscopy shows ulcer.
- EGD will allow visualization of ulcerated area.
- Abdominal x-rays show free air in perforation.

Treatment

- Administer antacids.
- Administer H2 blockers.
  - famotidine, ranitidine, nizatidine
- Administer PPI.
  - omeprazole, lansoprazole, rabeprazole, esomeprazole, pantoprazole
- Administer mucosal barrier fortifiers.
  - sucralfate
- Administer prostaglandin analogue.
  - misoprostol
- Adjust diet.
- Treat *H pylori* infection if present with combination therapy.
  - PPI plus clarithromycin plus amoxicillin, or
  - PPI plus metronidazole plus clarithromycin, or
  - Bismuth subsalicylate plus metronidazole plus tetracycline.

Nursing Diagnoses

- Acute pain
- Risk for imbalanced nutrition: less than what body requires
- Risk for imbalanced nutrition: more than what body requires

> ## NURSING INTERVENTION
>
> - Monitor vital signs.
> - Monitor intake and output.
> - Assess abdomen for bowel sounds, tenderness, rigidity, rebound pain, guarding.
> - Monitor stool for change in color, consistency, blood.
> - **Explain to the patient:**
>   - Diet modification to avoid acidic foods, caffeine, peppermint, alcohol.
>   - Eat more frequent, small meals.
>   - Avoid NSAIDs.
>   - Stop smoking.

16. Ulcerative Colitis

What Went Wrong

Ulcerative colitis is an inflammatory disease of the large intestine that affects the mucosal layer beginning in the rectum and colon and spreading into the adjacent tissue. There are ulcerations in the mucosal layer of the intestinal wall, and inflammation and abscess formation occur. Bloody diarrhea with mucous is the primary symptom. There are periods of exacerbations and remissions. Symptom severity may vary from mild to severe. The exact cause is unknown, but there is increased incidence in people of northern European, North American, or Ashkenazi Jewish origins. The peak incidences are from mid-teen to mid-twenties and again from mid-fifties to mid-sixties.

Prognosis

Patients with ulcerative colitis may have an increase in symptoms with each flare-up of the disease. Malabsorption of nutrients can cause weight loss and health problems. Some patients will need surgery to resect the affected area of the large intestine, resulting in a colostomy, ileal reservoir, ileoanal anastomosis, or ileoanal reservoir. There is an increased risk of colon cancer in patients with ulcerative colitis. The patient is also at risk for developing toxic megacolon or perforating the area of ulceration.

Hallmark Signs and Symptoms

- Weight loss
- Abdominal pain

- Chronic bloody diarrhea with pus due to ulceration
- Electrolyte imbalance owing to diarrhea
- Tenesmus—spasms involving the anal sphincter; persistent desire to empty bowel

Common Test Results

- Anemia—low hemoglobin and hematocrit due to blood loss and chronic disease.
- Elevated ESR owing to inflammation.
- Electrolyte disturbance because of diarrhea and poor absorbance of nutrients.
- Double-contrast barium enema shows areas of ulceration and inflammation.
- Sigmoidoscopy or colonoscopy shows ulcerations and bleeding.

Treatment

- Keep stool diary to identify irritating foods.
- Low-fiber, high-protein, high-calorie diet.
- Administer antidiarrheal medications.
  - loperamide
  - diphenoxylate hydrochloride and atropine
- Administer salicylate medications to reduce inflammation within the intestinal mucosa.
  - sulfasalazine
  - mesalamine
  - olsalazine
  - balsalazide
- Administer corticosteroids during exacerbations to reduce inflammation.
  - prednisone
  - hydrocortisone
- NPO for bowel rest during exacerbations.
- Administer anticholinergics to reduce abdominal cramping and discomfort.
  - dicyclomine
- Surgical resection of the affected area of large intestine.

Nursing Diagnoses

- Acute pain
- Diarrhea
- Impaired skin integrity
- Disturbed body image

NURSING INTERVENTION

- Monitor intake and output.
- Monitor stool output, frequency.
- Weigh patient regularly.
- Sitz bath.
- Vitamins A and D ointment or barrier cream applied to skin.
- Witch hazel to soothe sensitive skin.
- Monitor for toxic megacolon (distended and tender abdomen, fever, elevated WBC, elevated pulse, distended colon).
- **Explain to the patient:**
  - Home care for new ostomy patients or refer to enterostomal therapist for education.
  - Proper skin care of perianal area to avoid skin breakdown.
  - Avoid fragranced products which can be irritating.
  - Dietary modification, and which foods to avoid.
  - Medication use, schedule, and side effects.
  - Importance of follow-up care.
  - Wound care for postoperative patients.

REVIEW QUESTIONS

1. **Treatment of the patient with appendicitis includes:**

   A. Transfusion to replace blood loss.

   B. Bowel prep for cleansing.

   C. Surgical removal of appendix.

   D. Medications to lower pH within the stomach.

2. **Patients with a paralytic ileus typically have:**

   A. Intravenous fluid replacement and a nasogastric tube connected to suction.

   B. Surgical correction of the problem.

    C. Endoscopic injection of botulinum toxin or esophageal dilation.

    D. Endoscopy to allow biopsy followed with broad-spectrum antibiotics.

3. **On assessment of the abdomen in a patient with peritonitis, you would expect to find:**

    A. A soft abdomen with bowel sounds every 2 to 3 seconds.

    B. Rebound tenderness and guarding.

    C. Hyperactive, high-pitched bowel sounds, and a firm abdomen.

    D. Ascites and increased vascular pattern on the skin.

4. **Buildup of bile salts may cause the systemic symptom of:**

    A. Hypotension.

    B. Pruritus (itching).

    C. Ecchymosis (bruising).

    D. Urticaria (hives).

5. **The patient with gastroesophageal reflux disease should be taught:**

    A. To avoid coffee, tea, or other caffeine-containing beverages.

    B. To take H2 blockers, such as ranitidine, as directed.

    C. To avoid acidic foods such as citrus or tomato.

    D. All of the above.

6. **Patients with gastric ulcer typically exhibit the following symptoms:**

    A. Epigastric pain worse after eating and weight loss.

    B. Epigastric pain worse before meals, pain awakening patient from sleep, and melena.

    C. Decreased bowel sounds, rigid abdomen, rebound tenderness, and fever.

    D. Boring epigastric pain radiating to back and left shoulder, bluish-gray discoloration of periumbilical area, and ascites.

7. **Chronic hepatitis C may be treated with:**

    A. Sulfasalazine.

    B. Interferon and ribavirin.

    C. Metronidazole or ciprofloxacin.

    D. Acetaminophen.

8. **A patient presents with abdominal pain that is initially periumbilical but over time moves to the right lower quadrant area. This pain is most likely due to:**

    A. Appendicitis.

    B. Crohn's disease.

    C. Cholecystitis.

    D. Diverticulitis.

9. **Patients with GI bleeding may experience an acute or chronic blood loss. The patient is experiencing hematochezia. The physician recognizes this as:**

A. Vomiting of bright red or maroon blood.

B. Black, tarry stool.

C. Coffee ground emesis.

D. Red- or maroon-colored stool rectally.

10. **An inflammatory bowel disorder in which the patient develops abdominal pain, bloody diarrhea, tenesmus, and weight loss is:**

A. Crohn's disease.

B. Diverticulitis.

C. Ulcerative colitis.

D. Appendicitis.

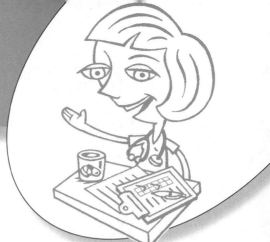

Chapter 8

Endocrine System

At the end of this chapter, the student will be able to:

- Identify normal anatomy and physiology related to the endocrine system
- Discuss the disease-causing pathologic changes within the endocrine system
- List four signs or symptoms of specific endocrine disease
- Recognize expected nursing and medical management of endocrine disease

KEY CONCEPTS

1. Addison's disease
2. Cushing's syndrome
3. Diabetes insipidus
4. Diabetes mellitus
5. Goiter
6. Hyperparanthyroidism
7. Hypoparanthyroidism
8. Hyperpituitarism
9. Hypopituitarsim
10. Hyperthyroidism
11. Hypoparanthyroidism
12. Hyperprolactinemia
13. Metabolic syndrome
14. Pheochromocytoma
15. Primary aldosteronism
16. Syndrome of inappropriate secretion of antidiuretic hormone

KEY TERMS

Acromegaly
Aldosterone
Antidiuretic hormone (ADH)
Catecholamines
Chvostek's sign
Cortisol
Cortisone
Epinephrine
Gigantism
Glucocorticoids
Graves' disease
Hydrocortisone
Insulin
Mineralocorticoids
Myxedema
Norepinephrine
Parathyroid hormone (PTH)
RAIU
Triiodothyronine(T3)
Thyroid-stimulating hormone (TSH)
Thyroxine (T4)
Thyrotropin-releasing hormone (TRH)
Trousseau's sign
Vanillylmandelic acid (VMA)

How the Endocrine System Works

The endocrine system is composed of several glands, scattered throughout the body (see Fig. 8–1). The glands release hormones which are chemical messengers, substances that control and regulate the activity of target cells and organs. In addition, these hormones influence growth, development, digestion, and regulate metabolism and reproduction. The glands generally release the hormones into the blood due to a stimulus, another hormone, or a threshold.

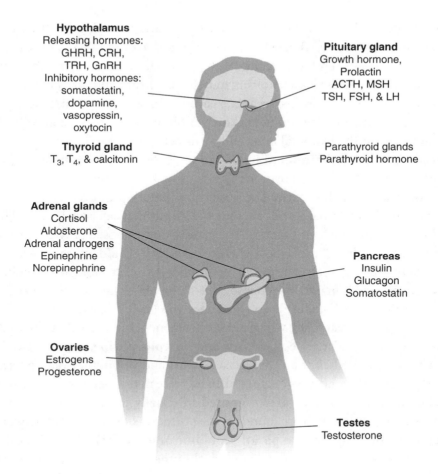

Hypothalamus
Releasing hormones:
GHRH, CRH,
TRH, GnRH
Inhibitory hormones:
somatostatin,
dopamine,
vasopressin,
oxytocin

Pituitary gland
Growth hormone,
Prolactin
ACTH, MSH
TSH, FSH, & LH

Thyroid gland
T_3, T_4, & calcitonin

Parathyroid glands
Parathyroid hormone

Adrenal glands
Cortisol
Aldosterone
Adrenal androgens
Epinephrine
Norepinephrine

Pancreas
Insulin
Glucagon
Somatostatin

Ovaries
Estrogens
Progesterone

Testes
Testosterone

FIGURE 8–1 • Anatomy of the endocrine system. The endocrine organs are located throughout the body with their function controlled by hormones delivered through circulation, produced locally or by direct neuroendocrine stimulation. Integration of hormone production from endocrine organs is under regulation by the hypothalamus.

Source: Reproduced with permission from: Molina PE: *Endocrine Physiology*, 3rd ed. New York, NY: McGraw-Hill; 2010. Fig. 1–1.

The signal to turn off the hormone production is regulated by a process called direct feedback. Direct feedback is necessary to maintain homeostasis. The body receives feedback about changes in hormone levels and impacts organs or body systems to adjust the hormone production to tell the body to return to homeostasis. When the concentration of the substance reaches a threshold, the gland and its production are turned off. The glands, the hormones they produce, and the effects are stated as next.

The thyroid gland is located in the anterior neck, overlying the trachea. It makes three hormones: **thyroxine (T4), triiodothyronine (T3)**, and calcitonin, which affect the blood calcium and phosphate release from the bones. Thyroid hormones affect metabolism, muscles, the heart, and many other body organs and systems. They help regulate carbohydrate metabolism, lipids, proteins, and growth and development. Anterior pituitary glands are controlled by hormones from the hypothalamus and by direct feedback. The anterior pituitary secretes **thyroid-stimulating hormone (TSH)**, follicle-stimulating hormone (FSH), luteinizing hormone (LH), growth hormone, prolactin, and adrenocorticotropic hormone. The posterior pituitary produces oxytocin and vasopressin. The adrenal glands are bilateral glands that cap each kidney. They are located in the retroperitoneum. The glands are composed of two parts: the cortex and the adrenal medulla. The cortex secretes: (1) **aldosterone**, which is responsible for renal reabsorption of sodium and excretion of potassium; (2) **cortisol,** which maintains glucose control, increases hepatic gluconeogenesis (the making of glucose), and manages the body's stress response; and (3) androgens (testosterone), which are sex hormones. The adrenal medulla produces, stores, and secretes epinephrine and **norepinephrine**, which are called **catecholamines**. When they are released, heart and respiratory rate increase, blood pressure rises, airways dilate, and an increase in the metabolic rate is seen.

The parathyroid glands are composed of usually four, sometimes six or more, small glands which are found on the posterior side of the thyroid gland. Their function is to produce **parathyroid hormone (PTH)**. PTH, also called parathormone, maintains the calcium level in the blood. It also regulates the phosphorus level in the body. If the serum calcium level falls, PTH is released, which causes bones to break down, releasing calcium into the blood. It also causes the kidneys to decrease the calcium released in the urine and increases phosphate excretion.

Just the Facts

1. Addison's Disease

What Went Wrong

Addison's disease is inadequate secretion of hormones from the adrenal cortex, **glucocorticoids** (which help control glucose, suppress the immune response, aid in stress response), **mineralocorticoids** (help maintain electrolyte balance), androgens and estrogens (which control sexual development and function) resulting from damage to the adrenal cortex. Autoimmune destruction of the adrenal gland and tuberculosis are two common causes of Addison's disease. Hemorrhage or tumors are also possible causes. A patient can experience Addisonian crisis when infection, surgery, or other stressful events result in a decrease in the production of cortisol and aldosterone. Addisonian crisis is a medical emergency.

Prognosis
With ongoing treatment, patients can expect a normal lifespan.

Hallmark Signs and Symptoms
- Weakness and fatigue due to insufficient cortisol
- Weight loss owing to insufficient cortisol
- Loss of appetite, nausea and vomiting, and oral (buccal) mucosa lesions
- Orthostatic hypotension because of poor fluid status from aldosterone deficiency
- Bronzing of the skin as a result of hyperpigmentation from the autoimmune disease

Common Test Results
- Increased blood urea nitrogen (BUN) due to dehydration.
- Increased serum potassium from changes in aldosterone secretion.
- Decreased serum cortisol being secreted from the adrenal cortex.
- Decreased serum glucose from decreased corticosteroids.
- Positive 24-hour urine aldosterone level owing to less aldosterone being secreted.
- Positive adrenocorticotropic hormone (ACTH) stimulation test; ACTH acts on the adrenal cortex to stimulate adrenal hormone secretion. An infusion of ACTH is given, and the test is positive if the infusion fails to raise the cortisol level.
- Abnormal adrenal glands appear on CT scan.

Treatment
- Administer **cortisone** or **hydrocortisone** to replace cortisol.
- Administer fludrocortisone to regulate sodium and potassium balance.
- Maintain fluid balance.

Nursing Diagnoses

- Fatigue related to disease state
- Risk for deficient fluid volume
- Disturbed body image due to disease state

NURSING INTERVENTION

- Monitor fluids and electrolytes.
- Weigh the patient daily.
- Suggest bone density test for osteoporosis due to the decrease in mineralocorticoids.
- **Explain to the patient:**
  - Medication must be taken every day.
  - Wear a medical alert bracelet.
  - Keep an emergency supply of medication available. Self-injection of medication may be necessary during stressful times as Addisonian crisis may develop. Symptoms include abdominal pain, difficulty breathing, hypotension, and altered level of consciousness.

---

2. Cushing's Syndrome

What Went Wrong

The adrenal cortex secretes an excess of glucocorticoids or the pituitary gland an excess of ACTH as a result of either a pituitary tumor, pituitary hyperplasia, adrenal tumor, or from ongoing glucocorticoid therapy. An excess of ACTH stimulates the release of cortisol.

Prognosis

Patients can expect a normal lifespan once the tumor is removed; however, tumors may recur. If untreated, Cushing's may lead to progressive symptoms, even death.

Hallmark Signs and Symptoms

- Moon face (round, full appearance of face) during excess cortisol production
- Buffalo hump (fat pad located in the upper back) from excessive corticosteroids

- Osteoporosis from an excess of corticosteroids, which weaken the bones
- Absence of menstruation (amenorrhea) from the effects of excess steroids
- Changes in mental status from excessive steroids
- Striae (purple stretch marks) on abdomen, breasts, and thighs
- Skin changes (infections or acne, easy bruising) due to excess cortisol
- Muscle weakness
- Women experience hirsutism (excessive hair growth) on face, neck, chest, and abdomen
- Men experience impotence, decreased fertility, and sex drive

Common Test Results

- Dexamethasone suppression test: a dose of glucocorticoid is given to test the hypothalamus-pituitary-adrenal axis. If there is suppression with the dose, it indicates a pituitary origin of the excess cortisol. If no suppression occurs, the etiology is an adrenal or ectopic tumor.
- Increased cortisol in 24-hour urine collection from excess production.
- Presence of a pituitary tumor or adrenal tumor on a CT scan; the tumor will show on a CT scan.
- Increased blood glucose due to overproduction of steroids.
- Increased sodium owing to excess fluid loss.
- Decreased potassium.

Treatment

- Surgical removal of the pituitary tumor or adrenal tumor.
- Radiation treatments targeting a pituitary tumor.
- Cortisol replacement may be necessary during recovery.

Nursing Diagnoses

- Disturbed body image related to illness
- Excess fluid volume due to excess water and sodium reabsorption
- Risk for infection owing to immunosuppression and inadequate primary defenses

NURSING INTERVENTION

- Daily weighing to monitor fluid status.
- Monitor input and output to ensure adequate hydration.
- Monitor for elevated blood glucose levels and the presence of urinary glucose and acetone as elevated levels of corticosteroids may produce hyperglycemia.
- Allow for adequate rest to allow the body to stabilize.
- Avoid trauma to the skin because elevated levels of corticosteroids can delay wound healing.
- Bone densitometry to assess for osteoporosis as corticosteroids can leech calcium from the bone.
- Following surgery:
  - Assist in early ambulation, deep breathing, coughing to facilitate mucous mobilization, and decrease risk for emboli.
  - Monitor incision site for drainage, erythema, and signs of infection.
- **Explain to the patient:**
  - Maintain a high-calorie, high-calcium diet to aid in wound repair and replace calcium.
  - Administer pain medication as needed.

3. Diabetes Insipidus

What Went Wrong

Antidiuretic hormone (ADH) is produced within the hypothalamus and then stored in the pituitary until needed. Either a decrease in the production of an ADH by the hypothalamus or a decrease in the release of ADH by the pituitary compromises the ability of the kidneys to concentrate urine. This results in the excretion of large amounts of diluted urine. The patient then drinks large volumes of fluid to replace the fluids lost due to increased urine output. If the kidneys develop difficulty in responding to the ADH, the condition is referred to as nephrogenic diabetes insipidus. The condition may be owing to damage or injury of the hypothalamus such as head tumor, trauma, infection, or surgery. Elevated calcium levels or medications (such as lithium) may also cause diabetes insipidus.

Prognosis

Treatment will eliminate the symptoms of diabetes insipidus and the patient can expect a normal lifespan.

Hallmark Signs and Symptoms

- Increased urine volume as the kidneys fail to concentrate urine.
- Increased thirst as the body attempts to replace lost fluid.

Common Test Results

- Normal blood glucose indicating that diabetes insipidus is not a complication of diabetes mellitus.
- Low specific gravity in urine due to increased fluid in the urine.
- Increased BUN, indicating dehydration because the concentration of solutes to fluid is rising.
- Electrolytes indicate dehydration; Na and Cl will rise as the concentration increases.
- Vasopressin challenge test. Those patients with diabetes insipidus will note a decrease in output and thirst.
  - If urine output decreases and urine specific gravity increases, then the problem is with the pituitary gland and kidneys are normal.
  - If urine output remains unchanged and urine specific gravity remains low, then the pituitary gland is normal and the problem is with the kidneys.
- Presence of a pituitary tumor or hypothalamus tumor may appear on an MRI.

Treatment

- Administer replacement ADH hormone such as vasopressin or desmopressin to return normal urination.
- Administer a diuretic such as hydrochlorothiazide to decrease urination.
- Place the patient on a low-salt diet to reduce urine production in the kidneys.
- Increase fluid intake until urination returns to normal.

Nursing Diagnoses

- Risk for impaired urinary elimination
- Impaired oral mucous membrane related to inadequate oral secretions
- Deficient fluid volume due to excessive fluid loss or inadequate fluid intake

NURSING INTERVENTION

- Maintain fluid and electrolyte balance.
- Monitor intake and output.
- Monitor for signs of dehydration.
- Weigh the patient each day using the same scale, at the same time of day, wearing similar clothing.
- **Explain to the patient:**
  - Medication must be taken every day.
  - Wear a medical alert necklace/bracelet to alert healthcare providers that you have diabetes insipidus.

4. Diabetes Mellitus

What Went Wrong

Our body converts certain foods into glucose, which is the body's primary energy supply. Insulin from the beta cells of the pancreas is necessary to carry glucose into cells where it is used for cell metabolism. Diabetes mellitus occurs when beta cells either are unable to produce insulin (type 1 diabetes mellitus) or produce an insufficient amount of insulin (type 2 diabetes mellitus). Type 2 diabetes mellitus can also be due to the body's inability to utilize the insulin that has been produced. This is referred to as insulin resistance. In these patients, the serum insulin level tends to be elevated. As a result, glucose does not enter cells but remains in the blood. Increased glucose levels in the blood signal to the patient to increase intake of fluid in an effort to flush glucose out of the body through the kidneys. Patients then experience increased thirst and increased urination. Cells become starved for energy because of the lack of glucose and signal to the patient to eat, causing the patient to experience an increase in hunger. There are three types of diabetes mellitus. These are type 1 (where patients are insulin-dependent) where beta cells are destroyed by an autoimmune process; type 2 (where patients may or may not need to take insulin) where beta cells produce insufficient insulin or the body is unable to utilize the insulin (insulin resistance) that has been produced; and gestational diabetes mellitus (DM that occurs during pregnancy).

Prognosis

Patients with type 1 and type 2 diabetes mellitus are at risk for complications such as vision loss (diabetic retinopathy), damage to blood vessels and nerves (diabetic neuropathy), and kidney damage (nephropathy). However, complications can be minimized by maintaining a normal blood glucose level through consistent monitoring, administering insulin, taking oral or injectable medications, and following an American Diabetic Association diet. Patients with gestational diabetes mellitus will recover following pregnancy; however, they are at risk for developing type 2 diabetes mellitus later in life.

Hallmark Signs and Symptom

- Type 1:
  - Fast onset because no insulin is being produced.
  - Increased appetite (polyphagia) because cells are starved for energy, signals a need for more food.
  - Increased thirst (polydipsia) from the body attempting to rid of glucose.
  - Increased urination (polyuria) from the body trying to rid of glucose.
  - Weight loss since glucose is unable to enter cells.
  - Frequent infections as bacteria feeds on the excess glucose.
  - Delayed healing because elevated glucose levels in the blood hinder the healing process.
- Type 2:
  - Slow onset because some insulin is being produced.
  - Increased thirst (polydipsia) from the body attempting to rid itself of glucose.
  - Increased urination (polyuria) from the body trying to rid itself of glucose.
  - *Candida* infection as bacteria feeds on the excess glucose.
  - Delayed healing because elevated glucose levels in the blood hinder the healing process.
  - Some patients are asymptomatic and diagnosed when blood work detects elevated glucose.
- Gestational:
  - Asymptomatic
  - Some patients may experience increased thirst (polydipsia) from the body attempting to rid itself of glucose.

Common Test Results

- Fasting plasma blood glucose test with a serum glucose level of 126 mg/dL (7.0 mmol/L) on two different tests.
- Oral glucose tolerance test (OGTT) with a plasma glucose of 200 mg/dL (11.1 mmol/L) 2 hours after ingesting 75 g oral glucose.
- Random plasma glucose at or above 200 mg/dL (11.1 mmol/L) in a symptomatic patient.
- Glycosylated hemoglobin A1c 6.5% or higher on two separate tests. This test is unreliable in settings where the patient's red blood cell (RBC) turnover is affected, such as hemolytic anemia, iron deficiency anemia, and pregnancy.
- Increased glucose in urine (glucosuria). This is not a reliable diagnostic test as the renal threshold (of blood glucose level) varies from patient to patient. Once the renal threshold is breached, there will be + glucose in the urine. This test may be used to help monitor glucose control during exacerbations.

Treatment

- Type 1:
  - Regular monitoring of blood glucose.
  - Administer insulin to maintain normal blood glucose levels (see Table 8–1).
  - Maintain a diabetic diet.
  - Administer:
  - Rapid-acting insulin: given with meals (onset in 10 to 30 minutes; peak action between 30 and 90 minutes; duration of action between 1 and 5 hours, depending on drug).
    - aspart
    - lispro
    - glulisine
  - Short-acting insulin: for short-term glucose control (onset in 30 to 60 minutes; peak action in 2 to 5 hours; duration of onset is 5 to 8 hours).
    - Regular insulin

TABLE 8–1 Insulin Guide					
Drug	Appearance	Onset	Peak	Duration	Compatibility
Rapid-acting	Clear	10-30 minutes	30-90 minutes	1-5 hours	All insulin except lente. Aspart is not compatible.
Short-acting	Clear	30-60 minutes	2-5 hours	2-8 hours	
Intermediate-acting	Cloudy	1-2.5 hours	3-12 hours	18-24 hours	Regular insulin
Long-acting	Cloudy	4-6 hours	6-20 hours	20-36 hours	Regular

- Intermediate insulin: provides glucose control for about half the day (onset between 1 and 2.5 hours; peak action between 3 and 12 hours; duration between 18 and 24 hours, depending on drug)
  - NPH
  - lente
- Long-acting insulin: for all day coverage (onset between half the day to 3 hours; peak onset between 6 and 20 hours, except glargine; duration of action between 20 and 26 hours)
  - ultralente
  - detemir
  - glargine
- Combination products also available.
- Type 2:
  - Maintain ideal body weight through diet and exercise.
  - Regular monitoring of blood glucose.
  - Administer oral sulfonylureas to stimulate secretion of insulin from the pancreas (see Table 8–2).
  - Administer oral biguanides to reduce blood glucose production by the liver.
    - metformin

TABLE 8–2 Type 2 Diabetes Medications

Drug	Potential initial A1c reduction	Comments

• Oral sulfonylureas
  • chlorpropamide (first generation)
  • glyburide (second generation)
  • glipizide (second generation)
  • glimepiride (second generation)
  • tolbutamide (first generation)
  • tolazamide (first generation)
	up to 1%-2%	Chlorpropamide—use caution with renal or hepatic patients

• Oral biguanides • metformin	up to 1%-2%	Decreases glucose production in liver; decreases intestinal absorption of glucose and improves insulin sensitivity; care in patients with renal impairment

• Thiazolidinediones
  • pioglitazone
  • rosiglitazone
	up to 1%-2%	Combats insulin resistance by making cells more sensitive, decreases glucose released from liver; cardiac risk, especially with rosiglitazone

• Oral alpha-glucosidase inhibitor
  • acarbose
  • miglitol
	up to 1/2%-1%	Delays glucose absorption and digestion of carbohydrates; lowers blood sugar; reduces plasma glucose and insulin

• Oral meglitinides
  • repaglinide
  • nateglinide
		Glucose-dependent stimulation of pancreas to release more insulin

• Oral DPP4 inhibitors
  • sitagliptin
  • saxagliptin
  • linagliptin
		Glucose-dependent stimulation of secretion of insulin from pancreas, reduces glucose production; does not cause weight gain

• Injected incretin mimetics
  • exenatide
  • pramlintide
		Synthetic form of naturally occurring hormones. Assists pancreatic insulin production in setting of hyperglycemia; regulates liver production of glucose; decreases appetite; slows glucose transit from stomach to intestine

- Administer thiazolidinediones to sensitize peripheral tissues to insulin.
  - rosiglitazone
  - pioglitazone
- Administer meglitinides to stimulate section of insulin from the pancreas.
  - repaglinide
  - nateglinide
- Administer dipeptidyl peptidase-4 (DPP-4) inhibitors to stimulate insulin production.
  - sitagliptin
  - saxagliptin
  - linagliptin
- Administer alpha-glucosidase inhibitors to delay absorption of carbohydrates in the intestine.
  - acarbose
  - miglitol
- Administer incretin mimetics to assist insulin production in the pancreas and help regulate liver production of glucose. It also decreases appetite and increases the time glucose remains in the stomach before entering the small intestine for absorption.
  - pramlintide (amylin analog)
  - exenatide
- Gestational:
  - Regular monitoring of blood glucose.
  - Maintain weight through diet and exercise.
  - Most oral diabetes medications are contraindicated in pregnancy.
  - Administer insulin if diet and exercise fail to control blood glucose levels.

Nursing Diagnoses

- Risk for imbalanced nutrition: less than what body requires
- Risk for injury related to sensory alterations
- Risk for delayed surgical recovery

- Knowledge deficit for disease process
- Body image disturbance
- Nutrition self-care deficit

NURSING INTERVENTION

- **Explain to the patient:**
  - The disease and the importance of maintaining normal glucose levels.
  - Blood glucose monitoring.
  - Diet and food choices, including portion sizes.
  - Encourage exercise.
  - Discuss coping skills to reduce stress.
  - Teach self-injection of insulin.
  - Urge smoking cessation.
  - Self-care.
  - Acute management (sick day rules).
  - Prevention of complications, such as hyperglycemia and hypoglycemia.
  - Importance of daily medications.
  - Hypoglycemia signs, symptoms, and interventions.
  - Sweating, lethargy, confusion, hunger, dizziness, and weakness are all signs and symptoms of hypoglycemia.
  - Management of hypoglycemia: glucose tablets, or 4 ounces of fruit juice, several hard candies, or a small amount of a carbohydrate.
  - The signs and symptoms of hyperglycemia: fatigue, headache, blurry vision, and dry itchy skin.
  - Management of hyperglycemia: a change in medication or dosage, increase in regular exercise, more careful food intake and meal planning, an increase in the number of fingersticks, and discussion with the MD/NP/PA.
  - Glucagon injection for hypoglycemic events.

5. Goiter

What Went Wrong

A lack of iodine in the patient's diet (endemic, simple goiter) causes the thyroid gland to become enlarged. This is seen less today because iodine is added to table salt. The thyroid gland can also become enlarged by ingesting large amounts of goitrogenic drugs or goitrogenic foods that decrease production of thyroxine, such as strawberries, cabbage, peanuts, peas, peaches, and spinach.

This results in sporadic simple goiter. A simple goiter is not caused by inflammation or neoplasm.

Prognosis
Prognosis is good if treated and patients go on to live normal lives.

Hallmark Signs and Symptoms
- Difficulty in swallowing (dysphagia) due to a large thyroid pressing on the esophagus
- Enlarged thyroid gland
- Respiratory distress from the large gland causing pressure on the trachea
- A tight feeling in the throat from a large gland
- Coughing

Common Test Results
- Decreased or normal serum T4 level caused by an underactive thyroid.
- Increased serum TSH, by the pituitary gland, attempting to stimulate or shut off production of the thyroid in making thyroid hormone.
- Radioactive iodine uptake (**RAIU)** tests uptake normal or increased—a radioactive isotope is injected into a vein. A scan of the thyroid is done to visualize the thyroid more completely.
- Ultrasound enables sound waves to bounce off the gland, giving the size and location of any nodules.

Treatment
- If increased TSH, administer hormone replacement with levothyroxine (T4), desicated thyroid, or liothyronine (T3).
- If the thyroid gland is overactive, then administer small doses of Lugol's solution or potassium iodide solution.
- If the simple goiter cannot be reduced through medication, then a thyroidectomy is performed during which all or part of the thyroid is removed.

Nursing Diagnoses
- Imbalanced nutrition: less than what body requires; related to inadequate intake in relation to metabolic needs

- Fatigue related to sleep deprivation
- Hyperthermia related to increased metabolic rate

NURSING INTERVENTION

- Avoid goitrogenic foods or drugs in sporadic goiter since they decrease thyroid hormone production.
- Use iodized salt to prevent and treat endemic goiter since the thyroid needs iodine to make thyroid hormone.
- **Explain to the patient:**
  - The need for lifelong thyroid replacement after thyroidectomy and radioactive iodine treatment.
  - The need for intermittent laboratory work to monitor the thyroid.
  - Visits to the primary care practitioner to monitor size of thyroid gland.

---

6. Hyperthyroidism

What Went Wrong

There is an overproduction of T3 and T4 by the thyroid gland that can be caused by hyperthyroidism (Graves' disease), which is an autoimmune disease where the body's immune system attacks the thyroid gland. Other causes can be a benign tumor (adenomas) resulting in an enlarged thyroid gland (goiter), inflammation, taking too much levothyroxine, or an overproduction of TSH by the pituitary gland, which may be caused by a pituitary tumor.

Prognosis

The prognosis is good if the cause of hyperthyroidism is treated; however, hyperthyroidism is a chronic disease. Signs such as bulging eyes (exophthalmos) are not reversible. Furthermore, thyroid surgery may result in complications.

Hallmark Signs and Symptoms

- Enlarged thyroid gland (goiter), possibly caused by tumor
- Protrusion of the eyeballs (exophthalmos) due to lymphocytic infiltration which pushes out the eyeball (see Fig. 8–2)
- Sweating (diaphoresis); excess thyroid hormone raises the metabolic rate
- Increased appetite owing to increased metabolism
- Nervousness because of high levels of thyroid hormone

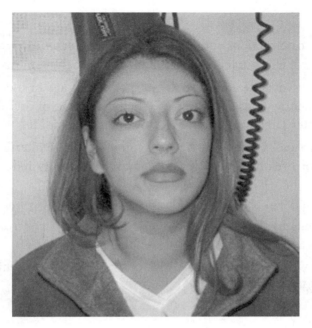

FIGURE 8−2 • Patient displaying common findings of Graves' disease: lid retraction and mild proptosis (exophthalmos), particularly evident on the left eye and goiter.

Source: Reproduced with permission from: Usatine RP, Smith MA, Mayeaux EJ Jr, Chumley H, Tysinger J: *The Color Atlas of Family Medicine.* New York, NY: McGraw-Hill; 2008. Fig. 217−1.

- Weight loss due to increased metabolism
- Menstrual changes owing to elevated levels of thyroid hormone
- Difficulty concentrating
- Restlessness
- Diarrhea
- Elevated blood pressure

Common Test Results

- Increased serum T3.
- Increased serum T4.
- Low **TSH**.
- Increased TRH and TSH if pituitary gland is the cause of hyperthyroidism.
- Presence of antibodies if cause is **Graves' disease**.
- Thyroid scan reveals enlarged thyroid.

Treatment

- For mild cases and for young patients, administer antithyroid medication such as propylthiouracil and methimazole to block synthesis of T3 and T4.
- For Graves' disease and for patients 50 years of age or older, radioactive iodine therapy is used to decrease the production of thyroid hormones. Administer Lugol's solution, SSKI, or potassium iodide.
- For severe cases where the size of the thyroid gland interferes with swallowing or breathing, the thyroid gland is surgically reduced in size or removed.
- Administer beta blockers such as propranolol until hyperthyroidism diminishes to decrease sympathetic activity and control tachycardia, tremors, and anxiety.
- Patients will have an increased risk of osteoporosis. Screening should be done periodically.

Nursing Diagnoses

- Imbalanced nutrition: less than what body requires related to inadequate intake in relation to metabolic needs
- Fatigue related to sleep deprivation
- Hyperthermia related to increased metabolic rate

NURSING INTERVENTION

- Monitor vital signs.
- Provide cool environment.
- Protect the patient's eyes with dark glasses and artificial tears if the patient has exophthalmos.
- Provide a diet high in carbohydrates, protein, calories, vitamins, and minerals.
- Monitor for laryngeal edema following surgery (hoarseness or inability to clearly speak).
- Keep oxygen, suction, and a tracheotomy set near bed in case the neck swells and breathing is impaired.
- Keep calcium gluconate near the patient's bed following surgery. This is the treatment for tetany and is used to maintain the serum calcium level in normal range.

- Place the patient in a semi-Fowler's position to decrease tension on the neck following surgery.

- Support the patient's head and neck with pillows.
- Monitor for muscle spasms and tremors (tetany) caused by manipulation of the parathyroid glands during surgery.
- Check drainage and hemorrhage from incision line; red flags are frank hemorrhage and purulent, foul-smelling drainage.
- Monitor for signs of hypocalcemia (tingling of hands and fingers).
- Check for **Trousseau's sign** (inflate blood pressure cuff on the arm and muscles contract).
- Check for **Chvostek's sign** (tapping over the facial nerve causes twitching of the facial muscles). Both this sign and Trousseau's sign are positive when the parathyroid glands have been manipulated during thyroid surgery, in which case they secrete too much phosphorus and not enough calcium. Since muscles, that is the heart, need calcium for work, a low calcium level may cause muscle spasms which are easily detected by Chvostek's sign and **Trousseau's sign**. The treatment is IV calcium, administered quickly.

7. Hypothyroidism

What Went Wrong

Hypothyroidism (**myxedema**) is a lack of, or too little, thyroid hormone. It may be caused by Hashimoto's thyroiditis which is a chronic disorder caused by abnormal antibodies that attack the thyroid gland. Hypothyroidism can also be caused by decreased production of the TSH hormone from the pituitary gland, a side effect of surgery, inflammation of the thyroid gland, radiation therapy to the neck area, viruses, and treatment for hyperthyroidism. Medications such as amiodarone, lithium, propylthiouracil, or methimazole may also cause thyroid dysfunction.

Prognosis

Prognosis is excellent with replacement of thyroid hormones.

Hallmark Signs and Symptoms

- Fatigue due to slow metabolism
- Increased sensitivity to cold owing to slow metabolism
- Thin, brittle nails because of low levels of thyroid hormone, which helps growth and development

- Thick dry hair from lack of thyroid hormone
- Dry skin from lack of thyroid hormone
- Menstruation changes due to diminished levels of thyroid hormone
- Slow cognitive function as a result of slow metabolism
- Weight gain, low levels of thyroid hormone cause fatigue, sluggishness
- Constipation
- Joint or muscle pains
- As the disease progresses, you may also see:
  - Hoarseness or changes in voice, including slowing of speech
  - Puffiness in the face, hands, and feet
  - Thickening of the skin
  - Loss of the outer edge of the eyebrows

Common Test Results

- Increased TSH unless the cause is due to a decreased production of TSH by the pituitary gland.
- Decreased T3 and T4.
- Presence of thyroglobulin, indicating Hashimoto's thyroiditis.
- Presence of peroxidase autoantibodies in serum, indicating Hashimoto's thyroiditis.
- Increased cholesterol levels.

Treatment

- Replacement hormone; levothyroxine is the treatment of choice.
- Serum measurements of T3 and T4 will need to be performed after 6 to 8 weeks to determine if the patient is taking the correct dose.
- The patient needs to be aware that this is a lifetime replacement.

Nursing Diagnoses

- Risk for imbalanced nutrition: more than what body requires
- Hypothermia related to decreased metabolic rate
- Risk for constipation related to decreased motility of the GI tract

NURSING INTERVENTION

- Monitor vital signs.
- Provide a warm environment.
- Low-calorie diet.
- Increase fluids and fiber to prevent constipation.
- Take thyroid replacement hormone each morning to avoid insomnia.
- Monitor for signs of thyrotoxicosis (an increase in T3): nausea, vomiting, diarrhea, sweating, tachycardia, and palpitations.
- **Explain to the patient:**
  - Side effects of thyroid hormone replacement.
  - Review the signs of hyperthyroidism and hypothyroidism.
  - Contact healthcare provider if signs change.

8. Hyperparathyroidism

What Went Wrong

Overactivity of the parathyroid glands caused by a tumor results in too much PTH, resulting in hypercalcemia and hypophosphatemia. Excess calcium is reabsorbed by the kidneys and may result in kidney stones; however, malfunction in the feedback mechanism prevents detection of excessive calcium levels in the blood, thereby failing to adjust the secretion of PTH. Parathyroid tumors are usually benign.

Prognosis

Patients can expect a normal lifespan once the parathyroid tumor is removed.

Hallmark Signs and Symptoms

- Asymptomatic
- Increased serum calcium level
- Bone pain or fracture as a result of excreting calcium from bone
- Kidney stones
- Frequent urination due to increased calcium in the urine (hypercalciuria)
- Blurring of vision owing to cataract formation

Common Test Results

- Increased serum calcium level.
- Increased serum PTH.
- Increased alkaline phosphatase.
- Decreased serum phosphorus.
- Increased urine calcium.
- Presence of parathyroid tumor shows on ultrasound.
- Fine needle biopsy of the parathyroid tumor.
- Bone density testing may show loss of bone density.

Treatment

If the patient has no symptoms and near-normal or normal calcium levels, watchful waiting may be an option. Continued monitoring of blood levels and symptom status is recommended.

- Surgical removal of the parathyroid tumor.
- Administer bisphosphonates to lower serum calcium by increasing calcium absorption in the bone.
- IV normal saline to dilute serum calcium.
- Diuretic such as furosemide to excrete excess calcium in the urine.

Nursing Diagnoses

- Impaired urinary elimination
- Activity intolerance
- Fatigue related to sleep deprivation

NURSING INTERVENTION

- Monitor intake and output.
- Monitor for fluid overload.
- Monitor electrolyte balance.
- Force fluids.
- Give the patient acid-ash juices such as cranberry juice.
- Strain urine for kidney stones.
- Place the patient on a low-calcium and high-phosphorus diet.

- **Explain to the patient:**
  - Avoid over-the-counter calcium supplements.
  - Maintain daily activities.

9. Hypoparathyroidism

What Went Wrong

Hypoparathyroidism is diminished functioning of the parathyroid glands leading to low levels of PTH, which helps to control the blood levels of calcium, phosphorus, and vitamin D. When the PTH level is insufficient, the patient may develop low calcium and elevated phosphorus levels. The primary cause of hypoparathyroidism is destruction of the glands due to surgery in the anterior neck area. It may also be caused by an autoimmune cause. Parathyroidectomy is no longer a major cause since surgery now only removes the gland that is malfunctioning. Occasionally the gland(s) may be accidentally removed during thyroidectomy.

Prognosis

Prognosis depends on the promptness with which a diagnosis is made and treatment started.

Hallmark Signs and Symptoms

- Muscle cramps, muscle spasm, or tetany (muscle irritability) due to abnormal levels of calcium. Monitor for respiratory difficulty or arrhythmia if muscle involvement noted.
- Tingling of periorbital area, hands, and feet from abnormal calcium levels.
- Lethargy owing to low levels of PTH.
- Cataract development.
- Convulsions because of acute low calcium levels.

Common Test Results

- Decreased serum calcium due to low levels of PTH
- Increased serum phosphate because of low levels of PTH
- Decreased serum PTH from diminished secretion from the parathyroid glands
- Decreased urinary calcium from diminished PTH

- Positive Chvostek's sign owing to decreased calcium levels
- Positive Trousseau's sign due to decreased calcium levels

Treatment

- Initiate seizure precaution.
- Administer calcium gluconate by slow IV drip for acute hypocalcemia.
- Oral calcium—calcium gluconate, lactate, or carbonate.
- Large doses of vitamin D to help absorption of calcium.
- Aluminum hydroxide gel or aluminum carbonate gel (basic) to decrease phosphate levels.
- High-calcium, low-phosphorus diet.

Nursing Diagnoses

- Risk for imbalanced nutrition: less than what body requires
- Ineffective health maintenance
- Impaired urinary elimination

NURSING INTERVENTION

- If the parathyroids were damaged during neck surgery:
  - Keep tracheostomy set and injectable calcium gluconate at bedside for impaired respiration from swelling as well as for emergency administration of calcium.
  - Administer calcium to maintain the serum levels in a low normal range.
  - Calcium, phosphorus, and PTH level testing should be done every 3 months.

10. Hyperpituitarism

What Went Wrong

The pituitary gland produces an excessive amount of growth hormone. If hyperpituitarism (**acromegaly**) occurs before epiphyseal closure, the patient (infants and children) has **gigantism**, resulting in an overgrowth of all body tissues. If hyperpituitarism occurs after epiphyseal closure, which is rare, the patient has acromegaly resulting in bone thickening, growth in width (transverse growth), and enlarged organs (visceromegaly). Excess secretion of growth hormone is often due to a benign anterior pituitary adenoma. In some cases, the tissue overgrowth may be a carcinoma. Prolactin or thyroid hormones may also be affected.

Prognosis
Successful treatment can stop progression of the disease; however, physical changes that occur before treatment begins are permanent.

Hallmark Signs and Symptoms
- Increased body size caused by overproduction of growth hormone
- Hypertension
- Orthopedic complaints such as arthritis and carpal tunnel syndrome
- Cardiovascular changes such as heart enlargement, heart failure, arteriosclerosis, or hypertension
- Hypogonadism causing delayed or arrested puberty

Common Test Results
- Increased serum growth hormone as the pituitary gland is producing an excess of growth hormone.
- Increased prolactin; most pituitary tumors will cause on overproduction of one or more of the pituitary hormones.
- Increased glucose; diabetes is common in acromegaly.

Treatment
- Administer dopamine agonists such as bromocriptine and cabergoline to decrease the tumor size.
- Long-acting octreotide (an octapeptide) may be administered to help control acromegaly.
- Surgical removal of the pituitary tumor.
- Radiation (either external or gamma knife) to reduce adenoma size.
- Hormone replacement therapy following surgery.
- Antihypertensive medications to control blood pressure.

Nursing Diagnoses
- Disturbed body image related to illness or illness treatment

NURSING INTERVENTIONS
- Monitor blood pressure.
- Perform range of motion exercise to assure joint mobility.

- Provide emotional support.
- **Explain to the patient:**
  - Action of medications
  - Do not stop taking hormone replacement suddenly.

11. Hypopituitarism

What Went Wrong

Hypopituitarism results when the pituitary gland is unable to secrete a normal amount of pituitary hormones. Hormones released by the pituitary include adrenocorticotropic hormone or ACTH (which stimulates the adrenal gland to release cortisol); ADH (which helps control water lost through the kidneys); TSH (which stimulates the thyroid to release hormones that impact metabolism); growth hormone (which stimulates growth); FSH and LH (which both impact sexual function and fertility); prolactin (which stimulates milk production); and oxytocin (which stimulates uterine contraction and release of milk). Primary causes are pituitary tumors, inadequate blood supply to the pituitary gland, head trauma, infection, stroke, increased intracranial pressure (as in a bleed) radiation therapy, brain surgery, or surgical removal of a portion of the pituitary gland. Secondary causes affect the hypothalamus, which regulates the pituitary gland.

Prognosis

Patients require lifelong treatment and can expect a normal lifespan.

Hallmark Signs and Symptoms

- Fatigue caused by a decreased production of ACTH
- Lethargy and diminished cognition caused by a decreased production of TSH
- Sensitivity to cold due to low TSH, which stimulates thyroid hormone
- Decreased appetite and unintentional weight gain because of TSH deficiency
- Infertility owing to decreased luteinizing hormone (LH) and follicle—stimulating hormone (FSH) production
- Short stature due to diminished secretion of growth hormone
- Menstrual irregularities or amenorrhea caused by decreased production of FSH and LH
- Loss of libido because of decrease in sex hormones

Common Test Results

- Decreased ACTH usually due to a lesion of the pituitary.
- TSH deficiency owing to a mass, trauma, surgery, or idiopathic.
- Decreased prolactin due to a mass, causing diminished or lack of prolactin from the anterior pituitary.
- Presence of a pituitary tumor is shown on MRI.

Treatment

- Administer replacement hormones (estrogen, testosterone, corticosteroids, growth hormone, and/or thyroid hormone).
- Surgical removal of the pituitary tumor if it exists.

Nursing Diagnoses

- Disturbed body image associated with illness
- Sexual dysfunction related to disease

NURSING INTERVENTION

- Monitor weight daily because ADH and ACTH, from the pituitary, regulate fluid retention and excretion in the body.
- Monitor intake and output to ensure the balance is equal due to hormone regulation.
- **Explain to the patient:**
  - The need to take medication for the rest of the patient's life.
  - The need for frequent laboratory tests.

---

12. Hyperprolactinemia

What Went Wrong

There is an overproduction of the prolactin hormone that promotes lactation. Excessive secretion is usually caused by a pituitary tumor (prolactinoma) but may also be due to hypothyroidism, chronic kidney disease, and medications that affect the pituitary gland.

Prognosis

Prognosis is very good once a diagnosis is made and treatment of the underlying cause is started.

Hallmark Signs and Symptoms

- The primary symptom is decreased fertility.
- In women, symptoms may include decreased or absent menstruation, headache, mood changes, and galactorrhea, from hormone imbalance.
- Men may experience erectile dysfunction, diminished libido, gynecomastia, headache, and mood changes from too much hormone.

Common Test Results

- Increased serum TSH as hypothyroidism can be a contributing factor to hyperprolactinemia.
- Increased creatinine/BUN as renal failure can be a contributing factor.
- Serum human chorionic gonadotropin test for pregnancy (beta hCG) as pregnancy can cause hyperprolactinemia.
- Serum AST, ALT, and bilirubin may be increased as cirrhosis has been known to cause hyperprolactinemia.
- Serum testosterone, FSH, LH, prolactin, and estradiol may be decreased in hypogonadism.
- Pituitary tumor present in MRI.

Treatment

- Administer dopamine agonists.
  - bromocriptine
  - cabergoline to shrink pituitary tumor and return prolactin to normal levels
- Discontinue medications that may be causing the pituitary glands to over-produce prolactin.
  - amphetamines
  - estrogens
  - methyldopa
  - narcotics
  - protease inhibitors
  - risperidone
  - selective serotonin inhibitors

  - tricyclic inhibitors
  - verapamil
- Radiation therapy to reduce the pituitary tumor.
- Surgical removal of the pituitary tumor.

Nursing Diagnoses

- Disturbed body image associated with illness or illness treatment
- Sexual dysfunction related to disease (related to loss of libido, infertility, impotence)

NURSING INTERVENTIONS

- Monitor serum hormone levels to assure that medication is improving the patient's condition.

---

13. Metabolic Syndrome

What Went Wrong

Patients have a collection of symptoms that include high blood glucose, central obesity, high blood pressure, and high triglycerides based on family history. The patient typically develops **insulin** resistance (adequate or elevated levels of insulin produced but the insulin is unable to supply glucose into the cells) while the liver produces a higher level of glucose. This syndrome significantly increases risk of cardiovascular disease.

Prognosis

A diagnosis of metabolic syndrome puts one at high risk for the development of diabetes and heart disease. Changes in lifestyle must be made to decrease the chance of incurring these diseases.

Hallmark Signs and Symptoms

- Hypertension
- Abdominal obesity (men > 40 inches, women > 35 inches)
- Elevated triglycerides with low high-density lipoprotein (HDL) cholesterol

Common Test Results

- Decreased HDL
- Increased triglycerides
- Elevated fasting glucose
- Elevated serum insulin level

Treatment

- Administer statin to lower triglycerides and low-density lipoprotein (LDL).
- Administer niacin to raise HDL.
- Administer fibrates to lower triglycerides.
- Administer angiotensin-converting enzyme (ACE) inhibitors to lower blood pressure.
- Administer angiotensin receptor blockers to lower blood pressure.
- Administer insulin sensitizers to improve the effectiveness of insulin.
- Manage weight through diet and exercise.

Nursing Diagnoses

- Readiness for enhanced nutritional metabolic pattern
- Risk for injury related to hyperglycemia
- Readiness for enhanced activity program

NURSING INTERVENTIONS

- Monitor blood glucose.
- Encourage weight loss.
- **Explain to the patient:**
  - It is important to continue medication even if symptoms are not present.

---

14. Pheochromocytoma

What Went Wrong

A tumor on the adrenal medulla secretes excessive amounts of **epinephrine** and norepinephrine. It may involve one or both adrenal glands. Tumors most commonly occur during early to mid-adulthood. Epinephrine and norepinephrine affect the heart rate, blood pressure, and metabolism.

Prognosis

Patients who are diagnosed and treated early can expect a normal life with close follow-up, if the tumor is benign. Patients can expect a limited prognosis if the tumor is malignant. Metastasis may develop at any time. The patient's hypertension often resolves with removal of the tumor but may recur later in life.

Hallmark Signs and Symptoms

- Uncontrollable hypertension as a result of increased epinephrine and norepinephrine
- Headaches due to hypertension
- Palpitations and tachycardia owing to increased production of catecholamines
- Dilated pupils because of increased production of epinephrine and norepinephrine
- Irritability, nervousness, or hand tremor as a result of increased epinephrine and norepinephrine

Common Test Results

- Presence of elevated levels of catecholamines in serum
- Increased catecholamines, metanephrines, and **vanillylmandelic acid (VMA)** in 24-hour urine collection
- Presence of adrenal tumor shown in abdominal CT scan
- Adrenal biopsy to determine cell type if tumor present

Treatment

- Surgical removal of the adrenal tumor.
- Administer antihypertensive medication to help lower blood pressure.
- Administer beta blockers to diminish the effects of epinephrine and norepinephrine.
  - propranolol

Nursing Diagnoses

- Risk for delayed surgical recovery
- Ineffective tissue perfusion (cardiac)
- Anxiety

> ### NURSING INTERVENTION
>
> - Monitor blood pressure.
> - Administer medication to control hypertension.
> - Monitor urine for catecholamines.
> - Decrease stress.
> - **Explain to the patient:**
>   - Quit smoking to help lower blood pressure.
>   - Reduce caffeine to help lower blood pressure.

15. Primary Aldosteronism

What Went Wrong

The adrenal cortex secretes an excessive amount of aldosterone caused by either an adrenal tumor or a malfunctioning adrenal cortex. The majority of cases are due to a benign adrenal tumor, and it is more common between the ages of 30 and 50. Secondary aldosteronism is due to sources outside the adrenal gland producing aldosterone. Some medications, such as calcium channel blockers, can lower aldosterone levels which can confuse the diagnosis.

Prognosis

The patient can expect a normal lifespan, if diagnosed and treated early.

Hallmark Signs and Symptoms

- Increased blood pressure caused by the excess aldosterone
- Headache due to increased blood pressure
- Muscle weakness or numbness from decreased serum potassium
- Increased thirst (polydipsia) because of high levels of aldosterone
- Fatigue
- Increased urination (polyuria) due to high levels of aldosterone

Common Test Results

- Decreased serum potassium.
- Twenty-four-hour urine collection to monitor aldosterone, creatinine, and cortisol levels.
- Increased urinary aldosterone.

- Presence of an adrenal tumor on a CT scan.
- Abdominal CT may show adrenal mass.

Treatment

- Administer diuretics to control hypertension and raise potassium levels.
  - spironolactone
- Administer medications to block the effect of aldosterone.
  - eplerenone
- Surgically remove the adrenal tumor if present.

Nursing Diagnoses

- Risk for imbalanced fluid volume
- Risk for activity intolerance
- Impaired physical mobility

NURSING INTERVENTION

- Restrict sodium intake.
- Monitor intake and output.
- Weigh the patient daily.
- **Explain to the patient:**
  - Thirst, dry mucous membranes are caused by low sodium. Allow sips of water, ice chips.

---

16. Syndrome of Inappropriate Antidiuretic Hormone Secretion

What Went Wrong

Syndrome of inappropriate secretion of antidiuretic hormone (SIADH) is caused by too much ADH being secreted by the posterior pituitary gland. ADH is responsible for controlling the amount of water reabsorbed by the kidney; it prevents the loss of too much fluid. When too much water is detected, ADH production or secretion is halted. SIADH may be caused by damage to the hypothalamus or pituitary, inflammation of the brain, central nervous system disorders, or certain medications (such as selective serotonin receptor inhibitors [SSRIs], carbamazepine, cyclophosphamides, and chlorpropamide).

Certain cancers, especially small cell carcinoma of the lung, may produce ADH. Patients may develop euvolemic (normal volume) dilutional hyponatremia. There is a low sodium level with normal fluid volume.

Prognosis
If sodium (Na) levels are kept within normal limits, prognosis is excellent.

Hallmark Signs and Symptoms
- Headaches due to hyponatremia
- Nausea and vomiting owing to hyponatremia
- Confusion because of hyponatremia
- Personality changes or confusion due to hyponatremia
- Coma, seizures, or death as a result of hyponatremia

Common Test Results
- Hyponatremia (low serum sodium) due to the dilution.
- Urine osmolality elevated (> 150 mOsmol/kg) because of inappropriate concentration of urine.
- Urine sodium is greater than 20 mEq/L.
- BUN and creatinine levels are low to normal.

Treatment
- Fluid restriction
- Treat underlying cause

Nursing Diagnoses
- Risk for imbalanced fluid volume
- Excess fluid volume

> - Monitor electrolytes to determine sodium levels.
> - Restrict fluid because excess fluid dilutes sodium levels.
> - Weigh the patient daily using the same scale, at the same time of day with similar clothing.
> - Monitor intake and output.

REVIEW QUESTIONS

1. **Addison's disease frequently causes skin pigment changes. When teaching the patient about medications used for Addison's disease, it is important that he or she understands:**

   A. To take plenty of water (at least 8 ounces or 240 mL) with the medication.

   B. Proper subcutaneous injection technique.

   C. That they continue for life.

   D. That they can be stopped when symptoms abate.

2. **Alison is being treated for hyperthyroidism. In reviewing her laboratory results, the physician would expect to see:**

   A. Diminished thyroid hormone.

   B. Elevated thyroid hormone.

   C. Diminished PTH.

   D. Elevated PTH.

3. **Twenty-eight-year-old Alicia has recently been diagnosed with hyperthyroidism. Signs and symptoms of hyperthyroidism include:**

   A. Tachycardia, sweating, and tremors.

   B. Fatigue, lethargy, and weight gain.

   C. Muscle twitching, tetany, and galactorrhea.

   D. Scotoma, alopecia, and hirsutism.

4. **Adam has just been diagnosed with diabetes insipidus. The most common presenting sign is:**

   A. Body wasting.

   B. Hyperglycemia.

   C. Hypoglycemia.

   D. Increase in urination.

5. **You are providing patient teaching for 46-year-old Anthony about his new medication levothyroxine. Treatment for hypothyroidism includes:**

   A. Testosterone gel applied daily.

   B. Levothyroxine taken orally daily.

   C. Rapid-acting insulin injections taken with food.

   D. Propranolol taken daily until symptoms resolve.

6. **Antoinette has gone to her primary care provider for a routine physical. Some of her laboratory results indicated an endocrine disorder. In hyperparathyroidism which test results are typical?**

    A. Decreased WBC and increased alkaline phosphatase.

    B. Increased calcium and decreased phosphate.

    C. Decreased PTH and increased magnesium.

    D. Increased PTH and decreased calcium.

7. **Alexa, a 32-year-old woman, has been diagnosed with metabolic syndrome. Nursing interventions would include teaching her about the typical accompanying signs and symptoms, such as:**

    A. Weight loss, malar rash, and pharyngitis.

    B. Hypothyroidism, podagra, and elevated fasting glucose.

    C. Violaceous rash, pitting peripheral edema, and palpitation.

    D. Hypertension, low HDL, and elevated triglycerides.

8. **Annabelle has been referred to an endocrinologist for evaluation of the following symptoms: infertility, hypogonadism, and delayed puberty. Which hormone(s) from the pituitary is/are lacking in Annabelle?**

    A. FSH and LH.

    B. ACTH.

    C. TSH.

    D. Growth hormone.

9. **Anthony is being treated with medication for hypothyroidism. The physician explains to Anthony that his symptoms should resolve as the medication reaches an appropriate level. Presenting signs and symptoms of hypothyroidism include:**

    A. Fatigue and cold intolerance.

    B. Weight loss and hyperglycemia.

    C. Polydipsia and polyphagia.

    D. Tachycardia and diarrhea.

10. **Addie has recently been diagnosed with Cushing's syndrome. The symptoms for which the primary care provider most likely tested the patient include:**

    A. Buffalo hump, moon facies, and central obesity.

    B. Diarrhea, confusion, and exophthalmos.

    C. Weight loss, low blood pressure, and tachycardia.

    D. Nausea, low hemoglobin, and shortness of breath.

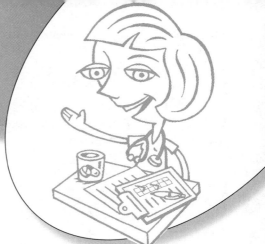

Chapter 9

Genitourinary System

LEARNING OBJECTIVES

At the end of this chapter, the student will be able to:

- Identify normal anatomy and physiology related to the genitourinary system
- Discuss the disease-causing pathologic changes within the genitourinary system
- List four signs or symptoms of specific genitourinary disease or injury
- Recognize expected nursing and medical treatment of genitourinary injury or disease

KEY CONCEPTS

1. Acute glomerulonephritis
2. Benign prostatic hypertrophy
3. Bladder cancer
4. Kidney cancer
5. Kidney stones
6. Prostate cancer
7. Pyelonephritis
8. Renal failure
9. Testicular cancer
10. Urinary tract infection

KEY TERMS

Azotemia
Bacilli Calmette-Guérin
Bladder biopsy
Cystoscopy
Glomerular filtration rate
Hematuria
Nephrectomy
Nephritic syndrome
Nephrolithiasis

Nocturia
Oliguria
Peripheral edema
Renal calculi
Transrectal ultrasound
Urinary frequency
Urinary hesitancy
Urinary urgency
Urography

How the Genitourinary System Works

The genitourinary system refers to the parts of the body involved in the production and transport of urine, as well as the surrounding structures (see Fig. 9–1). The kidneys are found in the posterior part of the upper abdominal area, relatively protected by the lower ribs. They are lateral to the spinal column. The left kidney is found higher than the right kidney due to the location of the liver within the abdomen. The renal artery supplies blood to the kidneys. The nephron is the functional unit of the kidney, the area where urine is formed. Within the nephron, there is a long tubule. This initially surrounds the glomerulus in an area called Bowman's capsule. Bowman's capsule narrows into a proximal convoluted tubule, which has many curves and eventually straightens into a downward loop of Henle, which makes a sharp turn to come back up into the cortex of the kidney. The initial upward portion of the loop of Henle is thin and then becomes thick, which is the distal convoluted tubule.

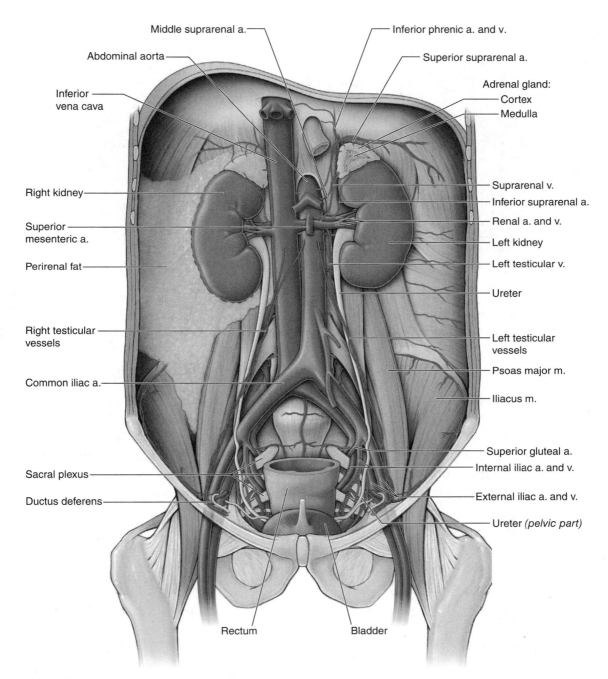

FIGURE 9–1 · Male anatomy of the renal system including kidneys, adrenals, and ureters.

Source: Reproduced with permission from: Morton DA, Foreman KB, Albertine KH: *The Big Picture: Gross Anatomy.* New York, NY: McGraw-Hill; 2011. Fig. 11–5.

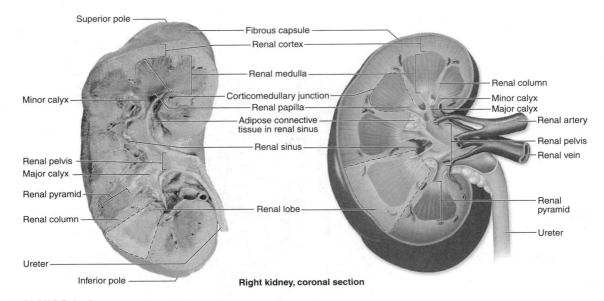

FIGURE 9−2 • Anatomy of a kidney.

Source: Reproduced with permission from: Mescher AL: *Junqueira's Basic Histology: Text and Atlas*, 12th ed. New York, NY: McGraw-Hill; 2010. Fig. 19–1.

The kidneys are responsible for filtering wastes from the bloodstream; they aid in the control of fluid and electrolyte balance, acid-base balance, blood pressure control through production of renin and red blood cell (RBC) through the production of erythropoietin (see Fig. 9–2). As urine is produced within the kidneys, it travels through the ducts (ureters) to the bladder. Once the body senses the urge to empty the bladder, the detrusor muscles contract and the sphincter at the bladder neck relaxes to aid in emptying the urine. The urine passes through the urethra to the outside. Male patients have a prostate gland located under the bladder, surrounding the urethra (see Fig. 9–3). Prostatic fluid is secreted from the gland into the urethra.

Just the Facts

1. Benign Prostatic Hypertrophy

What Went Wrong

The prostate gland is found just below the bladder in men, surrounding the urethra. As men age, the prostate enlarges, putting pressure on the surrounding structures and causing symptoms such as changes in urinary stream, frequent

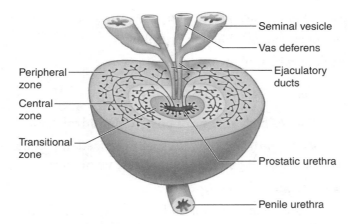

FIGURE 9−3 • The organization of the prostate gland.

Source: Reproduced with permission from: Mescher AL: *Junqueira's Basic Histology: Text and Atlas,* 12th ed. New York, NY: McGraw-Hill; 2010. Fig. 21–15.

urination, and urinary retention. The enlargement of the prostate causes narrowing of the urethra and upward pressure on the lower border of the bladder. Urinary retention may develop, as the body has a harder time emptying the bladder. Hydronephrosis and dilation of the renal pelvis and ureter are complications of the urinary retention due to overgrowth of the prostate.

Prognosis

The symptoms of benign prostatic hypertrophy (BPH) are the same as those for prostate cancer. It is important for the patients to have regular checkups to evaluate for risk of prostate cancer and conduct periodic screenings for prostate cancer. Renal function may be temporarily affected by hydronephrosis secondary to urinary retention.

Hallmark Signs and Symptoms

- **Urinary hesitancy**—difficulty initiating stream of urine due to pressure on the urethra and bladder neck
- **Urinary frequency**—need to urinate frequently owing to pressure on the bladder
- **Urinary urgency**—need to get to the bathroom quickly to urinate because of pressure on the bladder
- Nocturia—need to get up at night to urinate due to pressure on the bladder

- Decrease in force of urinary stream
- Intermittent stream of urination or dribbling
- Hematuria may be visible or microscopic

Common Test Results

- **Urography** shows high volume of post-void residual urine.
- Prostate-specific antigen (PSA) is usually elevated. It is concerning if the PSA level increases by doubling (or greater) within a year.
- Prostate ultrasound shows hypertrophy.
- Digital rectal examination reveals fullness of the prostate and loss of median sulcus (midline groove between the two lateral lobes of the prostate).
- Urinalysis may show microscopic hematuria.
- Blood urea nitrogen (BUN) and creatinine levels may elevate, if renal function is impaired.

Treatment

- Administer alpha$_1$-blockers for symptom relief.
  - doxazosin
  - tamsulosin
  - terazosin
- Monitor blood pressure; hypotension may be the side effect of some alpha$_1$-blockers.
- Administer finasteride to relieve symptoms by shrinking prostate gland.
- Monitor PSA levels periodically. Typical monitoring time frame is annual, may be more frequent if elevation is noted.
- Monitor renal function.
- Surgical removal of a portion of prostate tissue to relieve pressure.
- Continuous bladder irrigation postoperatively.
- Administer antispasmodics for patients experiencing bladder spasms.

Nursing Diagnoses

- Risk for impaired urinary elimination
- Urinary retention
- Risk for urge urinary incontinence

NURSING INTERVENTIONS

- Maintain the three-port catheter postoperatively. One port is for irrigation, another is for drainage, and the third to inflate a balloon that holds the catheter in position
- Monitor intake and output.
- Monitor vital signs for changes.
- Monitor postoperative patient's bladder irrigation:
  - Monitor the amount of fluid instilled and returned, and subtract the amount of fluid instilled from the amount returned to determine the actual urine output.
  - Document color of urinary output postoperatively; the greatest risk of hemorrhage is the first day after the operation.
  - Monitor for bladder spasms which may indicate blocked catheter drainage postoperatively.
- **Explain to the patient:**
  - Avoid caffeine, alcohol, decongestants, and anticholinergics which may increase symptoms of BPH.
  - Proper home care of the urinary catheter.
  - Monitor for signs of urinary tract infection.

2. Bladder Cancer

What Went Wrong

Bladder cancer is typically a nonaggressive cancer that occurs in the transitional cell layer of the bladder. It is recurrent in nature. Less frequently, bladder cancer is found invading deeper layers of the bladder tissue. In these cases, the cancer tends to be more aggressive. Exposure to industrial chemicals (paints, textiles), history of cyclophosphamide use, family history of nonpolyposis colorectal cancer, smoking, advanced age, smoking, and potentially the use of pioglitazone increase the risks of bladder cancer.

Prognosis

The more aggressive the cancer cell type, the greater the risk of metastasis of the disease. Patients may have advanced disease at the time of diagnosis. The more advanced the disease at the time of diagnosis and the more aggressive the tumor, the greater the risk of death for the patient.

Hallmark Signs and Symptoms

- Fatigue—due to chronic process
- **Hematuria**—blood in urine, may be microscopic
- Change in the urinary pattern—color, frequency, or amount of urine
- Urinary urgency, dribbling

Common Test Results

- Urinalysis shows RBCs in urine.
- **Cystoscopy** identifies tumor site and obtains biopsy.
- **Bladder biopsy** shows cancer cell type.
- Urine cytology may show abnormal cells.
- CT scan shows metastasis or invasion of tumor.

Treatment

- Surgical removal of tumor.
  - May be removal of superficial tumor from the bladder wall with a transurethral approach; removal of part or the entire bladder.
  - If the entire bladder is removed, a stoma is created on the surface of the abdomen or an ileal reservoir is created internally to collect the urine.
  - Instillation of **bacilli Calmette-Guérin (BCG)** into the bladder to decrease the chance of recurrence.
- Radiation therapy.
- Chemotherapy.

Nursing Diagnoses

- Risk of impaired urinary elimination
- Disturbed body image
- Fear
- Powerlessness

NURSING INTERVENTIONS

- Monitor vital signs.
- Monitor intake and output.

- Document the amount and color of drainage from all drains. If there is a bedside drainage bag (or possibly two), follow the tubing to see if it is urethral, suprapubic, or nephrostomy drainage. Record each drainage source separately.
- Monitor stoma for color and check adequate blood flow to tissue.
- Monitor abdomen for bowel sounds, pain, and distention.
- Monitor skin for signs of breakdown, redness.
- Monitor for side effects of medications.
- **Explain to the patient:**
  - Proper skin care postoperatively.
  - Catheterization of ileal reservoir if needed.

3. Acute Glomerulonephritis

What Went Wrong

Glomerulonephritis, also known as acute **nephritic syndrome**, is typically preceded by an ascending infection or occurs secondary to another systemic disorder. Infectious causes include group A beta-hemolytic *Streptococcus*, measles, mumps, cytomegalovirus, varicella, coxsackievirus, pneumonia due to mycoplasma, *Chlamydia psittaci*, or pneumococcal infection. Systemic disorders include systemic lupus erythematosus, viral hepatitis B or C, thrombotic thrombocytopenic purpura, or multiple myeloma. Exposure to hydrocarbon solvents increases the risk of developing glomerulonephritis.

Prognosis

Depending on the cause, the acute episode may completely resolve. Patients should be monitored during the occurrence; signs of renal function need to be checked.

Hallmark Signs and Symptoms

- Hematuria (urine may be dark, rust colored, or tea colored)
- **Peripheral edema**
- Elevated blood pressure, compared with patient's norm
- **Oliguria**—decrease in urine output
- Nausea, vomiting, and loss of appetite as renal function declines
- Malaise, fatigue, anorexia, muscle aches

Common Test Results

- Urinalysis shows protein, RBCs, and red blood cell casts.
- **Glomerular filtration rate** will be decreased.
- Twenty-four-hour urine collection for protein will be elevated.
- BUN level will be increased.
- Serum albumin will be decreased.
- Renal biopsy to determine the cause.

Treatment

- Monitor renal function.
- Monitor electrolyte levels.
- Monitor vital signs.
- Administer diuretics to remove excess fluids.
- Administer antihypertensive medication to control blood pressure.
- Monitor urinary output.
- Restrict fluid intake—measure output, intake should match 24-hour output plus 500 cc.
- Dietary restriction of sodium (salt), fluids, and potassium.
- Plasmapheresis if due to autoimmune cause.

Nursing Diagnoses

- Impaired urinary elimination
- Excess fluid volume

NURSING INTERVENTIONS

- Monitor vital signs.
- Monitor intake and output.
- Weigh daily.
- Assess respiratory system for lung sounds, difficulty breathing, crackles in lungs suggesting fluid overload.
- Assess cardiovascular status, heart rate, heart sounds, or presence of S_3 suggesting fluid overload.
- Assess extremities for edema.
- **Explain to the patient:**
  - About medications, disease process.

4. Kidney Cancer

What Went Wrong

Kidney cancer occurs when cancer cells create a tumor within the kidney. Exposure to chemicals, lead, and smoking all increase the risk of developing kidney cancer.

Prognosis

Identification of renal cancer is integral to a favorable outcome. Patients often have vague symptoms and may not seek healthcare until later in the disease when the cancer is well developed. Metastatic disease has the worst prognosis.

Hallmark Signs and Symptoms

- Weight loss (unintentional)
- Anemia due to altered erythropoietin production
- Hematuria (may be microscopic)
- Elevated blood pressure owing to increase in renin production
- Flank pain, dull, or aching occur in a less number of patients

Common Test Results

- CBC may show either anemia or erythrocytosis.
- Urinalysis shows RBCs.
- Erythrocyte sedimentation rate (ESR) may be elevated.
- Ultrasound shows renal mass.
- CT scan with contrast shows renal mass.
- MRI shows renal mass.

Treatment

- Surgical removal by **nephrectomy**
- Tumor destruction by radiofrequency ablation
- Chemotherapy

Nursing Diagnoses

- Fear
- Impaired skin integrity
- Risk of impaired urinary elimination

> ## NURSING INTERVENTIONS
>
> - Monitor vital signs for changes.
> - Monitor intake and output.
> - Monitor operative site for redness, swelling, and bleeding.
> - Monitor pain level postoperatively.
> - Hourly urine output monitoring for first 24 to 48 hours postoperatively. If a bedside drainage bag is present, follow the tubing up to see the site as multiple different drainage tubes can drain urine (nephrostomy, urethral, suprapubic).
> - Monitor hemoglobin and hematocrit as scheduled.
> - Monitor for signs of infection postoperatively.

5. Kidney Stones

What Went Wrong

Kidney stones, also known as **renal calculi** or **nephrolithiasis**, occur within the kidneys. Stones can also form elsewhere within the urinary tract. The patient may not have any symptoms from kidney stones until the stone attempts to move down the ureter toward the bladder. Patients develop crystals within the urine. A slow flow of urine gives the crystals time to form a stone. Crystals may be formed from calcium, uric acid, cystine, or struvite. Medications such as thiazide diuretics can increase the risk of kidney stone formation in some patients.

Prognosis

A stone may lodge in the ureter blocking the flow of urine. Hydronephrosis and swelling of the ureter may follow. Kidney stones typically recur, especially in those with a family history of nephrolithiasis.

Hallmark Signs and Symptoms

- Hematuria
- Unilateral spasms of pain in the flank area (renal colic). Pain may be severe.
- Pain may radiate to lower abdomen, groin, scrotum, or labia
- Nausea, vomiting, and sweating associated with the occurrence of pain
- Elevated blood pressure with pain

Common Test Results

- Urinalysis shows RBCs.
- Ultrasound shows stones.
- X-ray of kidneys, ureters, and bladder (KUB) shows stones.
- CT scan shows stones.
- MRI shows stones.

Treatment

- Provide pain relief.
  - narcotics such as morphine
  - non-narcotics such as ketorolac, a nonsteroidal anti-inflammatory drug (NSAID)
- Administer antispasmodics as adjuncts for pain control.
- Increase fluid intake to 3 L or more per day to flush through the urinary tract.
- Lithotripsy—shock waves are used to break the stone into very small pieces that can pass more easily.
- Stent placement to allow free flow of urine and passage of small stones or stone pieces.
- Surgical removal of stone.

Nursing Diagnoses

- Risk of impaired urinary elimination
- Acute pain

NURSING INTERVENTIONS

- Monitor intake and output.
- Monitor pain level and response to pain medications.
- Strain urine to obtain stone for analysis in the laboratory.
- **Explain to the patient:**
  - Adequate fluid intake.
  - Medications used to reduce the chance of recurrence.
  - Dietary modifications needed based on the content of stone.

6. Prostate Cancer

What Went Wrong

Cancer of the prostate typically is found in the peripheral area of the prostate gland. Nodules may be palpable on digital rectal examination. There is a greater incidence as men age. Routine screening for prostate cancer typically begins when men reach the age of 50. African-American men and those with a family history of the disease have a higher risk for prostate cancer and should begin screening at an earlier age. The symptoms of prostate cancer are the same as those of benign prostatic hypertrophy.

Prognosis

Prostate cancer is the most common cancer found in American men, and the second leading cancer-related cause of death. The number of cases of prostate cancer found on autopsy is even higher than those found clinically. Screening for prostate cancer has increased the number of cases identified.

Hallmark Signs and Symptoms

- Urinary hesitancy—difficulty initiating stream of urine due to pressure on urethra and bladder neck
- Urinary frequency—need to urinate frequently owing to pressure on bladder
- Urinary urgency—need to get to bathroom quickly to urinate because of pressure on bladder
- **Nocturia**—need to get up at night to urinate due to pressure on bladder
- Decrease in force of urinary stream
- Intermittent stream of urination
- Hematuria
- Palpable nodule on digital rectal examination
- Urinary retention owing to enlargement of the tumor blocking flow of urine
- Back pain as a result of metastasis

Common Test Results

- PSA elevates as tumor size increases.
- Digital rectal examination may reveal nodule.
- **Transrectal ultrasound** used to identify prostate cancer and determine the stage.

- MRI to identify prostate lesions and involvement of surrounding tissue or lymph nodes.
- Biopsy to identify cell type.
- Alkaline phosphatase elevates with metastasis to bone.

Treatment

- Radiation therapy
  - External beam
  - Brachytherapy—insertion of radioactive substance into prostate
- Surgery—radical prostatectomy
- Chemotherapy
- Cryosurgery—freezing of tissue with ultrasound guidance
- Watchful waiting—monitoring PSA and ultrasound depending on patient's age and cell type of cancer and any comorbidities
- Hormonal treatment to suppress natural androgen production
  - leuprolide
  - goserelin
  - estrogen
- Orchiectomy to reduce natural androgen production

Nursing Diagnoses

- Fear
- Impaired urinary elimination
- Pain

NURSING INTERVENTIONS

- Monitor vital signs.
- Monitor intake and output.
- Assess abdomen for signs of bladder distention due to urinary retention.
- Assess for pain in back.
- Assess skin for signs of redness or breakdown if undergoing radiation treatments.
- Monitor for side effects of medications.

7. Pyelonephritis

What Went Wrong

Pyelonephritis is an infection involving the kidneys. Inflammation of the tissue accompanies the infectious process. The most common bacteria are *Escherichia coli*, *Klebsiella*, *Enterobacter*, *Proteus*, *Pseudomonas*, and *Staphylococcus saprophyticus*. Typically the infection begins in the lower urinary tract and ascends upward. Identification of infections and initiation of treatment is important to prevent the infection from getting worse.

Prognosis

Older patients and patients with comorbidities have a greater chance of complications from pyelonephritis. Impaired renal function may complicate recovery in some patients. Septic shock may occur.

Hallmark Signs and Symptoms

- Flank pain (unilateral)
- Fever and chills due to infection
- Frequency, urgency, and dysuria owing to urinary tract infection
- Nausea, vomiting, and diarrhea because of infection
- Increased heart rate due to fever
- Costovertebral angle (CVA) tenderness

Common Test Results

- Urinalysis shows leukocytes, bacteria, nitrites, and RBCs; may see white blood cell (WBC) casts.
- Urine culture identifies the organism.
- Sensitivity shows which antibiotics the organism is most responsive to.
- CBC shows leukocytosis.

Treatment

- Administer antibiotics to treat infection—intravenous or oral depending on the severity of infection and comorbidities of the patient.
  - nitrofurantoin
  - ciprofloxacin

- levofloxacin
- ofloxacin
- trimethoprim-sulfamethoxazole
- ampicillin
- amoxicillin
- Administer antipyretics for fever.
- Administer fluids for dehydration due to vomiting and diarrhea.
- Administer phenazopyridine for relief of dysuria symptoms.
- Repeat urine culture after completion of antibiotic course.

Nursing Diagnoses

- Impaired urinary elimination
- Nausea
- Hyperthermia

NURSING INTERVENTIONS

- Monitor vital signs.
- Monitor intake and output.
- Assess for side effects of medication.
- **Explain to the patient:**
  - Phenazopyridine will cause orange-colored urine.

8. Renal Failure

What Went Wrong

A decrease in renal function can occur in an acute (sudden) or a chronic (progressive) manner. Acute renal failure can be broken down into prerenal, renal, and postrenal. Prerenal causes result from diminished renal perfusion. Hypovolemia due to blood or fluid losses, diuretic use, third-spacing of fluids, reduced renal perfusion owing to NSAID use or congestive heart failure (CHF) can cause prerenal failure. Renal failure in acute care patients most commonly results from acute tubular necrosis. Drug-related reactions, particularly to antibiotics, may cause an allergic interstitial nephritis. Pyelonephritis or glomerulonephritis may also cause renal failure. Postrenal failure is due to some type of urinary tract obstruction, bladder outlet obstruction, stone, prostate hypertrophy, or compression of the ureter because of abdominal mass.

Chronic renal failure is an irreversible disease due to damaging effects on the kidneys which may be caused by diabetes mellitus, hypertension, glomerulonephritis, HIV infection, polycystic kidney disease, or ischemic nephropathy.

Prognosis

In acute renal failure, kidneys start working following intensive treatment and rectifying the underlying condition that caused the problem. In chronic renal failure, the patient can die as a result of complications of the disease.

Hallmark Signs and Symptoms

- **Azotemia**—elevated BUN and creatinine
- If hypovolemic (prerenal), tachycardia, orthostatic hypotension, dry skin, and mucous membranes
- Weight loss owing to chronic disease
- Abdominal bruit renal artery stenosis which may result in ischemic nephropathy
- Peripheral edema with third spacing of fluids
- Decreased urinary output
- Uremic pruritus—see excoriations from scratching
- Anemia of chronic disease—kidneys produce erythropoietin

Common Test Results

- Creatinine elevated.
- BUN/creatinine ratio elevated.
- Urinalysis may show casts (hyaline or granular in acute prerenal; RBC, WBC in renal), proteinuria.
- Glomerular filtration rate decreases in chronic disease. May not be symptomatic until GFR drops to below 70 mL per minute.
- Creatinine clearance decreases.
- Renal ultrasound shows decrease in renal size in chronic renal failure; dilation and fluid buildup in postrenal failure.

Treatment

Treatment needs to address the underlying disease process. What will correct one cause may make another cause worse.

- Administer intravenous fluids to correct hypovolemia.
- Administer inotropic agents for patients with CHF to enhance cardiac output.
- Administer antibiotics for pyelonephritis.
- Stent placement or catheter (urethral, suprapubic, nephrostomy) to allow for drainage of urine if blockage present.
- Dialysis.
- Administer erythropoietin to treat anemia.
- Restrict potassium, phosphate, sodium, and protein in the diet.
- Administer phosphate binders to reduce phosphate levels.
- Administer sodium polystyrene sulfonate to reduce potassium levels.
- Monitor electrolyte levels.
- Control blood pressure.
- Control blood glucose levels.

Nursing Diagnoses

- Impaired urinary elimination
- Ineffective tissue perfusion (renal)
- Fear

NURSING INTERVENTIONS

- Monitor vital signs for changes in heart rate or blood pressure.
- Monitor intake and output.
- Assess intravenous site for redness, swelling, or pain.
- Check dialysis access site for signs of infection.
- Check arteriovenous shunt (AV shunt) for thrill (palpable turbulence of blood flow; gently feel for flow of blood through shunt) and bruit (audible turbulence of blood flow; listen with a stethoscope for sound of blood flow through shunt).
- No contrast dye tests.
- No nephrotoxic medication.
- Monitor patient very closely.

9. Testicular Cancer

What Went Wrong

Cancer involving the testicle typically occurs in men in their teens or twenties. It is the most common form of cancer in this age group. The cancer is hormonally dependent and tends to metastasize fairly quickly to lungs or to bone. A painless nodule may be found by the patient. There is an increased incidence in patients with a history of cryptorchism.

Prognosis

Prognosis is better for patients with solitary nodules that have not had a chance to metastasize. If detected in the early stage, it is one of the most treatable cancers. Tumors that have already metastasized to other locations have a poorer prognosis. The diagnosis will also have varying degrees of psychological impact on the patient.

Hallmark Signs and Symptoms

- Painless enlargement of the testis
- Palpable mass on the surface of testis
- Unilateral feeling of heaviness in the scrotum
- Testicular pain due to bleeding within the testis in a small percentage of patients
- Back pain owing to metastasis
- Cough or shortness of breath because of pulmonary metastasis

Common Test Results

- Scrotal ultrasound shows mass on testis.
- CT scan of pelvis, abdomen, and chest may be needed to check for metastasis.
- Human chorionic gonadotropin (hCG) elevated.
- Alpha fetoprotein (AFP) elevated.
- Lactate dehydrogenase (LDH) elevated.
- CBC shows anemia later in disease.

Treatment

- Orchiectomy.
- Chemotherapy, combination medications.
- Radiation therapy to reduce the chance of recurrence.

- Monitor tumor markers periodically.
- Monitor follow-up CT scans periodically.
- Depending on treatments planned, some patients may want to bank sperm, if fertility will be a concern after treatment.

Nursing Diagnoses

- Fear
- Anxiety
- Disturbed body image

NURSING INTERVENTIONS

- Monitor vital signs.
- Monitor intake and output.
- Assess patient's coping abilities.
- Teach patient testicular self-examination.

---

10. Urinary Tract Infection

What Went Wrong

Urinary tract infection occurs when an infecting organism, typically gram-negative bacteria such as *E coli*, enters the urinary tract. Inflammation of the local area occurs, followed by infection as the organism reproduces. Often the bacteria are present on the skin in the genital area and enter the urinary tract through the urethral opening. The organism can also be introduced during sexual contact. The infection occurs as an uncomplicated, community-acquired infection in this setting. Patients with a urinary catheter in place may also develop an infection due to the presence of the catheter which allows a pathway for the bacteria to enter the bladder. Instrumentation of the urinary tract, eg, cystoscopy, also allows a pathway for bacteria to enter the bladder. Some of the instruments are not completely sterilized between patients; they are treated with a high-level disinfectant due to fiberoptics and lenses within because they would not withstand the high temperatures needed to sterilize. These infections would be considered nosocomial.

Prognosis

Urinary tract infections that are identified are typically treated and resolved. Some bacteria have become resistant to certain antibiotics, so testing the urine to be sure the infection has cleared after treatment is a good idea. Infections that are left untreated can progress and travel upward through the urinary tract to involve the kidneys or become a systemic infection or sepsis, especially in elderly or infirm patients.

Hallmark Signs and Symptoms

- Frequency due to irritation of bladder muscles
- Urgency owing to irritation of bladder muscles
- Dysuria because of irritation of mucosal lining
- Feeling of fullness in suprapubic area
- Low back pain

Common Test Results

- Urinalysis shows leukocytes, nitrites, and RBCs.
- Urine culture and sensitivity indicate the infecting organism and the appropriate antibiotic to treat the infection.

Treatment

- Administer antibiotics.
  - nitrofurantoin
  - ciprofloxacin
  - levofloxacin
  - ofloxacin
  - trimethoprim-sulfamethoxazole
  - ampicillin
  - amoxicillin
- Encourage fluids to make urine less concentrated.
- Administer phenazopyridine for symptoms of dysuria.
- Repeat urine testing after antibiotics are completed.

Nursing Diagnoses

- Risk of impaired urinary elimination
- Risk of urge urinary incontinence

NURSING INTERVENTIONS

- Monitor intake and output.
- Monitor vital signs for changes, signs of fever.
- Encourage fluid intake.
- Encourage cranberry juice to acidify urine.
- **Explain to the patient:**
  - Phenazopyridine will cause orange-colored urine.

REVIEW QUESTIONS

1. **Symptoms of prostate cancer include:**
   A. Nocturia and intermittent stream of urination.
   B. Diminished force of urinary stream and urgency.
   C. Difficulty initiating stream of urine and frequency.
   D. All of the above.

2. **Teach a patient at risk for testicular cancer to:**
   A. Restrict potassium, phosphate, sodium, and protein in diet.
   B. Self-catheterize ileal reservoir.
   C. Perform testicular self-examination.
   D. Monitor change in color of urine.

3. **One of your patients is awaiting laboratory results for kidney function. The patient has recently recovered from a streptococcal throat infection. The patient has most likely developed symptoms of:**
   A. Pyelonephritis.
   B. Nephrolithiasis.
   C. Chronic renal failure.
   D. Glomerulonephritis.

4. **Dialysis is used to treat patients with:**
   A. Acute glomerulonephritis.
   B. Renal failure.
   C. Nephrolithiasis.
   D. Pyelonephritis.

5. **Patients with nephrolithiasis or kidney stones need to increase fluid intake. This is to:**

   A. Concentrate the urine.

   B. Help flush the stones through the urinary tract.

   C. Crystallize the struvite from the renal tubules.

   D. Break down the stones into smaller pieces that will more easily pass through the urinary tract.

6. **Care of the postoperative nephrectomy patient includes:**

   A. Assessing the wound site for redness, swelling, or drainage.

   B. Giving diuretics to enhance urinary output.

   C. Monitoring urinary output every 2 hours.

   D. Encouraging intake of cranberry juice to acidify the urine.

7. **Acute renal failure due to a decrease in circulating blood volume causing diminished renal perfusion is treated with:**

   A. Intravenous fluids.

   B. Inotropic agents.

   C. Erythropoietin.

   D. Diuretics.

8. **You are caring for a patient who has had a transurethral resection of the prostate for benign prostatic hypertrophy. There is a continuous bladder irrigation set up. You would notify the physician if you noted:**

   A. Any signs of hematuria.

   B. A decrease in the amount of blood in the urine.

   C. A change from clear red output to thicker, bright red output.

   D. The development of uremic pruritus.

9. **Patients with bladder cancer typically exhibit symptoms of:**

   A. Weight loss and low back pain.

   B. Fatigue and anemia.

   C. Hematuria and change in urinary pattern.

   D. Difficulty initiating urinary stream and nocturia.

10. **A physician is caring for a patient with a urinary tract infection. The physician would expect the plan of care to include:**

    A. Antibiotics and phenazopyridine.

    B. Erythropoietin and stent placement.

    C. Hormonal therapy and intravenous fluids.

    D. Hourly urine output measurements and antibiotics.

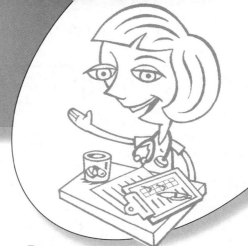

Chapter **10**

Integumentary System

At the end of this chapter, the student will be able to:

- Identify normal anatomy and physiology related to the integumentary system
- Discuss the disease-causing pathologic changes within the integumentary system
- List four signs or symptoms of specific integumentary disease or injury
- Recognize expected nursing and medical treatment of integumentary injury or disease

KEY CONCEPTS

1. Burns
2. Cellulitis
3. Dermatitis
4. Pressure ulcers
5. Skin cancers
6. Wounds and healing

KEY TERMS

Atopy
Basal cell carcinoma
Braden scale
Cryosurgery
Debrided
Eczema
Erythema
Eschar
Fibroblastic phase
First-degree burn
Hydrocolloids
Hyperpigmentation

Immunosuppressant
Lymphedema
Melanoma
Mohs surgery
Proliferative phase
Pruritis
RAST testing
Second-degree burn
Squamous cell
Third-degree burn
Vesicles

How the Integumentary System Works

The outside covering of the body, or the skin, serves three major purposes. It prevents dehydration, regulates body temperature, and protects the body against invasion by microbes. When this barrier is broken, whether by surgical incision, wound, cut, or scrape, the primary defense is no longer intact. Superficial breaks in the skin may be treated on an outpatient basis. However, deeper wounds, and those involving the face and neck, may need more intense care with IV antibiotics.

The skin is composed of three layers (see Fig. 10–1). The outermost layer of the skin is the epidermis. The epidermis does not have its own blood supply. It relies on the blood supply to the deeper layers of the skin. It is divided into the outermost squamous epithelium and the underlying layer where melanin and keratin are formed. Epidermal cells are formed in the lower layer and work their way to the surface. The dermis is the middle layer. This layer has a good blood supply, and it

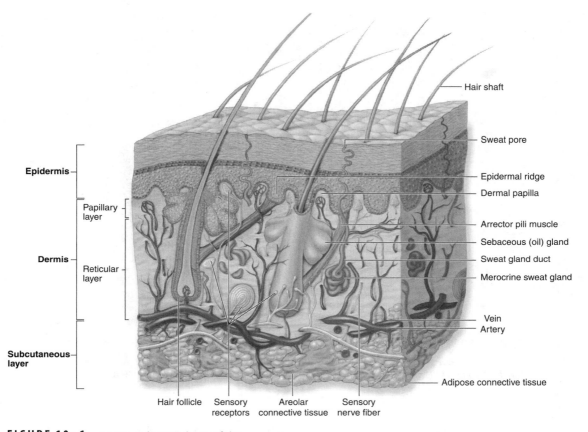

Hair shaft

Sweat pore

Epidermal ridge

Dermal papilla

Arrector pili muscle

Sebaceous (oil) gland

Sweat gland duct

Merocrine sweat gland

Vein

Artery

Adipose connective tissue

Epidermis

Papillary layer

Dermis

Reticular layer

Subcutaneous layer

Hair follicle   Sensory receptors   Areolar connective tissue   Sensory nerve fiber

FIGURE 10–1 · Layers and appendages of skin.

Source: Reproduced with permission from: Mescher AL: *Junqueira's Basic Histology: Text and Atlas*, 12th ed. New York, NY: McGraw-Hill; 2010. Fig. 18–1.

contains connective tissue, sebaceous glands, hair follicles, and sweat glands. The deepest skin layer, the subcutaneous layer, is composed primarily of fat.

Skin manifestations are described using the following terms: macules are small, flat-topped lesions, less than 1 cm in diameter, similar to a freckle. Papules are elevated lesions, also smaller than 1 cm in diameter (see Fig. 10–2A). A plaque is raised lesion that is greater than 1 cm in diameter (see Fig. 10–2B). A wheal is a raised area filled with fluid and usually temporary, such as in hives (see Fig. 10–2C). A vesicle is a fluid-filled blister less than 1 cm in diameter, often seen in shingles. Bullae are larger than 1 cm in diameter and are fluid-filled blisters. A pustule is an elevation containing purulent material. A nodule is a solid lesion, up to 1 cm in diameter (see Fig. 10–2D). A tumor is larger than 1 cm in diameter, and it is solid. Petechiae are smaller than 1 cm in diameter and are usually round areas of deposits of blood. A purpura is a large petechia.

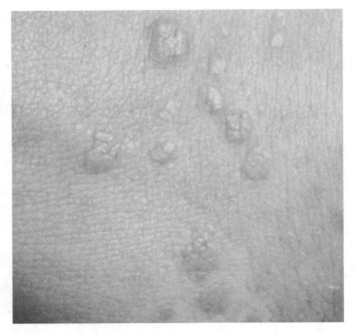

FIGURE 10−2A · Multiple, well-defined papules of varying sizes.

Source: Reproduced with permission from: Goldsmith LA, Katz SI, Gilchrest BA, Paller AS, Leffell DJ, Wolff K: *Fitzpatrick's Dermatology in General Medicine*, 8th ed. New York, NY: McGraw-Hill; 2012. Fig. 5–1.

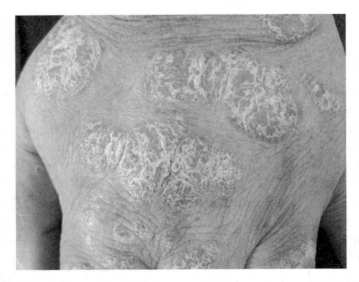

FIGURE 10−2B · Well-demarcated pink plaques with a silvery scale representing psoriasis vulgaris.

Source: Reproduced with permission from: Goldsmith LA, Katz SI, Gilchrest BA, Paller AS, Leffell DJ, Wolff K: *Fitzpatrick's Dermatology in General Medicine*, 8th ed. New York, NY: McGraw-Hill; 2012. Fig. 5–2.

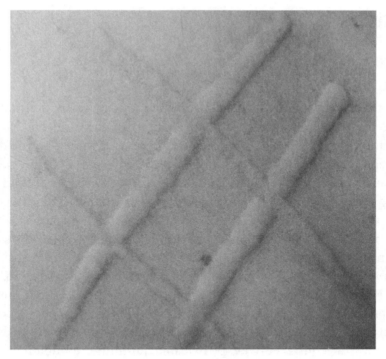

FIGURE 10–2C · Sharply demarcated wheal with a surrounding erythematous flare occurring within seconds of the skin being stroked.

Source: Reproduced with permission from: Goldsmith LA, Katz SI, Gilchrest BA, Paller AS, Leffell DJ, Wolff K: *Fitzpatrick's Dermatology in General Medicine*, 8th ed. New York, NY: McGraw-Hill; 2012. Fig. 5–5.

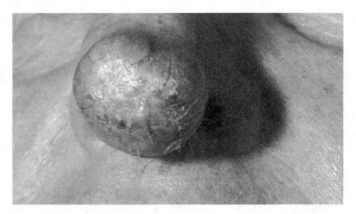

FIGURE 10–2D · Nodular basal cell carcinoma with well-defined, firm nodule with a glistening surface through which telangiectasia can be seen.

Source: Reproduced with permission from: Goldsmith LA, Katz SI, Gilchrest BA, Paller AS, Leffell DJ, Wolff K: *Fitzpatrick's Dermatology in General Medicine*, 8th ed. New York, NY: McGraw-Hill; 2012. Fig. 5–3.

Just the Facts

1. Burns

What Went Wrong

Burns are damage to the skin and body tissues caused by thermal injury (flames, heat, cold), friction, radiation (sunburn), chemicals, or electricity. Burns are generally divided into three categories, depending on the damage. First-degree burns are those with injury to the outer layer of skin called the epidermis. They will be red, and painful, with some swelling. A second-degree burn is when the epidermis is burned, as well as the next layer, the dermis. Severe pain, white and reddened areas, swelling, blisters, and perhaps drainage will be seen. A third-degree burn goes through all the layers of the skin and could involve underlying tissues. It is often painless due to the destruction of the nerves in the area. The area will look black (termed eschar) and/or reddened. Many drugs may make the skin more sensitive to the sun (photosensitive), producing the effect of sunburn with little exposure. Common medications with this effect include: amiodarone, carbamazepine, furosemide, naproxen, oral contraceptives, piroxicam, quinidine, quinolones, sulfonamides, sulfonylureas, tetracyclines, and thiazides, among others.

The rule of nines is used to determine the degree of damage, based on the body surface area involved (see Fig. 10–3). The head comprises 9% of the body surface. The anterior and posterior chest and abdomen each comprise 9% of the body surface. The mid to lower back (including buttocks) comprises 9% of the body surface. Each arm is 9% of the body surface area. Each leg accounts for 18% of the body surface area. The groin accounts for the final 1% of the body surface area.

Prognosis

Prognosis depends on the severity of the burn plus the amount of surface area involved. When large portions of the face, chest, hands, feet, genitalia, or joints have sustained a large second- or third-degree burn, prompt medical attention is necessary. Serious burns can lead to death. Burns covering the face, neck, or upper chest raise suspicion for smoke inhalation. If smoke inhalation has occurred, or if the nasal hairs are singed, or if quantities of soot are present around the face, assess for adequacy of breathing and damage to the respiratory tract. Patients may seem fine initially following smoke inhalation but rapidly deteriorate as swelling occurs within the airways. Cardiopulmonary resuscitation (CPR) may need to be started. Infants and elderly patients with burns require prompt medical attention.

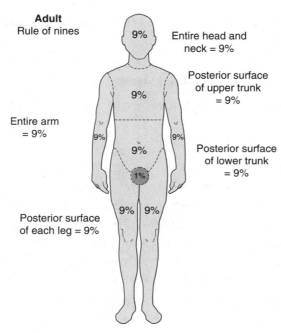

FIGURE 10-3 · The rule of nines, the estimation of body surface area in burns.

Source: Reproduced with permission from: McPhee SJ, Papadakis, MA: *Current Medical Diagnosis and Treatment 2010*, 49th ed. New York, NY: McGraw-Hill; 2010. Fig. 37–2.

Hallmark Signs and Symptoms

- Redness, no break in the skin—indicates a first-degree burn from damage to the epidermis
- Deeper red, with clear fluid blisters—indicates a second-degree burn as the epidermis and dermis are burned
- Charred black or dry white—indicates death of the tissue from the burn (third-degree burn)

Common Test Results

- Pulse oximetry—a sensor is placed on the finger, toe, or earlobe to assess the amount of oxygen in the blood to ensure adequate oxygenation.
- Chest x-ray or bronchoscopy—fiberoptic tube inserted into the upper airways to assess damage from smoke inhalation.
- Pulmonary function tests—show how well the lungs are working. The patient breathes into a machine, a spirometer, which records changes in

the lung size with inhalation and exhalation and the time it takes to perform this test.

- Electrolyte testing—to determine essential nutrients that are at inappropriate levels, secondary to fluid loss and fluid shifting.
- Rule of nines—a method of measurement to estimate the total body surface area burned.

Treatment

The objective of burn treatment is to prevent infection, decrease inflammation and pain, and promote healing of the areas. Treatment choices depend on the degree of burn and the amount of body surface area that was burned. Any second-degree burn (>5% to 10% of surface area) and all third-degree burns are treated in a hospital, preferably within a specialized burn unit. All electrical burns and burns of the ears, eyes, face, hands, feet, and perineum require hospital care, as do chemical burns and burns in infants or the elderly.

- Check the area for any exposed electrical wires, if you are present at the scene. Do not approach the patient if it is not safe to do so.
- For minor burns—use cold water (notice) to decrease the temperature of the area for a first-degree burn or a small second-degree burn, and to cool the skin and stop the burning.
- For chemical burns, ensure that all of the chemicals have been flushed away.
- For electrical burns, look for entrance and exit wounds. The electrical current will follow the path of least resistance.
- Cover the area loosely with dry gauze. This will prevent contamination of the area.
- If the skin is broken (second-degree burn), use a topical antibiotic ointment such as silvadene to prevent a secondary bacterial infection before applying the gauze.
  - Administer pain medications (ibuprofen, acetaminophen, or possibly narcotics) as needed.
- For third-degree burns, the eschar needs to be debrided (cut away) to allow new tissue to grow.
- These wounds are often covered in moist sterile saline gauze, as new tissue grows best in this environment. When the gauze dries; it adheres to the dead tissue. The area is mechanically debrided when the gauze is removed.
- Oral antibiotics may be necessary.

- Administer pain medications (oxycodone, morphine) as needed, especially before dressing changes that may be painful.
- Prevent heat loss due to large areas of tissue exposed from lack of skin coverage.
- Maintain fluid levels since fluid loss is common from evaporation and wound drainage. Accurate fluid replacement is necessary within the first 24 to 36 hours. Large bore IV access should be maintained. A variety of formulas exist to determine the early fluid needs. The formulas typically involve the patient's weight and percentage of body surface area involved. The timing of the fluid replacement begins at the time of the burn, not the time of entry into the healthcare system. Ringer's lactate is frequently used for large volume fluid replacement.

Nursing Diagnoses

- Risk of fluid volume deficit
- Pain, discomfort
- Risk of altered body temperature

NURSING INTERVENTION

- Anticipate pain medication needs to make the patient more comfortable.
- Assist in the range of motion to avoid contracture development due to pain with movement.
- Encourage family visitation.
- Assist with activities of daily living.
- Isolation may be needed to protect the patient from bacteria, especially if a large amount of skin is not intact.
- Maintain large bore IV access.
- **Explain to the patient:**
  - To look for signs and symptoms of infection: fever, increased redness, increase in drainage, or change in color of drainage.

---

2. Cellulitis

What Went Wrong

Cellulitis is an infection of the skin, caused by bacteria that enter the skin through an opening or break in the skin. The legs are the most common site of cellulitis, although it may occur anywhere bacteria enter. The most common bacteria are *Streptococcus* and *Staphylococcus*. Bacteria may enter through fissures in the feet from fungal infections, through cracks in the dry skin, from insect bites, or cuts from shaving. Bacteria may also enter as the result of a bite (animal or human). These infections tend to have more than one organisms involved. The elderly, immunocompromised patients and patients with lymphedema, diabetes, or poor circulation are at greatest risk.

Prognosis

If treatment is started early, the prognosis is good. If the symptoms do not begin to resolve or the infection is on the face or widespread, hospitalization and IV antibiotics are needed. A severe cellulitis of deep tissue, necrotizing fasciitis, is caused by streptococcal bacteria and it is considered a medical emergency.

Hallmark Signs and Symptoms

- Hot, red skin over the area of infection
- Swollen and painful skin and tissue due to the infection

Common Test Results

- Complete blood count (CBC) to check for elevation of the white blood cell count
- Culture of the wound to identify the organism causing the cellulitis
- Ultrasound of the leg to rule out a deep vein thrombosis (DVT) as the cause of redness, swelling, and discomfort

Treatment

Treatment for a beginning infection is oral antibiotics. If fever and body aches accompany the infection, the face is involved, or if the area is extensive, hospitalization may be necessary. Empiric treatment is started immediately and is effective against the most common bacteria.

- cephalexin
- clindamycin
- dicloxacillin
- levofloxacin

For water-related infections

- For fresh water injuries, expect later generation (third or fourth) cephalosporins or fluoroquinolones

- For salt (or brackish) water, expect doxycycline, ceftazidime, or fluoroquinolone (levofloxacin or ciprofloxacin)

For dog bites

- amoxicillin/clavulanate orally
- clindamycin or metronidazole with doxycycline or trimethoprim/sulfamethoxazole orally
- rocephin parenterally
- fluoroquinolone with metronidazole; or ampicillin/sulbactam; or carbapenem parenterally

For cat bites

- amoxicillin/clavulanate orally
- clindamycin or metronidazole with doxycycline or cefuroxime or trimethoprim/sulfamethoxazole orally
- rocephin with metronidazole parenterally
- ampicillin/sulbactam parenterally
- fluoroquinolone with metronidazole
- carbapenem parenterally

For human bites

- amoxicillin/clavulanate orally
- clindamycin or metronidazole with doxycycline or trimethoprim/sulfamethoxazole orally
- cefazolin (first generation cephalosporin) parenterally
- ampicillin/sulbactam parenterally
- Tetanus booster if needed
- Drainage of abscess by a surgeon may be necessary
- Pain medications

Nursing Diagnoses

- Pain, discomfort
- Risk of infection
- Impaired skin integrity

NURSING INTERVENTION

- Wash the affected area daily. Do not use scented products as these may irritate the skin further.
- Use a topical antibiotic ointment and a dry dressing twice daily.
- Elevate the area if possible.
- Monitor for temperature, enlarging area of redness, increase in drainage.
- **Explain to the patient:**
  - The importance of good hygiene.
  - How to prevent openings in the skin by using proper skin care interventions.
  - Monitor feet and legs daily for cracks, fissures.
  - Use care in trimming nails, or visit podiatrist.
  - Use moisturizing lotions regularly.

3. Dermatitis

What Went Wrong

Dermatitis is inflammation of the skin as a result of contact with an irritating substance such as a chemical, foreign substance, medication, or contact with a plant, such as poison ivy. The skin may become reddened, irritated, and itchy. The usual causes are allergic reactions. Often the patient has a personal history or a family history of asthma, allergy, or eczema. Some later symptoms may be the result of scratching of the skin. Often the cause may be a drug reaction, the body's immune system reacting to a medication.

Prognosis

Resolution of the rash occurs within 1 to 2 weeks once the offending substance is identified and removed. However, if the patient is atopic, frequent exacerbations and remissions may occur with unknown etiology. The skin reaction is typically self-limiting.

Hallmark Signs and Symptoms

- Rash on the affected skin area from contact with the offending substance
- Pruritis from histamine release from mast cells
- Erythema and edema

- Vesicles where the substance came in contact with the skin
- Hyperpigmentation from irritation from scratching

Common Test Results

- Radioallergosorbent test (RAST) testing may be done to determine allergens.
- Patch testing or skin testing to determine if a localized reaction occurs after skin exposure to the allergy-causing substance.
- Skin biopsy.

Treatment

Treatment involves determining, if able, the triggers that began the flare, and avoidance of the same. Treatment aimed at each symptom will help to decrease discomfort. If the dermatitis is widespread, IV medications, steroids, or anti-histamines may be necessary to resolve the flare. Topical corticosteroid cream, gel, or lotions will decrease the symptoms.

Nursing Diagnoses

- Body image disturbance
- Risk of altered skin integrity
- Pain, discomfort

NURSING INTERVENTION

- Avoid irritants that caused the dermatitis to prevent recurrence.
- Allow for healing and prevent bacterial infections.
- Cool compresses.
- Use protective gloves and clothing.
- Wash hands often.
- **Explain to the patient:**
  - Keep the skin moist.
  - Keep nails short to diminish scratching.
  - Warm, not hot, showers.
  - Use mild soap without unnecessary additives, such as scent.
  - Apply moisturizers.

4. Pressure Ulcers

What Went Wrong

A pressure ulcer starts on the skin and often progresses to deeper tissue; it is caused by impaired circulation to the tissue from pressure sustained over a period of time. Without adequate blood flow and the nutrition it brings, the tissue will die. Those often affected are confined to a wheelchair or a bed, and are unable to move themselves, not reducing the pressure frequently enough. It can take as little as a few hours in one position for a stage one pressure ulcer to develop. The usual sites of pressure ulcers, or bedsores, are on bony prominences, such as the buttocks, sacrum, heels, knees, and hips. Friction from linens can impair the integrity of the skin as can the shear force, when the skin moves in one direction and the deeper structures do not move. Assessment tools are available to predict the risk of pressure ulcers developing. A commonly used scale is the Braden scale which includes such criteria as friction, the nutritional status of the patient, mobility and activity levels, moisture exposure of the skin, and any limitations of sensory perception.

Prognosis

Unfortunately, prognosis is poor. The very factors that caused the pressure ulcer are the same factors that interfere with healing. Resolution often is very involved and slow. Setbacks are common, such as wound infection, cellulitis, and sepsis, which can lead to death.

Hallmark Signs and Symptoms

- Stage I:
  - Firm warm areas of skin from poor circulation
  - Spongy, reddened tissue from increased pressure
  - The skin remains intact and the redness is not blanchable
- Stage II:
  - Partial thickness (down to the dermis) opening in the skin with surrounding erythema from pressure
  - Affected skin may be shiny or appear as a shallow ulcer
- Stage III:
  - The ulcer is deep, down through the dermis, with red base and often some drainage

- May be able to see subcutaneous tissue (fat)
- May have undermining or tunnel formation
- Stage IV:
  - A full thickness ulcer involving muscle, bone, tendons, or ligaments with visible signs of tissue death
  - Undermining or tunneling more common
  - Exposure of bone increases risk of associated osteomyelitis

Common Test Results

- Culture to check for causative bacteria.
- CBC to evaluate the hemoglobin and hematocrit for oxygen-carrying capabilities
- Albumin and prealbumin levels to check on nutrition
- Chemistry to evaluate fluid status

Treatment

Treatment is based on relieving pressure and providing adequate nutrition. Wound treatment is aimed at preventing infection and encouraging healing. Stage I and stage II wounds may heal with conservative treatments. However, stage III and stage IV wounds often require surgical debridement and skin grafting. Treatment choice depends on the stage of the wound.

- Clean wound with soap and water or saline.
- Debridement to clean away dead, devitalized, and infected tissue. Debridement methods include surgery, topical enzymatics, and mechanical debridement.
- Dressings to protect the wound and keep it moist, which promotes healing.
  - Hydrocolloids that keep moisture in.
  - Nonadherent dressings to prevent tissue loss with removal.
  - Bulk dressings to absorb copious drainage.
  - Semipermeable dressings which allow for transfer of gases but are impermeable to liquids.
- Antibiotic ointment for infected wounds.
- Oral antibiotics.

- Specialized mattresses to decrease the pressure on the skin.
- Whirlpool treatments.

Nursing Diagnoses

- Impaired skin integrity
- Impaired physical mobility
- Nutrition altered: less than what body requires

NURSING INTERVENTION

- Prevention is the key to pressure ulcers.
- Mobility or repositioning of patients unable to move themselves; every 1 to 2 hours.
- Proper nutrition to encourage healing.
- Adequate fluid intake.
- Remove pressure from stage I areas.
- Use pillows to aid in positioning to reduce pressure on bony prominences.
- Use specialized wheelchair cushions to reduce pressure.
- Daily skin inspection.
- Stop smoking in order to increase oxygen to tissues.
- Daily measurement of wounds to assess status including length, width, and depth.

---

5. Skin Cancers

Cancers of the skin are the most common type of cancer. The incidence of skin cancer is one of the fastest growing. Early detection is of the utmost importance because a cure is obtainable in the early stages. Heredity may also be a factor. Skin cancer is usually divided into three major subtypes: basal cell, the most common; squamous cell, which is the second most common; and melanoma, the most fearsome. Basal cell carcinomas are directly related to sun damage, with most lesions occurring in sun-exposed areas. This type recurs frequently. Squamous cell carcinomas are often due to sun exposure, may be difficult to distinguish from some other benign changes in the skin, and spread more readily. Melanoma is the most deadly form of skin cancer; it usually occurs in sun-exposed areas such as on the face or upper back. A mnemonic to aid in melanoma characteristics may be helpful: ABCDE. A—asymmetrical shape; B—borders that are irregular; C—change in color; D—diameter larger than 6 mm (the size of a pencil eraser); and E—elevation.

What Went Wrong

New skin cells are made in the epidermis, which then push the older cells toward the surface where they are shed. Solar exposure can interrupt this process, causing cells to divide at an unusual rate, which may lead to a cancer. Those individuals with a large amount of exposure to ultraviolet radiation, which appears to be cumulative, are more at risk to develop cancerous tumors. Exposure to greater amounts of x-rays also increase the risk for skin cancers, as does arsenic which is a metal found in the environment and in our food. People who take immunosuppressant medications are at a greater risk for skin cancers as are fair-skinned people and those with a family history of skin cancer.

Prognosis

If the lesion is identified and treated early, prognosis is excellent. Follow-up care with frequent skin assessments is mandatory. Basal cell cancers are unlikely to have a poor prognosis. Squamous cell tumors may spread if left unchecked. Melanoma is staged by determining thickness of the lesion, and the extent to which it has spread. Stage 0 is a confined tumor. The other stages mean the cancer has spread to other tissues and organs.

Hallmark Signs and Symptoms

A wound that does not heal raises suspicion for skin cancer, especially if it occurs in a sun-exposed area.

- Basal cell—pearly white, waxy-appearing papule or a flat, brown patch
- Squamous cell—firm red nodule; a flat scaly lesion; a change in a scar
- Melanoma—any mole that is new, that has changed, and/or that meets any of the ABCDE criteria

Common Test Results

- Biopsy with an interpretation by a pathologist.
- CT, MRI, or PET scan to determine if metastasis has occurred.

Treatment

Treatment is dependent on the type of cancer, location, and size of the tumor.

- Surgical excision involves removing the tumor and surrounding healthy tissue to ensure all the cancerous tissue has been extracted. In melanoma, a sentinel node biopsy may also be done. A sentinel node is detected when dye is injected near the tumor site. The dye will travel toward the lymphatic system. The first node to uptake the dye is the sentinel node. This is the direction that cancerous cells would most likely travel.
- Cryosurgery in which the cells are killed by freezing with liquid nitrogen.
- Mohs surgery where the tumor is removed layer by layer. Each surface area is evaluated microscopically, to ascertain that no cancer cells are present in the remaining tissue.
- Laser treatments to vaporize the cancer cells.
- Topical creams and ointments.
- Radiation used to kill cancer cells in melanoma.
- Chemotherapy, using drugs to kill the melanoma cells.
  - Ipilimumab is used for the treatment of advanced melanoma. It has been shown to prolong survival.
  - Vemurafenib is used for metastatic or inoperable melanoma that tests positive for the genetic mutation called serine/threonine-protein kinase B-raf (BRAF V600E).

Nursing Diagnoses

- Impaired skin integrity
- Body image disturbance

NURSING INTERVENTION

- **Teach the patient:**
  - Stay out of the sun when its rays are the strongest.
  - Avoid tanning salons.
  - Wear sunscreen.
  - Wear sun-protective clothing.
  - Check the skin regularly for new moles, as well as changes in existing moles, freckles, and birthmarks.
  - Medications may make the skin more sensitive to sunlight.

6. Wounds and Healing

A wound is any break in the skin. It may be intentional, as with surgery, or unintentional, as a result of trauma. Types of wounds include surgical, penetrating (such as a knife), crushing, burn, lacerations, bites, (human, animal), ulcers, and pressure ulcers. Immediately after a wound occurs, inflammation begins with platelet aggregation. Next, leukocytes travel to the area for infection surveillance. A proliferative phase starts when the epidermal cells move toward the wound, and cover the approximated wound edges, usually by the third day. The fibroblastic phase occurs with collagen and fibroblasts entering the area, forming a connection that will eventually develop into a scar.

Wound healing occurs in various ways. Primary or the first intention happens when edges are closely approximated and new tissue, or granulation, knits the close edges together. Wound healing by secondary intention occurs in a larger wound where the edges are further apart. This is often intentional when the wound is infected, dirty, or from a bite. The granulation tissue builds across the surface of the wound forming a large clot and sequentially, a larger scar. Third intention is a wound that initially begins to heal as a second intention, or open, wound and is later closed.

Prognosis

Prognosis depends on the size, location, and cause of the wound. Items that need to be assessed in patients with wounds include chronic disease, such as diabetes, impaired circulation; nutrition; hydration status; and immunosuppression, such as corticosteroid or chemotherapeutic agents. Epithelialization of wound occurs within 48 hours, wound strength is 60% of previous strength within 4 months.

Hallmark Signs and Symptoms

- Pain from injury to nerves.
- Drainage from injury to tissues and cells migrating to the site of injury.
- Bleeding from injury to blood vessels.
- Foreign body—look for penetrating objects.
- Deeper tissue trauma—assess for non-intact tendons, ligaments, and pieces of bone.
- Debris—look for dirt, fragments.

- Signs and symptoms of infection include increased erythema; purulent, foul-smelling drainage; and fever.
- Wounds may be accompanied by pain, drainage, bleeding, infection, a foreign body, or deeper tissue trauma. Assessment of the wound, including deeper structures if necessary, is imperative.

Common Test Results

- CBC to assess for leukocytoses for infection
- Chemistry to assess hydration status

Treatment

- Assess circulation distal to the site if the wound is in a limb. Check distal pulses.
- Tetanus prophylaxis as needed. A booster is indicated if the last one was not within the past 10 years.
- Irrigation of the wound with large amounts of saline to flush away all dirt, debris, and foreign bodies.
- Wound closure, either by sutures, steri strips, adhesive, or dressings.
- Dirty wounds are usually left open to heal by secondary intention. This allows any discharge to drain and makes it easier to identify signs of infection.
- Antibiotics if necessary, usually 7 to 10 days.

Nursing Diagnoses

- Impaired tissue integrity
- Risk of infection
- Impaired skin integrity

NURSING TREATMENT

- **Explain to the patient:**
  - Disease process.
  - Signs of infection, ie, swelling, redness, increase in pain, fever, chills, drainage, bleeding, foul odor, or reopening of wound.
  - Medication, including indication for, frequency of use, and side effects.

- Demonstrate proper dressing change techniques, including frequency, proper hand washing, cleansing of wound, and application of topical if ordered.
- Adequate nutrition and hydration.
- Elevation of the affected limb, if indicated.
- Rest, decrease in activities.
- Proper immunization schedules

REVIEW QUESTIONS

1. When assessing a suspicious skin lesion, you are looking for A—asymmetry, B—irregular borders, C—variegated colors, D—diameter, and E—:
   A. Edema.
   B. Erythema.
   C. Elevation.
   D. Ever-changing.

2. Patient teaching for risk reduction of skin cancer should include:
   A. Having suspicious moles checked by a dermatologist.
   B. Daily sun exposure every ½ hour.
   C. Daily sun exposure of 1 hour to build tolerance.
   D. Applying moisturizer.

3. A patient with a second-degree burn has a greater risk for:
   A. Constipation.
   B. Infection.
   C. Hypotension.
   D. Hyperglycemia.

4. When staging a pressure ulcer, a stage II ulcer is recognized as:
   A. Redness, with no break in the skin.
   B. Shallow ulcer with reddened base.
   C. Dermis involvement with eschar.
   D. Bone visible with no drainage.

5. Appropriate treatment for a patient with cellulitis includes:
   A. Petrolatum and vitamins A and D ointment.
   B. Antibiotics, such as cephalexin, and over-the-counter analgesics.
   C. Weight-bearing exercises and diuretics, such as furosemide.
   D. Wet to dry dressings and steroids.

6. **A physician is caring for a patient with an infected wound. The physician would expect:**

    A. To prepare for sutures, to close the wound.
    B. The use of steri strips, to hold the edges together.
    C. To leave the wound open.
    D. To cover with a loose, fluffy dressing.

7. **Steps to prevent a pressure ulcer may include:**

    A. Not disturbing the patient.
    B. Changing the position of a bed-bound patient every 4 to 6 hours.
    C. Vigorously rubbing the skin with alcohol.
    D. Avoiding pressure on the heels of a bed-bound patient.

8. **For a patient with a mild dermatitis rash, physician would encourage:**

    A. Washing the area with an antiseptic soap frequently to keep the area clean.
    B. The use of an antifungal ointment.
    C. Talcum powder to soothe the inflamed skin.
    D. The use of a mild steroidal cream.

9. **A postoperative patient develops cellulitis in the leg. Nursing treatments would include:**

    A. Keeping both the legs elevated as much as possible.
    B. Encouraging ambulation as much as possible to help the blood flow.
    C. Application of ice four times a day for an hour each to reduce inflammation.
    D. Application of moisturizing lotion three times daily to keep the skin moist.

10. **To clean a wound, it is best to use:**

    A. Hydrogen peroxide to bubble away the debris.
    B. Tap water.
    C. Saline.
    D. It is best not to disturb a healing wound.

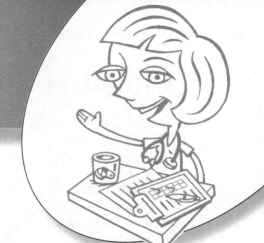

Chapter **11**

Fluids and Electrolytes

LEARNING OBJECTIVES

At the end of this chapter, the student will be able to:

- Identify normal anatomy and physiology affecting the balance of fluids and electrolytes
- Discuss pathologic changes affecting homeostasis
- List four signs or symptoms of specific electrolyte disorders
- Recognize expected nursing and medical treatment of fluid and electrolyte disorders

KEY CONCEPTS

1. Dehydration
2. Hypercalcemia
3. Hypocalcemia
4. Hyperkalemia
5. Hypokalemia
6. Hypermagnesemia
7. Hypomagnesemia
8. Hypernatremia
9. Hyponatremia
10. Hyperphosphatemia
11. Hypophosphatemia
12. Metabolic acidosis
13. Metabolic alkalosis

KEY TERMS

Acid-base balance
Aldosterone
Angiotensin
Antidiuretic hormone (ADH)
Diffusion
Edema
Extracellular
Hypertonic
Hypotonic

Interstitial space
Intracellular
Isotonic
Natriuretic peptides
Osmolarity
pH
Renin
Third space

How Fluids and Electrolytes Work

Fluids and Electrolytes and Acid-Base Balance

Fluids and electrolytes play a vital role in maintaining the proper function of many of the important systems in our body. Mechanisms such as the beating of our heart, the movement of our skeletal muscles, and nerve conduction, which allows us to sense something hot or painful, rely on the proper balance and placement of these elements. This finely tuned balance of fluids and electrolytes along with acid-base balance maintains the body in perfect homeostasis which is crucial for our survival.

Many health problems disrupt this balance. This section will first discuss the normal role and function of fluid and electrolytes and acid-base balance and then discuss those conditions that occur as a result of an imbalance of this mechanism.

Fluids

Fluids play an important role by providing a mechanism of transportation of many vital substances both to and from the cells of the body. Some of these substances include proteins, hormones, glucose, and electrolytes. This section will focus on electrolytes.

Fluids in the body are categorized mainly in relation to the cell. Fluid is either in the cell (intracellular fluid—ICF) or outside of the cell (extracellular fluid—ECF). The extracellular component is further divided into two compartments that hold fluid within the vascular space (intravascular) or within the tissues (interstitial). Roughly two-thirds of the body's fluids are in the intracellular component and one-third in the extracellular component (see Fig. 11–1).

As a function of	TBW	ICF	ECF	IF	IVF
Total weight	60%	40%	20%	15%	5%
TBW		67%	33%	25%	8%
ECF compartment				75%	25%

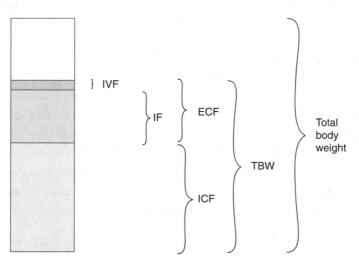

FIGURE 11–1 · Relation of fluid compartment to body weight and each other. ECF = extracellular fluid; ICF = intracellular fluid; IF = interstitial (extravascular) fluid; IVF = intravascular fluid; TBW = total body water.

Source: Reproduced with permission from: Tintinalli JE, Stapczynski JS, Ma OJ, Cline DM, Cydulka RK, Meckler GD: *Tintinalli's Emergency Medicine: A Comprehensive Study Guide,* 7th ed. New York, NY: McGraw-Hill; 2011. Fig. 21–1.

When we speak of fluids, we are mainly speaking of water which constitutes the bulk of all body fluids. A balance should be maintained to keep concentrations of water and electrolytes in the proper amount and concentration for normal function. The cell walls are semipermeable to allow for movement (diffusion) of molecules to maintain this balance. Water will move from an area of high concentration (of water) to an area of low concentration (of water). Areas of high water concentration also have low amounts of solute (electrolytes), and areas of low water concentration have high amounts of solutes (electrolytes). This movement of water from an area of higher concentration to an area of lower concentration through a semipermeable membrane is called osmosis and the pressure exerted by this mechanism is called osmotic pressure. The pressure exerted by the concentration of solute (electrolytes or plasma proteins) within these compartments also exerts their own pull on water—this is called oncotic pressure.

Another important concept to understand is the concept of osmolality. Osmolality is the amount of total milliosmoles of solute (electrolytes) per unit of total volume of solution. It is often expressed as (m/Osm/L). Each area of the body has precise ranges of osmolality. This is important to know because if the osmolality changes it tells us if there is fluid excess or deficit (see Fig. 11–2).

For example, if there is a disease process or injury that causes an increased osmolality in the ECF (meaning a very high concentration and ratio of electrolytes to water) water will move out of the cells and into ECF (specifically the interstitial component), causing edema. This may result in a systemic fluid/water deficit as too much fluid is being lost from the circulation into the interstitial space. Edema results when too much fluid travels into the interstitial space. Peripheral edema collects in dependent areas (the feet and ankles of ambulatory patients), or near the sacrum, buttocks, and hips of bedridden patients. Conversely, if the disease or injury causes a decreased osmolality in the ECF compartment (that is a low concentration of electrolytes to water), this will cause water to move into the cells. This can cause such conditions such as pulmonary congestion or encephalopathy. We call this a fluid/water overload.

The normal osmolality of plasma (an extracellular area) is 270 to 300 mOsm/L. If a laboratory report lists a person's plasma osmolality of 350 mOsm/L, this would indicate that they are in a fluid deficit state. We can correct this by administering the proper type of intravenous solution—when the patient's osmolality is above normal, expect an intravenous fluid that will help to correct the imbalance, such as 0.46% normal saline. Intravenous fluids are available as either

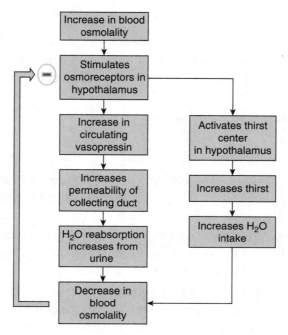

FIGURE 11–2 • Feedback loop that ensures homeostasis of blood osmolality. An increase in blood osmolality triggers the thirst mechanism as well as renal conservation of water via the release of vasopressin from the hypothalamus. Both outcomes decrease blood osmolality back toward the normal range, which feeds back to terminate hypothalamic signaling.

Source: Reproduced with permission from: Barrett KE, Barman SM, Boitano S, Brooks HL: *Ganong's Review of Medical Physiology.* New York, NY: McGraw-Hill; 2012. Fig. 16–4.

hypotonic (low osmolality), hypertonic (high osmolality), or isotonic (normal osmolality). A chart listing the different solutions and their osmolality and tonicity follows.

IV Fluids		
Solution	Osmolarity (mOsm/L)	Hypo-, Iso-, or Hypertonic
0.9% saline (normal saline, NS)	308	Isotonic
0.45% saline (1/2 normal saline)	154	Hypotonic
5% dextrose in water (D_5W)	272	Isotonic
10% dextrose in water ($D_{10}W$)	500	Hypertonic
5% dextrose in Ringer's lactate	525	Hypertonic
5% dextrose in 0.45% saline	406	Hypertonic
5% dextrose in 0.9% saline	560	Hypertonic
Ringer's lactate	273	Isotonic

Electrolytes

Electrolytes are those chemicals that carry an electric charge. They include the positively charged cations such as sodium (Na^+), potassium (K), magnesium (Mg^{2+}), calcium (Ca^{2+}), and the negatively charged anions (A^-) such as chloride (Cl^-), phosphate (HPO_4^{2-}), and bicarbonate (HCO_3^-).

In the intracellular area, Na is the major cation and Cl is the major anion.

Hormonal Regulation of Fluids and Electrolytes

Aldosterone is secreted by the adrenal cortex in response to sodium changes. Wherever sodium goes, water follows. Aldosterone signals the tubules within the nephrons in the kidneys to reabsorb sodium and therefore water. This increases blood osmolarity. Aldosterone also aids in control of potassium levels.

Renin is secreted by the kidneys in responses to changes in sodium or fluid volume. In the circulation, renin acts on a plasma protein called renin substrate (also called angiotensinogen), converting it to angiotensin I. In the pulmonary circulation, angiotensin-converting enzyme converts angiotensin I to angiotensin II. This causes vascular constriction and aldosterone secretion.

Antidiuretic hormone (ADH) is produced in the hypothalamus and stored in the posterior pituitary. It is released when there is a change in the osmolarity of the blood. ADH acts on the renal tubules, causing them to reabsorb more water, which decreases blood osmolarity. When the osmolarity gets too low, the release of ADH is not needed and the water is excreted in the urine.

Natriuretic peptides are hormones secreted by the cardiomyocytes in response to increases in blood volume and blood pressure. When atrial natriuretic peptide (ANP) and brain natriuretic peptide (BNP) are secreted, kidney reabsorption of sodium is inhibited and the glomerular filtration rate is increased. Blood osmolarity is decreased and urine output is increased.

Acid-Base Balance

As discussed earlier, this mechanism also serves a crucial role in maintaining a balance in our body for survival.

Maintaining acid-base balance will keep the pH level within the normal range of 7.35 to 7.45. The lungs and kidneys are integral in maintaining the normal acid-base balance. The body constantly monitors the pH level and makes adjustments in an attempt to correct any abnormalities. Acidosis results when the pH drops below 7.35 and alkalosis occurs when the pH rises above 7.45. Acidosis (acid is a small word) results in a lower number whereas alkalosis (alkali is a bigger word) results in a higher number. $pHCO_3$ is regulated by the kidneys. pCO_2

is regulated by the lungs. If the patient develops acidosis, there will be a low pH and either a drop in $pHCO_3$ (metabolic) or a rise in pCO_2 (respiratory). If the patient develops alkalosis, there will be an increase in pH and either an increase in $pHCO_3$ (metabolic) or a drop in pCO_2 (respiratory). (You can remember which way the numbers move in respiratory and metabolic acidosis and alkalosis by using the mnemonic Respiratory Opposite, Metabolic Equal [ROME]. In respiratory acidosis, the pH will be low and in a respiratory cause the pCO_2 will rise [opposite directions] but in a metabolic cause the $pHCO_3$ will be low [equal directions]. The same relationship occurs with alkalosis. An increased pH will have a low pCO_2 in respiratory causes [opposite directions] and in a metabolic cause the $pHCO_3$ will increase [same direction].) In an attempt to maintain as normal an internal environment as possible, the body will attempt to compensate for the changes that are occurring. The lungs are able to correct much more rapidly than the kidneys.

Just the Facts

1. Hyponatremia

What Went Wrong

Hyponatremia is an abnormally low amount of sodium in the blood. Low levels of sodium may be due to loss of sodium from the body, movement of sodium from the blood to other spaces, or dilution of sodium concentration within the plasma. Some causes include increased excretion or abnormal loss or excretion of sodium, water imbalance, hormonal imbalance (such as excess ADH), ecstasy (3,4-methylenedioxymethy-lamphetamine) use, hypothyroidism, renal failure, diuretics, diarrhea, vomiting, and wound drainage, burns, or excessive perspiration.

Prognosis

Identification and correction of the underlying cause is important in treatment of hyponatremia. Water restriction of all patients with hyponatremia will help to prevent further dilution of the plasma concentration of sodium. Seizure and death may occur if the electrolyte imbalance is not identified and corrected.

Hallmark Signs and Symptoms

- Hypotension, especially orthostatic (with position changes—from lying to sitting) due to a decrease in cardiac output in setting of hypovolemia

- Nausea
- Diarrhea owing to increased gastrointestinal motility
- Increased bowel sounds because of increased gastrointestinal motility
- Malaise or excessive activity
- Muscle weakness
- Decreased deep tendon reflexes
- Personality changes due to cerebral edema and increased intracranial pressure
- Altered level of consciousness
- Seizure

Common Test Results

- A blood serum sodium level is less than 135 mEq/L (normal sodium level is 135 to 145 mEq/L).
- Spot urine for sodium level.

Treatment

- Water restriction.
- Administer saline solution IV slowly if the patient has fluid deficit (hypovolemic)—administer slowly.
  - furosemide if fluid-overloaded
  - Treat underlying cause to correct problem

Nursing Diagnoses

- Deficient fluid volume
- Excess fluid volume
- Risk for disturbed thought processes
- Decreased cardiac output

NURSING INTERVENTION

- Record fluid intake and output to monitor fluid status.
- Monitor vital signs.
- Weigh the patient daily.
- Monitor laboratory results.

- Monitor for signs of dehydration: decreased skin turgor (elasticity), dry mucous membranes, decreased sweating, neurologic changes.
- Appropriate oral hygiene for dry mucous membranes.
- Proper skin care is especially important if the patient is experiencing diarrhea or dehydration.
- **Explain to the patient:**
  - Fluid restriction and dietary modifications.
  - Increase sodium in the diet appropriately, considering comorbidities.

2. Hypernatremia

What Went Wrong

Hypernatremia is an abnormally high amount of sodium in the blood. Fluid volume may be altered as a result of changes in the levels of sodium. A mild rise in sodium levels causes tissue that is normally excitable to become more irritable, for example, cardiac muscle. The osmolarity of extracellular fluid also increases as the sodium level increases. This is in attempt to correct the sodium level by bringing more fluid from the cells into the extracellular area. These dehydrated, more irritable cells have a decreased ability to respond to stimuli.

Causes may include insufficient water intake (patients who are NPO), insufficient sodium excretion due to hormone imbalance, renal failure, corticosteroids, increased sodium intake or increased water loss because of fever, hyperventilation, increased metabolism, and dehydration owing to sweating, vomiting, or diarrhea.

Prognosis

Identification and correction of the cause is necessary to return the patient to a normal fluid and electrolyte balance. IV fluids are carefully monitored during this treatment period to avoid overcorrection of the sodium level, causing hyponatremia. If the sodium level is severely elevated, the patient may need hemodialysis. Hypervolemia associated with hypernatremia in some patients may cause heart failure and pulmonary edema.

Hallmark Signs and Symptoms

- Weight gain due to fluid retention
- Restlessness, irritability, and agitation owing to increase in neural activity with normal or low fluid volume

- Decreased level of consciousness because of a decrease in neural activity with hypervolemia
- Muscle twitching due to irregular muscle contractions
- Muscle weakness bilaterally
- Blood pressure increased—compare with normal for the patient
- Decreased myocardial contractility, resulting in less effective pumping action of heart muscle
- Distended neck veins in hypervolemic patients
- Less cardiac output, especially with hypovolemic patients
- Increased thirst in an attempt to increase fluid intake

Common Test Results

- A blood serum sodium level is greater than 145 mEq/L. The normal sodium range is 135 to 145 mEq/L.
- Spot urine for sodium level.

Treatment

Hypotonic IV fluids are typically given to correct hypernatremic patients who are volume depleted. Diuretics are also used to help correct the sodium balance.

- Administer 0.225% sodium chloride, 0.33% sodium chloride, or 0.45% sodium chloride to correct fluid and sodium status.
- Administer diuretics to remove excess fluids and promote sodium loss.
  - furosemide, bumetanide

Nursing Diagnoses

- Disturbed thought process
- Risk for skin breakdown
- Excess fluid volume
- Deficient fluid volume

NURSING INTERVENTION

- Monitor vital signs, check pulse rate and rhythm, check blood pressure, and compare with prior.
- Weigh daily and compare.

- Record fluid intake and output to check the balance of fluid.
- Note color and clarity of the urine.
- Monitor IV site for patency, signs of infiltration such as redness or induration.
- Consult with a dietician.
- **Explain to the patient:**
  - Restrict salt in the diet.
  - Fluid intake restriction.
  - Proper oral hygiene to avoid irritation due to fluid restriction.
  - Monitor laboratory values.

3. Hypocalcemia

What Went Wrong

Hypocalcemia is an abnormally low level of calcium in the blood. Decreased levels of calcium may be due to inadequate intake or absorption (vitamin D deficiency, malabsorption), excess loss (associated with burns, renal disease, diuretics, or alcoholism), endocrine disorders (such as hypoparathyroidism), decreased serum albumin, hyperphosphatemia, or sepsis.

Prognosis

Identification and correction of the cause is necessary to return the patient to a normal fluid level and electrolyte balance. As the calcium level becomes more abnormal, the risk to the patient is greater. Seizures and cardiac arrhythmias may develop, which may become life-threatening.

Hallmark Signs and Symptoms

- Irritability
- Paresthesia of lips (circumoral) and extremities
- Muscle spasm and cramping
- Tetany—intermittent painful tonic spasms, usually involving the arms and legs
- Abdominal pain due to muscle cell cramping within the gastrointestinal tract
- Laryngospasm and stridor (abnormal high-pitched breathing sound) as airway becomes narrowed

- Seizures owing to irritation of nervous system tissue
- Cardiac arrhythmias because of increased excitation of cardiac muscle cells
- Prolonged QT interval will predispose to ventricular arrhythmias
- Contraction of facial muscle after tapping facial nerve anterior to ear (Chvostek's sign) due to increased excitation of nerve and muscle cells
- Carpal spasm after inflation of blood pressure cuff to upper arm—occludes brachial artery and applies pressure to nerves (Trousseau's sign)

Common Test Results

- Blood serum calcium level of less than 9 mg/dL.

Treatment

- Maintain intravenous access.
- High-calcium diet to replenish lost calcium.
- Administer vitamin D if the patient has deficiency; helps with absorption of calcium.
  - ergocalciferol (vitamin D$_2$)
- Administer calcium gluconate 10% IV (emergency treatment for seizure, tetany, cardiac arrhythmia).
- Administer calcium chloride (emergency treatment).

Nursing Diagnoses

- Imbalanced nutrition: less than what body requires
- At risk for injury

NURSING INTERVENTION

- Monitor vital signs for changes.
- Monitor intake and output.
- Monitor neurologic status for change, irritability, and disorientation.
- Monitor cardiovascular status for changes, irregularity of heartbeat, pulse deficit (difference between heartbeat and peripheral pulse checked at the same time), and cardiac rhythm.

- Monitor for signs of hypercalcemia when administering medication (can over-medicate with calcium).
  - Nausea
  - Vomiting
  - Anorexia
- Monitor laboratory results.
- **Explain to the patient:**
  - Avoid dependence on laxatives—these medications can alter bowel patterns, causing altered absorption and excess elimination of calcium and other electrolytes.
  - Avoid dependence or overuse of antacids—these medications cause excess intake of calcium (or other electrolytes, depending on composition).

4. Hypercalcemia

What Went Wrong

Hypercalcemia is an abnormally high amount of calcium in the blood. Excess intake of calcium (such as supplements or antacids) or altered excretion of calcium (such as in patients with renal failure or those taking thiazide diuretics) may cause hypercalcemia. Patients may also develop elevated calcium levels with prolonged immobility, glucocorticoid use, hyperthyroidism, hyperparathyroidism, lithium use, dehydration, or malignancies with metastasis to the bone.

Prognosis

Correction or treatment of the underlying disorder is necessary to correct the abnormal calcium level. High calcium levels cause altered excitability of heart, skeletal, and smooth muscle tissues of the gastrointestinal tract, and nervous tissues.

Hallmark Signs and Symptoms

- Increased heart rate initially.
- Bounding peripheral pulses.
- Bradycardia later as electrical conduction is slowed.
- Sinus arrest then cardiac arrest due to altered response of cardiac tissue to normal stimuli.

- Shallow respirations owing to skeletal muscle weakness.
- Muscle weakness because of changes in neuromuscular response to normal stimuli.
- Cardiac arrhythmias.
- Nausea and vomiting as a result of a decrease in peristaltic activity.
- Constipation due to a decrease in peristaltic activity.
- Dehydration.
- Kidney stones form as excess calcium deposits in kidneys; it may be excreted in urine.

Common Test Results

- Blood calcium level is greater than 10.5 mEq/L.
- Increased calcium level in urine.
- Electrocardiography (EKG) shows shortened ST segment and widened T-waves.

Treatment

Medications are typically used to reduce calcium levels. When levels are highly elevated or patients are having life-threatening problems, dialysis may also be utilized to reduce calcium levels.

- Stop all calcium-containing medications (supplements, antacids).
- Monitor cardiac rhythm.
- Maintain intravenous access.
- Administer 0.9% normal saline solution to ensure adequate hydration status; sodium aids in urinary excretion of calcium.
- Administer loop diuretics to enhance the excretion of calcium.
  - furosemide
- Administer plicamycin, a calcium binder, to lower calcium levels.
- Administer calcitonin, phosphorus, bisphosphonates (etidronate, pamidronate—to inhibit calcium resorption from the bone).

Nursing Diagnoses

- Ineffective breathing pattern
- Decreased cardiac output
- Impaired urinary elimination

NURSING INTERVENTION

- Monitor vital signs for changes.
- Monitor cardiovascular status for irregularity of heart rhythm, pulse deficit.
- Monitor intake and output.
- Assess muscle strength—hand grips, foot pushes bilaterally for strength and equality.
- Assess abdomen for bowel sounds, distention, and pain.
- Encourage mobilization, assist with ambulation if necessary to decrease bone resorption due to immobility.
- Assist with range-of-motion (ROM) exercises.
- Low-calcium diet to reduce intake.
- Strain urine for stones.
  - Monitor laboratory results.
- **Explain to the patient:**
  - Avoid calcium supplements.
  - Avoid calcium-based antacids.
  - Weight-bearing exercise is important to avoid bone resorption.

5. Hypokalemia

What Went Wrong

Hypokalemia is a lower-than-normal level of potassium in the blood. A balance between the amount of potassium within the cell (intracellular) and outside the cell (extracellular) is necessary. This allows the resting potential of the cell membrane to be maintained. When there are low potassium levels, a greater-than-normal stimulus is needed to depolarize the cell membrane. Many cells become more sluggish, especially nerve cells. However, cardiac cells become more excitable. Fluid losses due to diuretics or diarrhea, endocrine disorders (such as hyperthyroidism, hyperaldosteronism), insufficient intake of potassium, and low magnesium levels can all contribute to low potassium levels. Dietary intake is the main source of potassium, so patients with poor nutritional intake or prolonged NPO status are also at risk for hypokalemia.

Prognosis

Low potassium levels may range from minor to life-threatening. The more abnormal the level, the greater the chance the patient will develop a cardiac arrhythmia. Correction or treatment of the underlying cause is necessary to help restore the electrolyte balance.

Hallmark Signs and Symptoms

- Muscle weakness owing to need for greater stimulation of cell due to low potassium level
- Muscle cramps
- Malaise and lethargy
- Decrease in deep tendon reflex response because of lack of response of nerve tissue to normal stimuli
- Anorexia and constipation as a result of decrease in peristaltic activity
- Palpitations due to cardiac arrhythmias caused by excitability of cardiac muscle
- Rhabdomyolysis (destruction or degeneration of muscle tissue) in severe hypokalemia
- Cardiac arrest in severe hypokalemia

Common Test Results

- Serum potassium level is less than 3.5 mEq/L.
- EKG shows the development of U-waves, ST depression, premature ventricular contractions, and AV block.

Treatment

- Correct fluid imbalance.
- Stop or change medications that contribute to potassium loss, if possible (eg, loop diuretics).
- Encourage potassium-rich foods.
- Administer potassium supplements.
- Administer potassium in intravenous fluids.
- Avoid glucose in fluid which will shift potassium into cells.
- Potassium concentration is not more than 40 mEq/L in peripheral lines.
- Monitor cardiac rhythm.

Nursing Diagnoses

- Activity intolerance
- Decreased cardiac output
- Fatigue

NURSING INTERVENTION

- Monitor vital signs for change.
- Monitor cardiac system for rate, rhythm, and pulse deficit.
- Monitor intake and output.
- Monitor laboratory results.
- Monitor intravenous site for redness, swelling, warmth, and pain.
- **Explain to the patient:**
  - About medication and diet changes.
  - Foods rich in potassium (bananas, tomatoes, orange juice).

6. Hyperkalemia

What Went Wrong

Hyperkalemia is an elevated level of potassium in the blood. Dietary intake is the main source of potassium. Patients are at risk for hyperkalemia when there is excessive ingestion of potassium-rich foods or salt substitutes, they are on medications that cause potassium retention (ACE inhibitors, angiotensin receptor blockers, potassium-sparing diuretics such as amiloride or spirono-lactone, NSAIDs, trimethoprim, pentamidine), or there is excess release of potassium from the cells (hemolysis, acidosis, low insulin levels, beta-blocker use, digoxin overdose, succinylcholine, or rhabdomyolysis).

Prognosis

As potassium levels rise, the risk of cardiac arrhythmias also increases. An extreme elevation creates a medical emergency. Correction or treatment of the underlying cause is necessary to help restore the electrolyte balance.

Hallmark Signs and Symptoms

- Weakness and dizziness due to neuromuscular changes
- Abdominal distention
- Nausea, vomiting, and diarrhea owing to change in membrane potential on the GI system
- Palpitations because of arrhythmias
- Arrhythmias as a result of changes in normal cardiac conduction
- Cardiac arrest

Common Test Results

- Potassium level is greater than 5 mEq/L.
- EKG shows peaked T-waves, widened QRS-waves, ventricular asystole, and cardiac arrest.

Treatment

The treatment choices will depend on the severity of the potassium elevation. Decreasing further intake, enhancing renal excretion, and cellular uptake are all goals of treatment.

- Monitor cardiac rhythm.
- Administer intravenous insulin and glucose to move potassium from extracellular fluid to intracellular fluid.
- Administer calcium gluconate intravenously.
- Administer $NaHCO_3$ to move potassium from extracellular fluid to intracellular fluid.
- Administer diuretics to remove potassium from the body.
- Administer Kayexalate to remove potassium from the body via the GI tract.
- Monitor electrolyte levels.
- Restrict potassium intake.
- Dialysis for severe elevations.

Nursing Diagnoses

- Decreased cardiac output
- Risk for imbalanced fluid volume
- Activity intolerance
- Altered bowel elimination

NURSING INTERVENTION

- Monitor vital signs.
- Monitor cardiac rhythm.
- Monitor cardiovascular status for regularity of rhythm, rate, heart sounds, and peripheral pulses.
- Monitor abdomen for bowel sounds, distention, and pain.

- Monitor intravenous site for redness, swelling, and pain.
- Monitor laboratory results.
- **Explain to the patient:**
  - About medications and diet.
  - Avoid foods that are high in potassium.
  - Avoid salt substitutes (most are potassium-based).

7. Hypomagnesemia

What Went Wrong

Hypomagnesemia is a lower-than-normal magnesium level in the blood. Low serum levels of magnesium can be due to lack of sufficient intake or absorption (malnutrition, vomiting, diarrhea, celiac disease, Crohn's disease), excess excretion of magnesium (renal loss, chronic alcohol intake, diuretic use, aminoglycoside antibiotics, antineoplastics), or intracellular movement of magnesium (ascites, hyperglycemia, insulin administration). The cell membranes become more excitable in the setting of low magnesium levels. Patients may also have associated imbalances of potassium and calcium.

Prognosis

Correction of the magnesium level is necessary for normal electrolyte balance to the patient. Correction or treatment of the underlying condition may be necessary to correct the magnesium level. Nerve impulse transmission is increased in patients with hypomagnesemia. As the magnesium level drops, the patient may develop seizures or cardiac arrhythmias.

Hallmark Signs and Symptoms

- Painful paresthesia (numbness and tingling)
- Hyperactive deep tendon reflexes—using a reflex hammer, strike tendon at the specific site to elicit response (patellar tendon, Achilles tendon, brachioradialis, bicep, or tricep)
- Muscle twitching
- Seizures due to irritability of nervous tissue in the brain
- Confusion owing to central nervous system (CNS) irritability
- Headaches

- Mood changes or irritability
- Decreased appetite, nausea, and constipation owing to decreased gastrointestinal motility
- Decreased bowel sounds and abdominal distention
- Arrhythmia, ectopic beats, ventricular arrhythmias
- Contraction of facial muscle after tapping facial nerve anterior to ear (Chvostek's sign) due to increased excitation of nerve and muscle cells if concurrent hypocalcemia
- Carpal spasm after inflation of blood pressure cuff to upper arm—occludes brachial artery and applies pressure to nerves (Trousseau's sign) if concurrent hypocalcemia

Common Test Results
- Blood serum magnesium level is less than 1.5 mEq/L.
- EKG shows depressed ST segments and tall T-waves.

Treatment
- Administer magnesium sulfate intravenously to increase levels.
- Monitor deep tendon reflexes.
- Monitor cardiac rhythm.
- Increase magnesium in the patient's diet.
- May need to correct calcium and potassium concurrently.

Nursing Diagnoses
- Impaired gas exchange
- Risk for injury
- Decreased cardiac output

NURSING INTERVENTION
- Monitor intake and output.
- Monitor vital signs for changes.
- Monitor cardiovascular status for changes in heart rhythm and pulse deficit.
- Monitor laboratory results.

> • **Explain to the patient:**
>   • Eat whole grains, legumes, fish, and dark green leafy vegetables that are high in magnesium.
>   • Do not take laxatives.

8. Hypermagnesemia

What Went Wrong

Hypermagnesemia is a greater-than-normal amount of magnesium in the blood. Patients with poor renal function or long-term abuse of magnesium-containing compounds have difficulty excreting magnesium. The excess of magnesium in the blood causes the cell membranes to become less excitable than normal, requiring greater stimuli than would normally be needed to cause a required effect. As the magnesium level continues to rise, the cell membrane becomes more resistant to its natural stimuli.

Prognosis

Correction of the magnesium level is necessary to prevent life-threatening complications. Patients are at significant risk for cardiac arrest as the magnesium levels continue to rise.

Hallmark Signs and Symptoms

• Bradycardia due to slowed cellular response to normal stimuli
• Hypotension owing to vasodilation
• Drowsiness or lethargy
• Weakness
• Less-than-normal deep tendon reflexes
• Confusion
• Urinary retention
• Cardiac arrest when level severely elevated

Common Test Results

• Blood serum magnesium level is greater than 2.5 mEq/L.
• EKG shows widened QRS complex and prolonged PR intervals.
• *Blood urea nitrogen* (BUN) elevation if there is renal insufficiency.

Treatment

- Administer magnesium antagonist intravenously.
  - calcium chloride
- Administer loop diuretic to reduce the magnesium level.
  - furosemide
- Dialysis—hemodialysis or peritoneal, to remove excess magnesium (especially in patients with renal failure).
- Reduce magnesium in the diet (avoid meat, legumes, dark green leafy vegetables, fish, whole grains, nuts).
- Increase fluid intake to maintain hydration.

Nursing Diagnoses

- Impaired gas exchange
- Risk for injury
- Reduced cardiac output

NURSING INTERVENTION

- Monitor intake and output.
- Monitor vital signs for changes.
- Monitor cardiovascular status for changes in heart rate and rhythm.
- Monitor laboratory reports for electrolyte balance.
- **Explain to the patient:**
  - Avoid foods high in magnesium.
  - Avoid magnesium-based medications.

---

9. Metabolic Acidosis

What Went Wrong

The acid-base balance of the blood is thrown off, causing it to become more acidic. There is an arterial pH of less than 7.35. There may be an overproduction of hydrogen ions (lactic acidosis in fever or seizures, diabetic ketoacidosis, starvation, alcohol or aspirin intake), deficient elimination of hydrogen ions (renal failure), deficient production of bicarbonate ions (renal failure, pancreatic insufficiency), or excess elimination of bicarbonate ions (diarrhea).

Prognosis

Correction or treatment of the underlying cause is necessary to help restore the acid-base balance.

Hallmark Signs and Symptoms

- Lethargy due to increased hydrogen ion concentration in blood
- Muscle weakness bilaterally owing to neuromuscular manifestations
- Tachycardia early in acidosis; later, cardiac electrical conduction slows, causing bradycardia and increasing risk for heart block or arrhythmia
- Hypotension because of vasodilation
- Rapid, deep breathing (hyperventilation) as the body attempts to compensate

Common Test Results

- Arterial blood gas (ABG) showing pH less than 7.35 and bicarbonate less than 22 mEq/L, normal $PaCO_2$
- Ketones in urine possible
- Potassium level elevated
- Chloride level normal or elevated

Treatment

- Administer intravenous fluids for hydration as necessary.
- Monitor ABG levels.
- Administer supplemental oxygen as necessary.
- Administer bicarbonate if bicarbonate levels are low.
- Correct the underlying condition that is causing the imbalance.
- Administer insulin and fluids in diabetic ketoacidosis.
- Mechanical ventilation if necessary.
- Hemodialysis if necessary to restore normal balance in system or remove offending substance.

Nursing Diagnoses

- Disturbed thought processes
- Ineffective breathing pattern

> ## NURSING INTERVENTION
>
> - Monitor intake and output.
> - Monitor vital signs for changes.
> - Monitor laboratory test results.
> - Monitor ABG results.

10. Metabolic Alkalosis

What Went Wrong

The acid-base balance of the blood is basic because of either a decrease in acidity or an increase in bicarbonate. Alkalosis is often associated with decreased levels of potassium or calcium. Metabolic alkalosis may be due to excess intake of antacids, blood transfusions, long-term parenteral nutrition, prolonged vomiting or nasogastric suctioning, Cushing's disease, use of thiazide diuretics, or excess aldosterone.

Prognosis

Correction or treatment of the underlying cause is necessary to help restore the acid-base balance.

Hallmark Signs and Symptoms

- Muscle weakness due to neuromuscular changes and hypokalemia
- Muscle cramping and twitching owing to electrolyte changes
- Anxiety and irritability
- Tetany and seizures, as alkalosis worsens
- Positive Chvostek's sign because of hypocalcemia
- Positive Trousseau's sign due to hypocalcemia
- Increased reflexes as a result of neuromuscular irritability
- Increased heart rate and myocardial irritability

Common Test Results

- ABG showing pH greater than 7.45, bicarbonate greater than 28 mEq/L, pCO_2 elevated
- Serum potassium low, chloride low

Treatment

- Monitor ABGs and electrolyte levels.
- Administer fluids and electrolytes as necessary.
- Administer supplemental oxygen if necessary.
- Administer electrolyte replacement as indicated.

Nursing Diagnoses

- Risk for injury
- Disturbed thought process

NURSING INTERVENTION

- Monitor vital signs for changes.
- Monitor cardiovascular status for changes in heart rate and rhythm.
- Monitor intake and output.
- Assess intravenous site for signs of infiltration.
- Check neurologic status for changes.

---

11. Hypophosphatemia

What Went Wrong

Hypophosphatemia is a lower-than-normal amount of phosphorus in the blood. Chronic alcohol use, chronic obstructive pulmonary disease, and asthma medications (loop diuretics, corticosteroids, adrenergic agonists, xanthine derivatives) are associated with low phosphate levels. Vitamin D is important in the intestinal absorption of phosphate. Parathyroid hormone stimulates the release of phosphate from the bone tissue. An overproduction can lead to hypophosphatemia.

Prognosis

Correction or treatment of the underlying cause is necessary to help restore the electrolyte balance. Proper treatment cannot be given without identification of the underlying cause.

Hallmark Signs and Symptoms

- Muscle weakness due to impairment in oxygen delivery to the tissues
- Rhabdomyolysis with breakdown of muscle tissue
- Paresthesia (tingling sensations)

- Hemolytic anemia owing to fragility of RBCs
- Encephalopathy (irritability, confusion, disorientation, seizures, coma)
- Respiratory failure or trouble weaning from the ventilator because of changes in oxygen delivery to cells
- Weakening of bone structure seen in chronic, severe hypophosphatemia due to phosphate leaving bones
- Petechiae as a result of poorly functioning platelets

Common Test Results

- Phosphorus is less than 1.7 mEq/L in blood serum.
- Spot urine sampling for diminished phosphate.
- Parathyroid (PTH) levels elevated.
- In anemia, low hemoglobin and hematocrit.
- Elevated creatine kinase in rhabdomyolysis.

Treatment

- Administer potassium phosphate to replace phosphate.
- Oral potassium phosphate for mild to moderate loss, or intravenous for severe loss.
- Monitor for hypotension if intravenous replacement of phosphate.
- Monitor serum phosphate, calcium, potassium, and magnesium levels every 6 to 8 hours during initial replacement.
- Diet high in phosphorus for chronic hypophosphatemia.

Nursing Diagnoses

- Risk for injury
- Imbalanced nutrition

NURSING INTERVENTION

- Monitor intake and output.
- Monitor vital signs; may see hypotension with intravenous phosphate infusion.
- Monitor laboratory results.
- **Explain to the patient:**
  - Diet of turkey, skim milk and milk products, and dried fruits.

12. Hyperphosphatemia

What Went Wrong

Hyperphosphatemia is a higher-than-normal amount of phosphorus in the blood. Patients may develop increased phosphate levels as a result of renal insufficiency, increase in phosphorus intake (supplements, laxatives, enemas, excess vitamin D), hypoparathyroidism, rhabdomyolysis, or as a result of cell destruction from chemotherapy. As phosphate levels increase, calcium levels decrease.

Prognosis

Correction or treatment of the underlying cause is necessary to help restore the electrolyte balance.

Hallmark Signs and Symptoms

- Asymptomatic
- Symptoms of underlying disorder, such as renal disease
- May see symptoms of coexisting electrolyte disorders, such as hypocalcemia

Common Test Results

- Phosphorus level is greater than 4.6 mEq/L in blood serum.

Treatment

- Administer medications orally in divided doses during the day to bind phosphate.
  - calcium acetate
  - aluminum hydroxide
  - lanthanum
- Dialysis to remove excess phosphate.
- Diet low in phosphorus to avoid excess intake.
- Monitor laboratory report for correction of electrolytes.

Nursing Diagnoses

- Risk for injury
- Imbalanced nutrition

> ## NURSING INTERVENTION
>
> - Monitor intake and output.
> - Monitor vital signs.
> - Monitor laboratory results.
> - **Explain to the patient:**
>   - No over-the-counter medications (ie, laxatives) that contain phosphorus to avoid recurrence
>   - Medication use and schedule

13. Dehydration

What Went Wrong

Dehydration is a state of having less-than-normal body fluids, due to an excess loss of fluids or an inadequate intake of fluids. Dehydration may be actual or relative. A relative dehydration exists when the amount of fluid and electrolytes in the body is correct, but the placement is not correct. If fluid shifting has occurred and the fluid is now in the interstitial areas rather than in the circulating blood volume, the patient may actually be experiencing a relative dehydration. Even though there is adequate fluid within the body, it cannot be utilized at this time. More commonly, dehydration is actual and due to loss of fluid from the body or lack of adequate hydration.

Prognosis

Adequate replacement of fluids with the appropriate fluid type is essential to ensure adequate circulating blood volume.

Hallmark Signs and Symptoms

- Thirst as the body wants more fluids
- Poor skin turgor due to fluid loss
- Tachycardia—heart rate increases to circulate remaining volume faster
- Tachypnea—respiratory rate increases in an attempt to obtain more oxygen
- Decreased urinary output—less volume available to leave the body
- Increased BUN as volume depletes
- Hypotension owing to a decrease in circulating blood volume

Common Test Results

- BUN elevated
- Elevated hemoglobin and hematocrit as blood hemoconcentrates

Treatment

- Intravenous and oral fluid replacement.
- Monitor serum electrolytes, BUN, creatinine, urine electrolytes.
- Monitor cardiac rhythm if there is an electrolyte disturbance.

Nursing Diagnosis

- Deficient fluid volume
- Risk for impaired urinary elimination
- Impaired oral mucous membrane

NURSING INTERVENTION

- Monitor vital signs; check for orthostatic hypotension.
- Monitor intake and output.
- Assess intravenous access site for signs of redness, swelling, or pain.
- Assess skin and mucous membranes for dryness.
- Assess cardiovascular status—heart rate, heart sounds, peripheral pulses.
- Assess respiratory status—lung sounds, respiratory rate.
- Encourage oral fluid intake.
- Increase frequency of mouth care.
- Monitor laboratory results.

REVIEW QUESTIONS

1. **Rocco was admitted to the hospital with a diagnosis of hypomagnesemia. He is complaining of painful paresthesia. Which of the following do you recognize as part of his treatment plan?**

   A. Dialysis and removal of legumes and whole grains from the diet.
   B. Monitoring cardiac rhythm and checking deep tendon reflexes.
   C. Monitoring urinary output and auscultating bowel sounds.
   D. Palpating peripheral pulses and checking pupil reactions.

2. Vince has been taking excessive amounts of over-the-counter antacid tablets. He has been exhibiting signs of irritability, anxiety, muscle cramping, and weakness, and has recently developed tetany. The physician has initiated seizure precautions. He recognizes that the patient is being monitored and treated for:

A. Hyperkalemia.

B. Hyperphosphatemia.

C. Metabolic acidosis.

D. Metabolic alkalosis.

3. Derek has recently converted his outdoor garage to a gym. He has been exercising frequently in his new gym due to the convenience, even in the extreme heat. He has started taking salt tablets. The physician thinks his current symptoms may be owing to hypernatremia. His physician recognizes these as:

A. Cardiac arrhythmias, palpitations, and sinus arrest.

B. Weakness, dizziness, abdominal distention, nausea, vomiting, and diarrhea.

C. Weight gain, irritability, muscle twitching, and decreased myocardial contractility.

D. Muscle cramps, malaise, constipation, rhabdomyolysis, and pupillary constriction.

4. Grace was diagnosed with hyperparathyroidism after a workup to determine the cause of her elevated calcium levels. The greatest concern in a patient with hypercalcemia would be:

A. Cardiac arrhythmia and sinus arrest.

B. Nausea and vomiting.

C. Constipation and dehydration.

D. Kidney stones and muscle weakness.

5. Bernadette's morning laboratory results have just come in. Her serum potassium level is currently 5.4 mEq/L. The physician recognizes this as:

A. Hypokalemia.

B. Hyperkalemia.

C. Hypocalcemia.

D. Hypercalcemia.

6. A physician is monitoring intravenous fluids for Tom who is currently being treated for metabolic acidosis. The physician monitors his signs and symptoms typical of metabolic acidosis which include:

A. Elevated blood pressure, bradycardia, elevated respiratory rate, and muscle twitching.

B. Hypotension, altered heart rate, elevated respiratory rate, and muscle weakness.

C. Hypertension, tachycardia, slowed respiratory rate, and muscle spasms.

D. Hypotension, hypoxia, irritability, and paresthesia.

7. **When performing a neurologic assessment on Ken, the physician notices that there is contraction of his facial muscle after tapping the facial nerve anterior to his ear. He recognizes this as Chvostek's sign. This is seen in:**

   A. Hyponatremia.

   B. Hypokalemia.

   C. Hypocalcemia.

   D. Hypomagnesemia.

8. **Liz is an elderly woman brought in by concerned family members. After physical examination, she was diagnosed with dehydration. What assessment findings would you expect to see?**

   A. Bradycardia, slowed respirations, low body temperature, and weight gain.

   B. Rales, peripheral edema, palpitations, and diaphoresis.

   C. Tachypnea, tachycardia, hypotension, poor skin turgor, and decreased urinary output.

   D. Malaise, lymphadenopathy, fever, shortness of breath, and nausea.

9. **Rob has a history of using ecstasy. He is exhibiting symptoms of hypotension, nausea, diarrhea, personality change, diminished level of consciousness, and decreased deep tendon reflexes. Laboratory results confirm physician's suspicion of hyponatremia. Treatment would include:**

   A. Water restriction.

   B. 0.33% sodium chloride intravenously.

   C. Use of salt substitute.

   D. Calcium carbonate orally.

10. **Brendan has chronic obstructive pulmonary disease, causing a constant state of respiratory acidosis. He has a history of chronic trimethoprim and NSAID use, leading to hyperkalemia. Which of the following are associated with hyperkalemia?**

    A. Irritability, circumoral paresthesia, muscle spasms, tetany, abdominal pain, laryngospasm, and prolonged QT intervals.

    B. Muscle cramps, malaise, diminished deep tendon reflexes, anorexia, constipation, palpitations, and rhabdomyolysis.

    C. Cardiac arrhythmia, nausea, vomiting, constipation, dehydration, kidney stones, muscle weakness, and sinus arrest.

    D. Weakness, dizziness, abdominal distention, nausea, vomiting, diarrhea, palpitations, and cardiac arrhythmias.

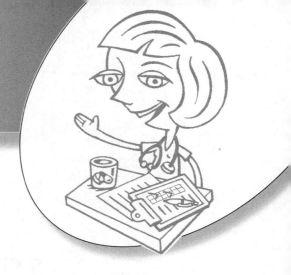

Chapter **12**

Mental Health

KEY CONCEPTS

1. Anorexia nervosa
2. Anxiety
3. Bipolar disorder
4. Bulimia nervosa
5. Delirium
6. Depression
7. Panic disorder
8. Schizophrenia

KEY TERMS

Affect
Cognition
Content of thought
Delusions
Impairment in judgment
Insight

Judgment
Mood
Paranoid ideation
Selective serotonin reuptake inhibitors
Suicidal ideation
Thought process

A Look at Mental Health

Alterations in mental health can be more difficult to diagnose because there is no definitive laboratory test or radiological study with which to isolate the disorder. Patients may initially seek treatment from primary care practitioners for a variety of complaints: anxiety, insomnia, generalized aches, or other somatic complaints.

A thorough patient history should include past medical conditions, any prior mental health conditions and their treatment course, current medications, social history (including habits, work, exercise, and substance use), cultural background, environmental factors, family history, and changes in libido, appetite, or sleep. Physical examination focuses on the chief complaint from the patient's point of view and traces the progression of symptoms in a chronological order from the time of onset. Mental status examination is completely focusing on the patient's appearance, activity and behavior, affect, mood, speech, content of thought, thought process, cognition, judgment, and insight.

The majority of patients are cared for on an outpatient basis. Hospitalization should be considered for those who:

- Are too sick to care for themselves.
- Present a serious threat to themselves or to others.
- Neglect to care for themselves.
- Are violent or have bizarre behavior.
- Have suicidal ideation.
- Have paranoid ideation.
- Have delusions.
- Have a marked impairment in judgment.

Patients with a coexisting mental health disorder are also admitted to a medical surgical floor only if the medical condition warrants medical treatment. Caring for the patient admitted with a medical or surgical condition does not preclude the need to care for the patient's depression or schizophrenia as well. Patients may also develop medical conditions as a result of their mental health issues. Patients with inadequate nutritional intake due to an eating disorder may have significant electrolyte imbalances or cardiac dysfunction.

Just the Facts

1. Anorexia Nervosa

Anorexia nervosa is a disease process that exists within the developed world, where access to adequate amounts of nutritious food is not an issue. An unrealistic expectation of body size may be part of the process, due to society's expectations as depicted in the media. There is an alteration of normal eating behaviors, resulting in a refusal to maintain body weight at or above that which is minimally expected.

What Went Wrong

Patients have a fear of gaining weight, even though they appear underweight to those around them. Patients may restrict the intake of calories or binge and purge to rid the body of the calories consumed. Anorexia affects women much more frequently than men, with onset typically in the teen or preteen years. The patient has an altered perception of body image.

Prognosis

There is an increased mortality rate for patients with untreated anorexia nervosa. The majority of these patients succumb to cardiovascular or renal problems. Patients may need to be treated periodically for electrolyte disturbances, cardiac rhythm disturbances, or renal dysfunction. The medical treatment of the patient needs to be incorporated with the cognitive-behavioral therapy to best meet the needs of the patient. The symptoms of disease may recur.

Hallmark Signs and Symptoms

- Disturbance in self-perception of body shape
- Refusal to maintain minimal normal body weight
- Abnormalities in eating behaviors
- Electrolyte imbalances due to nutritional deficiency
- Amenorrhea (absence of menstrual flow) or oligomenorrhea (very light menstrual flow) owing to lack of body fat
- Dental caries or periodontitis because of nutritional deficiency
- Temporal wasting, visible ribs, and other bony prominences as a result of lack of body fat
- Cardiovascular abnormalities due to electrolyte disturbance
- Gastrointestinal abnormalities owing to nutritional deficiency
- Dizziness because of lack of calorie intake
- Bradycardia (heart rate below 60 beats per minute)
- Hypotension (low blood pressure)

Common Test Results

- Cell blood count (CBC)—may see anemia of chronic disease if iron, B_{12}, and folate levels are not sufficient to keep up with red blood cell (RBC) production.
- Electrolytes—abnormalities of sodium (Na), potassium (K), chloride (Cl), and carbon dioxide (CO_2).
- Calcium—abnormality because stores are depleted and insufficient intake.
- Magnesium—abnormality because the stores are depleted and intake is insufficient.

- Phosphorus—abnormality as stores are reduced and there is insufficient intake.
- Blood urea nitrogen (BUN) elevated if fluid depleted.
- Thyroid-stimulating hormone (TSH) to rule out thyroid dysfunction as the cause of weight loss.
- FHS and LH to monitor hormone function to stimulate ovulation.
- Elevated amylase and normal lipase if vomiting.
- Electrocardiograph (EKG) shows abnormal heart rhythm.

Treatment

- Psychotherapy:
  - Interpersonal therapy
  - Cognitive-behavioral therapy
  - Family therapy
- Antidepressant medications—selective serotonin reuptake inhibitors (SSRIs).
- Medical treatment of electrolyte imbalance—replacement as needed.
- Monitor cardiac rhythm for rate and presence of arrhythmia.
- Calorie replacement; monitor for problems with initial refeeding.
- Monitor vital signs.
- Monitor weight.
- Monitor fluid and calorie intake.

Nursing Diagnoses

- Disturbed body image
- Imbalanced nutrition: less than what body requires
- Altered dentition

NURSING INTERVENTION

- Monitor vital signs.
- Monitor calorie intake.
- Monitor cardiac rate and rhythm.
- Monitor laboratory results; report abnormalities.

2. Anxiety

What Went Wrong

Patients exhibit symptoms when an imbalance develops between the number of open receptor sites and the number of available neurotransmitters. Neurotransmitters are released from one side of a synapse and land on a specific receptor site across the synapse. A second mechanism exists (a reuptake mechanism) to remove excess neurotransmitters left within the space between where they are released and where they fill the receptor sites. When there are insufficient neurotransmitters available to fill the open neurotransmitter receptor sites, the patient develops symptoms. Patients experience an uncontrollable feeling of anxiousness which is present more days than not.

Symptom onset is typically in late teens through early thirties. Anxiety is more common in women and in patients with a family history of anxiety.

Prognosis

Without proper treatment, the anxiety will continue, and symptoms may even progress. The patient's quality of life is adversely affected. Social functioning becomes impaired and in some cases the patient becomes more socially isolated. Physical symptoms continue, at times necessitating visits to a primary care provider or even the emergency room. With proper treatment, the symptoms are controlled, neurotransmitter balance is restored, and remission is achieved. The symptoms will typically recur at a later point, even when properly treated. It may be months or years after a successful course of treatment before the symptoms recur. The treatment that was effective in the past will typically be effective again in the future. A longer treatment course is recommended for subsequent treatment cycles when using selective serotonin reuptake inhibitors.

Hallmark Signs and Symptoms

- Fear, tension, and apprehension due to alteration in neurotransmission
- Persistent worry
- Trouble concentrating
- Irritability and restlessness
- Tachycardia, palpitations, and elevated blood pressure owing to autonomic nervous system stimulation
- Hyperventilation because of fear, elevated heart rate, and palpitations

- Sweating and tremors as a result of autonomic nervous system stimulation
- Sleep disturbance and fatigue due to alteration in neurotransmission
- Headache owing to nervous system irritability and lack of sleep

Common Test Results

- Normal laboratory results

Treatment

- Administer anxiolytics for acute treatment.
  - alprazolam, clonazepam, clorazepate, diazepam, lorazepam, oxazepam
- Monitor for respiratory depression or decrease in blood pressure.
- Have benzodiazepine antagonist (flumazenil) on hand to reverse the effect if needed.
- Administer antidepressants.
  - selective serotonin reuptake inhibitors—paroxetine
  - selective serotonin and norepinephrine reuptake inhibitors—venlafaxine
  - tricyclics
  - buspirone
- Administer beta blockers for symptom control.
- Psychotherapy.
- Cognitive-behavioral therapy.
- Relaxation techniques such as biofeedback.
- Desensitization—repeated exposures to graded doses of the object or situation that produces the anxiety.
- Group therapy.
- Family therapy.
- Emotive therapy.

Nursing Diagnosis

- Sleep pattern disturbance
- Anxiety
- Fear

- Impaired social interaction
- Ineffective role performance

NURSING INTERVENTION

- Monitor medication intake.
- Discuss patient's response to therapy.
- Monitor vital signs and watch for elevation in blood pressure with some medications.
- Monitor weight; some medications are associated with changes in weight.
- Monitor sleep; ask the patient about restful sleep during the night or difficulty falling asleep.
- **Explain to the patient:**
  - To avoid alcohol intake with benzodiazepine use

---

3. Bipolar Disorder

Patients suffering from mood disorders often have difficulty with interpersonal interactions. Substance abuse occurs as patients attempt to self-medicate.

What Went Wrong

Some patients experience episodes of depression alternating with episodes of mania or hypomania. These episodes may occur in a mixed or cyclic manner. There tends to be a high comorbidity with substance abuse in these patients. Depressive episodes tend to last longer than the manic episodes. During mania, the patients are overenthusiastic, elated, hyperactive, and often engage in activities that they later regret. Others may be drawn to the patient during manic episodes due to their outgoing, engaging behavior. Later the patient's behavior tends to alienate owing to mood swings, irritability, aggression, and grandiosity. There is a positive correlation between creative behavior and mood disorders. During the manic phase, the patient has grandiose ideas.

Prognosis

Proper medication treatment is necessary to control the symptoms of bipolar disorder. Initial diagnosis and treatment of depression without recognition of the coexisting mania can lead to the onset of mania due to the antidepressant treatment. It is important to treat both components of the disorder to effectively manage the patient. Ongoing treatment is often necessary to prevent the patient from cycling into another manic or depressive episode. Some patients may have psychotic symptoms as part of the disease process.

Hallmark Signs and Symptoms

- Elation
- Hyperactivity
- Increased irritability
- Flight of ideas
- Grandiosity
- Diminished need for sleep
- Rapid speech
- Easily distracted
- Excessive spending
- Hypersexuality
- Episodes of depression
- The patient may stray from the medication regimen because he or she feel weighed down

Common Test Results

- Laboratory results are normal.

Treatment

- Mood stabilizers:
  - lithium
  - valproic acid
  - carbamazepine
  - lamotrigine
- Antipsychotic medications:
  - olanzapine
  - risperidone
  - aripiprazole
- Psychotherapy

- Assess suicide risk
- Antidepressants

Nursing Diagnoses

- Powerlessness
- Social isolation
- Risk for loneliness
- Altered sexuality patterns

NURSING INTERVENTION

- Monitor the patient frequently when first admitted.
- Ask about suicidal ideation.
- Monitor medication intake.
- Discuss patient's response to therapy.

4. Bulimia Nervosa

The ideal body type depicted in the media has affected the perception of body image of many adolescents and young adults. Some patients may have an associated biologic vulnerability that makes this societal pressure more pronounced. Peer issues or family problems may compound this, setting the stage for development of symptoms.

What Went Wrong

Patients have recurrent episodes in which they eat a much larger quantity of food than would be expected within a given time frame; this is accompanied by a lack of control over eating, followed by some compensatory mechanism to prevent weight gain. This compensatory mechanism may include self-induced vomiting, excessive exercise, laxative use, diuretic use, enema use, or fasting. While eating disorders overall are much more common in women, men are more likely to have bulimia than anorexia.

Prognosis

Patients may need to be treated periodically for electrolyte disturbances, cardiac rhythm disturbances, or renal dysfunction. The medical treatment of the patient needs to be incorporated with the cognitive-behavioral therapy to best meet the needs of the patient. The symptoms of disease may recur.

Hallmark Signs and Symptoms

- Repeated binge eating followed by compensatory behavior (vomiting, excessive exercise, laxative use, fasting)
- Electrolyte imbalances
- Amenorrhea or oligomenorrhea due to loss of body fat
- Cardiovascular disturbance
- Erosion of enamel on back of teeth owing to repetitive vomiting
- Callus formation on knuckles from self-induced vomiting
- Gastrointestinal disturbances because of repetitive purging

Common Test Results

- Electrolytes—abnormalities of sodium (Na), potassium (K), chloride (Cl), and carbon dioxide (CO_2).
- Calcium—abnormality as stores are depleted and intake is insufficient.
- Magnesium—abnormality as stores are reduced and there is insufficient intake.
- Phosphorus—abnormality as stores are depleted and intake is not sufficient.
- Blood urea nitrogen elevated if fluid depleted.
- Elevated amylase and normal lipase if vomiting.

Treatment

- Psychotherapy:
  - Interpersonal therapy
  - Cognitive-behavioral therapy
  - Family therapy
- Medical treatment of electrolyte imbalance—replacement as needed.
- Monitor cardiac rhythm for rate and presence of arrhythmia.
- Monitor vital signs.
- Monitor weight.
- Monitor fluid and calorie intake.

Nursing Diagnoses

- Disturbed body image
- Imbalanced nutrition: less than what body requires
- Altered dentition

NURSING INTERVENTION

- Monitor vital signs.
- Monitor calorie intake.
- Monitor cardiac rate and rhythm.
- Monitor laboratory results; report abnormalities.

---

5. Delirium

What Went Wrong

Patients exhibit a global disturbance in cognitive functions that may develop rapidly, sometimes within hours. Symptom severity may vary during the course of the day, depending on the cause of symptoms. The patient with a sudden onset of disorientation and behavioral changes, especially the elderly patient, is often sent for a psychiatric evaluation.

Prognosis

Delirium is often due to an underlying infection, ischemic change, or metabolic disturbance. Rapid identification and intervention for the underlying cause is essential for the patient. Without proper treatment, the cause may prove to be fatal.

Hallmark Signs and Symptoms

- Confusion
- Disorientation
- Behavioral changes
- Inappropriate words or dress
- Agitation

Common Test Results

- Electroencephalogram (EEG) may show generalized slowing.
- White blood cell (WBC) elevated in bacterial infection.

- Glucose abnormalities in hyperglycemia or hypoglycemia.
- EKG abnormalities in myocardial ischemia or infarction.
- CT scan of the brain may show ischemic changes.
- Electrolyte abnormalities if causative.

Treatment

- Monitor vital signs.
- Monitor neurologic status, orientation, level of consciousness, eye opening, and pupil response.
- Treatment of underlying cause.
- Supplemental oxygen supply if hypoxic.

Nursing Diagnosis

- Risk for falls

NURSING INTERVENTION

- Protect the patient from injury.
- Monitor intravenous site for signs of infiltration.
- Perform neurologic checks.

6. Depression

Patients with depression have a persistent sense of sadness, more days than not, often associated with somatic complaints. The medical workups for varied physical complaints will be negative. Patients typically have a loss of interest in normal activities and alterations in sleep and eating habits. Up to one-third of patients will seek care from primary care providers. Patients can also present as unkempt, dirty, withdrawn, or unwilling to engage in conversation. They see life as a state of hopelessness. The patient's depression must be treated seriously since it can lead to suicide. A patient's request for help might be his or her last recourse.

What Went Wrong

Several different theories exist involving the cause of depression. Genetic factors may lead to changes in the normal functioning of neurotransmitters.

Neurotransmitters are released from one side of a synapse and land on a specific receptor site on the other side of the synapse. When a balance is maintained between the amount released and the amount needed to fill the receptor sites, normal function continues. When there is an imbalance, the neurotransmission is altered. Developmental factors can often be traced back to childhood. Personality disorders may begin during school age or adolescence. Psychosocial stressors are another factor linked to the development of depression. Major life changes such as the death of a family member, unemployment, or moving away from family and friends may lead to the onset of depression. A sense of sadness or grief is considered a normal response to this type of loss and should resolve as the person progresses through the normal stages of grieving. Depression, however, is not a normal response to loss. A grieving person will have a sustained sense of self-esteem, whereas a person with depression will have a sense of worthlessness.

Prognosis

Proper treatment can help control the symptoms of depression. Adequate treatment can cause remission of symptoms. It is not unusual for there to be a recurrence of symptoms at some point in the future, even with appropriate treatment.

Hallmark Signs and Symptoms

- Intense feeling of sadness
- Depressed mood
- Anhedonia (loss of interest in usual activities)
- Hopelessness or worthlessness
- Difficulty concentrating
- Indecision
- Changes in sleep (more or less than usual), eating (more or less than usual), and activity (more or less than usual)
- Social withdrawal and isolation
- Decreased libido
- Thoughts of death
- Physical complaints include headache, malaise, decreased libido, and changes in sleep, activity, and eating

Common Test Results

- Diagnostic testing results normal, unless coexisting disease present.

Treatment

- Ask the patient about suicidal thoughts.
- Ask the patient about the suicidal plan.
- Psychotherapy.
- Cognitive-behavioral therapy.
- Support groups.
- Antidepressant medications:
  - SSRIs
  - venlafaxine
  - nefazodone
  - bupropion
  - mirtazapine
  - tricyclics
  - monoamine oxidase inhibitors
- Electroconvulsive therapy (ECT) in refractory cases.

Nursing Diagnoses

- Hopelessness
- Risk for suicide
- Dysfunctional grieving
- Impaired social interaction
- Social isolation
- Disturbed self-esteem

NURSING INTERVENTION

- Monitor the patient frequently when first admitted.
- One-to-one observation if the patient is a suicidal risk.
- Develop a level of sensitivity and trust with the patient.
- Ask the patient about suicidal ideation; if the patient has a plan, or has attempted to carry out a plan.

- Monitor medication intake.
- Discuss patient's response to therapy.
- Monitor vital signs; watch for elevation in blood pressure with some medications.
- Monitor weight; some medications are associated with changes in weight.
- Monitor sleep; ask the patient about restful sleep during the night, and difficulty falling asleep.

7. Panic Disorder

What Went Wrong

Patients experience intermittent episodes that have a sudden onset and no predictable pattern, causing intense anxiety associated with pronounced physical symptoms. These episodes are short in duration and recurrent in nature. The disorder tends to present before the age of 25, is twice as common in women as it is in men, and tends to be familial. Some patients will choose to self-medicate with alcohol or other drugs in an attempt to escape the disease, diminish symptoms, or decrease the occurrence of the episodes. Others become dependent on tranquilizing medications. Panic attacks can impede a person's life and restrict activity, especially in anticipation of a panic attack.

Prognosis

With proper treatment, the frequency and intensity of the episodes will decrease. Some patients may not experience complete resolution of symptoms, even with appropriate medications.

Hallmark Signs and Symptoms

- Depersonalization, as if the symptoms are happening to someone else
- Sense of doom and fear of dying due to the intensity of the physical symptoms
- Fear of losing control owing to the unpredictable nature of the episodes
- Worry about future attacks because of the unpredictable nature of the episodes
- Change in behavior as a result of anxiety about being in a place where an attack might occur
- Palpitations, tachycardia, and chest pain

- Dyspnea
- Choking sensation
- Nausea
- Dizziness
- Diaphoresis
- Numbness

Common Test Results
- EKG normal
- Cardiac monitor normal
- Laboratory results normal
- Pulse oximetry normal

Treatment
- Cognitive-behavioral therapy
- Relaxation therapy
- Administer antidepressants
  - selective serotonin reuptake inhibitors
  - tricyclics
  - monoamine oxidase inhibitors
- Administer benzodiazepines as adjunctive treatment
  - clonazepam, alprazolam, lorazepam
- Provide reassurance to the patient

Nursing Diagnosis
- Powerlessness
- Fear
- Social isolation

NURSING INTERVENTION
- Provide reassurance to the patient.
- Reduce anxiety.
- Monitor vital signs.

8. Schizophrenia

What Went Wrong

The exact cause of schizophrenia is not known. There is a familial tendency to the disease, and genes have been identified that are associated with the disease. Dysfunction of the neurotransmitter dopamine seems to be partially responsible for the development of the symptoms of psychosis associated with schizophrenia. NMDA receptors may also be involved in the disease.

Prognosis

Patients with schizophrenia typically need long-term medication to control symptoms. Medication compliance can be difficult for some patients, whether due to accessibility of medications, side effects, symptoms of disease, or desire not to take daily medication. Symptom recurrence is likely.

Hallmark Signs and Symptoms

- Impairment in reality testing
- Flat affect
- Disorganized speech
- Disorganized thought process
- Unusual behavior
- Delusions
- Auditory hallucinations

Common Test Results

- Diagnostic tests normal

Treatment

- Antipsychotic medications:
  - clozapine
  - aripiprazole
  - ziprasidone
  - loxapine

- risperidone
- olanzapine
- quetiapine
- thiothixene
- Psychotherapy
- Behavioral therapy
- Structured environment

Nursing Diagnoses

- Impaired environmental interpretation syndrome
- Disturbed thought process
- Disturbed auditory sensory perception

NURSING INTERVENTION

- Monitor medication intake.
- Discuss patient's response to therapy.
- **Explain to the patient:**
  - Importance of medication compliance.

REVIEW QUESTIONS

1. **Ongoing treatment of Karen would include monitoring of:**

   A. Electrolyte levels.

   B. Thyroid studies, FSH, LH.

   C. Caloric intake.

   D. All of the above.

2. **Sam presents with impairment in reality testing, flat affect, delusions, and auditory hallucinations. What medical diagnoses would the physician expect to find in Sam's chart?**

   A. Biopolar disorder.

   B. Schizophrenia.

   C. Delirium.

   D. Anxiety.

3. Teresa was recently started on fluoxetine, a selective serotonin reuptake inhibitor for treatment of her depression. After just a few days she is hardly sleeping, hyperactive, easily distracted, and appears elated. You would expect her treatment to include:

A. Continuation of the selective serotonin reuptake inhibitor.

B. Switching to a tricyclic antidepressant.

C. Starting a mood stabilizer in place of the fluoxetine.

D. Adding a monoamine oxidase inhibitor.

4. Alex is a 78-year-old married man with sudden onset of confusion and disorientation. He is exhibiting combative behavior, which is upsetting to his wife because it is so unlike his normal, easy-going nature. A psychiatric consult has been called. He has no previous psychiatric history. The psychiatric suspects Alex has:

A. Delirium.

B. Psychosis.

C. Depression.

D. Panic disorder.

5. Felicia's family brings her in for an evaluation. They are concerned because she states that she is hearing voices. You recognize this as symptomatic of:

A. Bipolar disorder.

B. Panic disorder.

C. Schizophrenia.

D. Bulimia nervosa.

6. Mick arrived in the emergency room (ER) showing signs of fear, tension, apprehension, and persistent worry. He reports trouble concentrating. Mick is showing signs of:

A. Biopolar disorder.

B. Schizophrenia.

C. Delirium.

D. Anxiety.

7. Joan presents with signs and symptoms of bipolar disorder. What medication would you anticipate the physician prescribing to stabilize Joan's mood?

A. Aripiprazole.

B. Lithium.

C. Bupropion.

D. Tricyclics.

8. **Karen has been dieting and exercising daily. Her weight is well below the recommended minimum for her height. Assessment for Karen would include looking for:**

   A. Ecchymosis and extraocular movements.

   B. Temporal wasting and irregular heart rhythm.

   C. Peripheral edema and rales.

   D. Periorbital edema and chorea.

9. **Mandy is a 17-year-old adolescent girl. On physical examination you note partial erosion of her tooth enamel and callus formation on the posterior aspect of the knuckles of her hand. This is indicative of:**

   A. A connective tissue disorder and she should be referred to a dermatologist.

   B. Self-induced vomiting and she likely has bulimia nervosa.

   C. Self-mutilation and correlates with anxiety.

   D. A genetic disorder and her siblings should also be tested.

10. **Appropriate treatment for Alex would include:**

    A. Selective serotonin reuptake inhibitors.

    B. Monoamine oxidase inhibitors.

    C. Atypical antipsychotic medication.

    D. Identification and treatment of the underlying disorder.

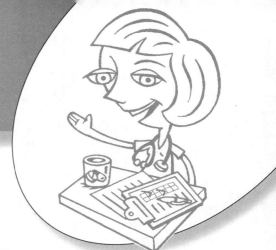

Chapter **13**

Perioperative Care

LEARNING OBJECTIVES

At the end of this chapter, the student will be able to:

- Identify the factors that contribute to surgical classifications
- List four potential postoperative complications with signs or symptoms
- Recognize expected nursing and medical treatment of the surgical patient

KEY CONCEPTS

1. Cardiovascular complications
2. Gastrointestinal complications
3. Infection
4. Respiratory complications
5. Surgical classifications
6. The intraoperative period
7. The postoperative period
8. The preoperative period

KEY TERMS

Anatomic location
Anesthesia
Degree of urgency
Extent of the surgery
Informed consent
Intraoperative
Postanesthesia care unit
Postoperative
Postoperative complications

Preoperative
Preoperative clearance
Preoperative teaching
Risk for injury
Reason for surgery
Surgical procedures
Surgical team
Transfer of the patient

Perioperative Care

The care of the surgical patient ideally begins when the patient is first informed of the need for surgery. The surgical procedure may be a sudden, unexpected event for the patient, resulting in stress and anxiety, such as necessary surgery following trauma, or may be something that the patient has planned, such as a liposuction, far in advance. The more time the patient has to prepare for surgery, both physically and emotionally, the better the patient is able to cope with the physiological stresses of the surgery. Nurses are in a position to care for the patient, provide necessary education, act as a patient advocate, and encourage health promotion behaviors.

Just the Facts

1. Surgical Classifications

The American Society of Anesthesiology categorizes surgical procedures based on the degree of risk to the patient. The urgency, location, extent, and reason for the procedure are all considered, as well as the patient's age; preexisting cardiovascular, respiratory, and neurologic status; endocrine disorders; malignancies; nutritional, fluid, and electrolyte status; abnormal laboratory findings; abnormal vital signs; and presence of infection. The risks of doing the surgery are weighed against the risks of not doing the surgery. There are some cases in which the risk of surgery is very high, but the patient may certainly die if the surgery is not performed (eg, patients with uncontrolled internal bleeding following a gunshot or stabbing). As a result, there may be preoperative consultation performed by cardiology or another specialty to evaluate the surgical risk, and make any testing recommendations before surgery.

The anatomic *location* of the surgery will affect the degree of risk to the patient. Surgical procedures performed within the thoracic cavity or skull are a greater risk to the patient than procedures performed on the extremities. Surgical procedures involving vital organs such as the heart, lungs, or brain carry a higher risk. The procedures that involve a greater potential for blood loss, such as vascular surgery, also involve greater risk.

The degree of *urgency* of the procedure is described as emergent, urgent, or elective. Emergent procedures need to be performed immediately after identifying the need for surgery. Examples include surgery to stop bleeding from trauma, shooting, or stabbing, or a dissecting aortic aneurysm. Urgent procedures are scheduled after the determination of surgical need is made. Examples include tumor removal and removal of kidney stones. Elective procedures are scheduled in advance at a time that is convenient for both patient and surgeon. Postponement of the surgery for several weeks or even months will not cause harm to the patient. Examples include joint replacement procedures and cosmetic procedures.

The *extent* of the surgery will affect the risk to the patient. The more extensive the surgical procedure, the greater the potential risk to the patient. More extensive surgical procedures cause more physical insult to the body and typically require a longer duration of anesthesia. The anesthesia can also cause stress to the patient's system, interact with medications in the patient's system, and must be metabolized out of the body.

The *reason* for surgery is another way that surgical procedures are classified. The purpose may be diagnostic, curative, restorative, palliative, or cosmetic. Diagnostic procedures are performed to obtain a biopsy for definitive diagnosis of a mass. Curative procedures are performed to remove a diseased area, such as a lumpectomy for breast cancer or an appendectomy. Restorative procedures are performed to restore function, such as joint replacements. Palliative procedures are performed primarily for comfort measures, such as tumor debulking. Cosmetic procedures are typically performed at the patient's request; at times some cosmetic procedures may fall into restorative (repairing damage or a congenital defect), curative, or diagnostic (in the setting of skin cancer).

Patients are classified within a range from 1, an otherwise normal, healthy patient, through 6, a patient who has been declared brain dead and is awaiting surgical recovery of organs for donation.

The perioperative period can be broken down into the *preoperative* (time before the surgery), *intraoperative* (time during the surgery), and the *postoperative* (time following the surgery until recovery) periods.

2. The Preoperative Period

The preoperative period, the time prior to surgery, is used to prepare the patient for surgery both physically and psychologically. Ideally there is time to correct as many abnormalities as possible prior to the surgical procedure. For patients having a scheduled procedure with a significant anticipated blood loss, this is the time to donate blood to be banked for use in their surgery and begin to take iron, folic acid, vitamin B_{12}, and vitamin C to aid in red blood cell (RBC) production. Preoperative clearance is given, informed consent is obtained, and preoperative teaching occurs during this time.

Preoperative Clearance

The patient's primary care provider typically gives preoperative clearance for surgery. This physician, nurse practitioner, or physician's assistant are familiar with the patient's medical history and current medications and are able to adequately assess the impending risk of the surgery to the patient. Things to consider when providing clearance for the patient include the type of surgical intervention planned, the potential for blood loss during surgery, the patient's age, general health and comorbidities, past medical and surgical history, current medications, use of herbal remedies or supplements, alcohol use, smoking history, substance use, allergies, family history including problems with surgery, and diagnostic testing results. Diagnostic studies often include a CBC (to identify anemia or signs of infection), a metabolic panel (to identify electrolyte imbalance, abnormal glucose, liver or renal function), a urinalysis (to identify infection, protein, glucose), PT/INR/PTT (to identify blood clotting disorders), an EKG (to identify abnormal cardiac rhythms or damage to myocardium), chest x-ray (to identify pulmonary pathology or enlargement of cardiac silhouette), or pulmonary function testing (for patients with respiratory disorders such as asthma or emphysema). Computerized tomography (CT) scans, magnetic resonance imaging (MRI) scans, positron emission tomography (PET) scans, or stress testing may be ordered for individual patients depending on their medical history, type of surgical procedure planned, and results of other diagnostic studies. At times, a consultation with a specialist, particularly cardiology specialist, may be warranted before clearance will be provided.

Informed Consent

An informed consent is obtained prior to any invasive or dangerous procedure. The reason for the surgery, type and extent of surgery to be performed, the risks of the procedure, the person to perform the procedure, alternative options and their associated risks, and the risks associated with anesthesia are all explained to the patient. It is the surgeon's responsibility to make sure this information is explained to the patient. The patient must be a competent adult in order for his or her signature to be valid. If the patient has been given medications that alter his or her ability to reason or to make judgments, the consent will not be valid. The nurse witnesses the patient's signature on the consent form.

Preoperative Teaching

Explaining normal preoperative routines to the patient can be very helpful, so the patient knows what to expect. The nurse needs to be familiar with the types of surgical procedures and what the expected postoperative course will entail. The extent of the procedure, type of incision, presence of any tubes or drains, and anticipated pain level after the surgery will help guide the type of teaching necessary for the patient.

Preoperatively the patient can expect to be nothing by mouth (NPO), or not allowed to eat or drink anything for several hours prior to the procedure. The time frame will depend on the extent and location of procedure, the type of anesthesia, and the scheduled time of surgery. An exception to this nothing-by-mouth rule would be for patients who need to take oral medications the morning of surgery. Cardiovascular, diabetic, and certain other medications may need to be taken even though the patient is not to eat or drink anything else.

An intravenous access site will be obtained prior to the surgery. Fluids can be administered to the patient in this way. The access also allows for giving the patient medications intravenously for rapid action. Fluids are routinely given in the operating room and in the immediate recovery period. The patient may have continued intravenous fluids for more extensive procedures.

Skin preparation may only involve washing of the surgical site in the operating room with an antimicrobial solution. Other patients may need to have removal of hair from the surgical site. This may be with a razor or a depilatory agent. It is important not to cut the skin if you are shaving a surgical site; small cuts or abrasions on the skin allow for potential sites of infection. Depilatory agents can be caustic on the skin of some patients, causing irritation or a rash. A small spot test away from the surgical area is a good idea in a patient with known skin sensitivity or history of allergies.

For patients having planned surgery involving the intestinal tract, a bowel preparation will be completed prior to the surgery. This is done to decrease the bacterial count within the intestinal tract. Cleansing of the bowel is also completed to empty the intestine of stool before the surgeon plans on cutting into either the small or the large intestine. Both of these preparations help to reduce the possibility of infection in the postoperative period. For patients who will have tubes or drains in place in the postoperative period, a simple explanation of what to expect can help to alleviate some anxiety.

Availability of pain medication in the postoperative period should be explained to the patient. In many instances, the patient is able to manage his or her own pain medication. For outpatient procedures, patients may be given a prescription for an oral pain medication prior to the procedure. This way the medication is available when the patient gets home from the surgery. For postoperative patients in the hospital, many patients have an intravenous patient-controlled analgesia, known as PCA, for pain treatment, where pain medication is delivered via a pump. Typically, a small basal dose of narcotic is delivered all the time. These patients also have the ability to press a button whenever they are experiencing pain. The pump will monitor the amount and timing of each dose of pain medication. If the patient is due for medication, a dose will be administered; if the patient is not due for medication, no dose will be administered. It is important to monitor the number of times the patient is in need of pain medication and how often the dose is actually being delivered. In cases where the patient is looking for medication much more frequently than it is being delivered, a dose adjustment may be necessary. The nurse should notify the surgeon about the increased demand for pain medication.

Transfer of the Patient

Most facilities have a preoperative checklist to assist the nurse to make sure that all the needed components have been checked prior to sending the patient to the OR. All pertinent documentation—the signed consent form, the patient's chart, and current laboratory results—accompanies the patient to the OR.

3. The Intraoperative Period

The intraoperative period is the time involved with the surgical procedure. The focus during this time is on asepsis and protection of the patient. Within the operative suite, the staff wears scrub suits. They change into the scrub shirt and pants when they get to the locker room within the surgical area. A surgical cap covers hair. Shoe covers are worn to prevent tracking bacteria or dirt from other areas into the ORs. Some staff members have shoes dedicated for use in the OR which may not need shoe covers unless they leave the operative suite.

The Surgical Team

Members of the surgical team include the surgeon, a surgical assistant, an anesthesiologist or anesthetist, a circulating nurse, a scrub nurse or surgical technician, and a holding area nurse. The *surgeon* is the doctor who will perform the surgery. The *surgical assistant* may be another surgeon, a surgical resident, an RN first assist, or a physician's assistant. The person providing anesthesia and monitoring the vital signs of the patient is either an *anesthesiologist* (a physician) or a certified registered nurse *anesthetist* (CRNA). The *circulating nurse* is a registered nurse who acts as the patient advocate, obtains the necessary supplies for the procedure, makes sure diagnostic studies, and blood products are available if necessary, prepares the operative table, positions the patient (padding bony prominences if necessary) appropriately for the surgery, and cleanses the skin in the operative area before positioning surgical drapes. The *scrub nurse* or *surgical tech* sets up the sterile field, assists with draping the patient, and hands sterile supplies into the operative field and takes used instruments from the surgeon. The circulating nurse and scrub nurse (or surgical technician) together count all instruments, sponges, and sharps used in the surgical field. The count is performed before, during, and after the procedure. The *holding area nurse* cares for the patients who have been brought into the OR suite but who are not yet ready to go into the OR. The holding area nurse may be managing several patients at one time and can also help to transport and transfer the patient.

Before entering the OR, the members of the surgical team scrub at the sink just outside the room in which the surgery will be performed. Prior to starting the scrub, the team member applies a mask with face shield or goggles. The surgical scrub is usually timed and covers the area from the fingertips to 2 inches above the elbows. The surgical scrub renders the skin clean, not sterile. After the scrub, the skin is dried with a sterile towel. A sterile gown and sterile gloves are applied. The gown is considered sterile in the front from 2 inches below the neck to the waist and from the elbow to the wrist. The circulating nurse applies the gown and gloves unassisted and then assists the other members of the team into their gown and gloves as they enter the room.

Risk for Injury

During the surgery, the patient is anesthetized and cannot tell you if there is pressure anywhere. The patient is positioned to allow for maximal access to the operative site. This sometimes causes unnatural positioning of the patient or the patient's extremities. The operative table is padded to decrease pressure on the patient. There may be additional padding added to areas of flexion or bony prominences to reduce the risk of pressure ulcer formation or nerve damage due to positioning.

Heat loss can occur during surgery. The patient is sent to the OR in a hospital gown, which may be pulled up or removed depending on the body location of the surgery. The body is draped for privacy so that only the surgical area is exposed. The temperature within the OR is kept rather cool because the air exchange rate is higher within the OR than in other rooms (to decrease bacterial counts), and the staff are wearing double layers of clothes. Warmers can be set up for the patients during certain procedures when heat loss is expected—a large, open operative site or a long duration of surgery.

At the end of the surgical procedure, the wound is closed. The closure is to hold the wound edges together and to prevent contamination. Closure may be achieved with sutures (either absorbable or nonabsorbable), staples, glue, or skin closure tape. Nonabsorbable sutures and staples will have to be removed in the postoperative period.

Drains may be inserted near the operative site if significant wound drainage is anticipated. Some drains are attached to suction, some have self-suction, and some will drain due to gravity. The wound site is covered with a sterile dressing before the patient is transferred out of the OR.

Anesthesia

Anesthesia can be administered through general or regional routes (for major procedures) or conscious sedation (for minor procedures). General anesthesia renders the patient unconscious and incapable of breathing on his or her own; pain reception is also blocked. These patients must be intubated and mechanically ventilated for the duration of the anesthesia. Regional anesthesia can be achieved through nerve blocks, or epidural or spinal anesthesia. Nerve blocks occur when an anesthetic agent is injected into an area immediately surrounding a particular nerve or nerve bundle. The nerve tissue becomes anesthetized, effectively causing the tissue that it supplies to become pain free. With epidural anesthesia, an anesthetic agent is injected into the epidural space surrounding the spinal column, usually in the lower lumbar area. The nerves become anesthetized as they leave the spinal column, causing the area of the body supplied by these nerves to become pain free. This anesthesia is most commonly associated with childbirth but is used for many surgical procedures. Spinal anesthesia is not commonly used; the anesthetic agent is injected into the spinal fluid. Patient positioning is very important, as gravity will cause the anesthetic agent to travel. The patient must remain flat after the procedure to prevent leakage of cerebrospinal fluid from the puncture site.

4. The Postoperative Period

After the surgery, the patient enters the postoperative period. The immediate postoperative period requires close monitoring as the patient emerges from anesthesia. The patient will then be transferred to either a same-day surgery area for discharge home that day or an inpatient surgical unit for care. After discharge from the hospital, the patient may need home care. Return to full activities may take several weeks.

Postanesthesia Care

The patient is transferred from the OR to the postanesthesia care unit (PACU) for close monitoring in the immediate postoperative period. Initial assessment is focused on the ABCs: airway, breathing, and circulation. Monitor the patient's airway, gas exchange, pulse oximetry, oxygen delivery, accessory muscle use, and breath sounds. The patient can develop stridor due to edema or bronchospasm. The cardiovascular status is checked next. Vital signs (pulse, respiratory rate, and blood pressure) are checked frequently until stabilized cardiac rhythm is monitored.

The surgical wound is checked for signs of drainage or bleeding. The dressing is checked. The drains are checked for output and patency. Tubes that need to be connected to suction (such as nasogastric tubes) are connected. Intravenous fluids are monitored.

Neurologic assessment is performed to check the level of consciousness. Following general anesthesia, the patient follows a predictable progression in the return to consciousness. Initially there is muscular irritability, and then restlessness followed by pain recognition and the ability to reason and control behavior. Pupil responses are monitored, looking for bilaterally equal responses to light. Motor responses are monitored, looking initially for purposeful response to painful stimuli and later for response to command. Pain treatment is begun during this time. As the anesthetic agent wears off, it is important to assess the patient's level of pain. This may be assessed through subjective information in patients who are conscious, or through more objective signs in patients who are still in semiconscious states. Monitor for changes in vital signs (elevated pulse and BP), changes in movement, and moaning. Expected pain levels can be estimated from the type of surgery and give a starting point for those patients as they begin to come out of the anesthesia.

Gastrointestinal status is monitored for the presence of nausea or vomiting. This may be a reaction or side effect to anesthesia. Check for abdominal distention and the presence of bowel sounds. Monitor drainage from the nasogastric tube; note the amount and color of drainage.

Monitor laboratory results as indicated. Electrolyte levels, hemoglobin or hematocrit levels, blood urea nitrogen (BUN) and creatinine, arterial blood gases (ABGs), or other studies may be necessary in the immediate postoperative period. The diagnostic studies necessary will depend on the patient's history, the estimated blood loss during surgery, and the type of procedure performed.

After the initial recovery time, the stable patient who is transferred from the PACU to the same-day surgical area continues to be monitored. Vital signs are taken, although not as frequently. Respiratory and cardiovascular functions are monitored. Cardiac rhythm may no longer need to be monitored, depending on the surgery and the patient's medical history. The dressing is checked for any drainage. Bowel sounds are checked. Clear fluids are given if the patient is not experiencing nausea. Patients are monitored for urinary output prior to being discharged to home.

Patients who are admitted to the hospital are transferred from the PACU to a surgical unit. Vital signs, respiration, and cardiovascular status are checked. The dressing is monitored for drainage; drainage tubes are monitored for output. Intravenous lines are monitored for signs of infiltration and proper flow rates. Bowel sounds are monitored.

Patients who are unstable or who have had extensive procedures are transferred to intensive care for close monitoring. Nurses who are used to caring for complex, unstable patients care for these patients. Occasionally, these patients will be transferred directly from the surgical suite to the ICU to be recovered in the critical care unit. Their vital signs and cardiac rhythms are closely monitored. Some patients will still be on mechanical ventilation.

Postoperative Complications

The focus of care that is common for all of these postoperative patients is identification of complications. Common complications involve the cardiac, respiratory, and gastrointestinal areas, and infections.

5. Cardiovascular Complications

What Went Wrong

Patients may develop cardiovascular complications due to the physiological stress of surgery, side effects of the anesthesia or other medications, or comorbidities. Myocardial infarction (MI), cardiac arrhythmias, or hypotension are likely during surgery or in the immediate postoperative period. When getting the patient out of bed for the first time after surgery, it is good practice to have the patient sit on the side of the bed for a minute or two before standing up to ascertain if the patient feels dizzy owing to a drop in blood pressure associated with position change. Deep vein thrombosis (DVT) is a later vascular complication associated with inflammation and decreased mobility after surgery.

Hallmark Signs and Symptoms

- Chest pain which may radiate to back, neck, jaw, or arm due to ischemia in MI
- Shortness of breath owing to altered cardiac output and tissue perfusion
- Dizziness or lightheadedness because of diminished cardiac output and cerebral tissue perfusion or cardiac arrhythmia
- Palpitations as a result of cardiac arrhythmia
- Cardiac arrhythmias due to myocardial irritability—possibly owing to ischemia, medication side effect, or electrolyte imbalance
- Low blood pressure because of diminished cardiac output
- Unilateral calf pain and lower extremity swelling owing to DVT

Common Test Results

- Elevated troponin levels in MI.
- EKG shows ST elevation or T-wave inversion with lack of oxygen delivery to myocardial tissue.
- Cardiac monitor or EKG shows arrhythmia.
- BP below normal level.
- Doppler ultrasound of extremity shows clot within blood vessel.

Treatment

- Monitor cardiac rhythm.
- Administer antiarrhythmic medications to stabilize cardiac rhythm.

- Administer intravenous fluids to expand circulating blood volume to raise blood pressure.
- Administer blood-thinning medications to decrease the likelihood of clot enlarging or additional clots forming.
  - heparin
  - low-molecular-weight-heparin
  - warfarin

Nursing Diagnoses

- Decreased cardiac output
- Ineffective cardiopulmonary tissue perfusion
- Ineffective peripheral tissue perfusion
- Impaired physical mobility

NURSING INTERVENTIONS

- Monitor vital signs for changes.
- Check blood pressure lying down and sitting up for orthostatic change.
- Monitor cardiovascular status for cardiac rhythm, heart sounds, peripheral pulses, capillary refill, and pulse deficit.
- Assess for peripheral edema.
- Ask patient about calf pain or tenderness.
- Monitor intravenous site for signs of infiltration.
- Encourage ambulation and leg exercises to prevent development of DVT.
- Monitor proper use of elastic stockings or sequential compression devices postoperatively.

6. Respiratory Complications

Patients with preexisting respiratory disorders, obesity, or thoracic or upper abdominal surgical procedures are at greater risk of developing respiratory complications postoperatively.

What Went Wrong

After surgery, patients are not as mobile. This lack of physical activity leads to diminished chest wall and diaphragmatic movement, resulting in a decreased amount of air exchange. Alveolar sacs can collapse, leading to areas of atelectasis. Pain medications can adversely affect respiratory status by decreasing respiratory drive. Patients at increased risk for respiratory complications may develop pneumonia in the postoperative period due to diminished airflow, increased respiratory secretions, and inflammatory processes. Patients with increased risk for clotting or DVT, or those with hypercoagulable states are at risk for developing a pulmonary embolism.

Hallmark Signs and Symptoms

- Shortness of breath due to diminished airflow and resultant decreased oxygenation
- Chest pain in the area of atelectasis owing to collapse of the alveolar sacs within that area of the lung
- Productive cough because of pneumonia
- Fever due to infection in pneumonia
- Sudden-onset chest pain and shortness of breath in pulmonary embolism as clot blocks arterial blood flow within the lung
- Diminished oxygen levels as gas exchange are impaired in atelectasis, pneumonia, or pulmonary embolism

Common Test Results

- Pulse oximetry shows diminished oxygenation.
- Chest x-ray shows the area of collapse in atelectasis, infiltrate in pneumonia, and wedge infiltrate in pulmonary embolism.
- CT scan shows alveolar collapse in atelectasis, area of infiltrate in pneumonia.
- Spiral CT or helical CT shows clot in pulmonary embolism.
- White blood cell (WBC) elevated in bacterial pneumonia.

Treatment

- Administer supplemental oxygen.
- Administer antibiotics for pneumonia—initially intravenously, then orally.
  - macrolides
  - fluoroquinolones

- Administer blood-thinning agents to prevent enlarging of clot or development of new clots in pulmonary embolism.
- Mechanical ventilation if necessary.

Nursing Diagnoses

- Ineffective breathing pattern
- Ineffective airway clearance
- Impaired gas exchange
- Ineffective cardiopulmonary tissue perfusion

NURSING INTERVENTIONS

- Monitor vital signs for changes.
- Monitor respiratory status: check respiratory rate, rhythm, and depth; check skin color; listen to breath sounds.
- Monitor pulse oximetry level for oxygenation.
- Monitor intravenous site for signs of infiltration.
- Encourage coughing and deep breathing exercises.
- Encourage incentive spirometer use.
- Encourage early ambulation.

7. Infection

The skin is the body's first line of defense against infection. During surgery this line of defense is penetrated. Even though the surgical procedure is performed in as aseptic an environment as possible, the possibility of infection still exists.

What Went Wrong

Wound infections can develop in the postoperative period. The wound may be contaminated before surgery, such as with penetrating trauma, or may become infected during healing. The surface of the skin has bacteria that are naturally present, referred to as normal flora. These bacteria may enter the wound and cause infection. Nosocomial infections can also occur at the surgical site, caused by bacteria found elsewhere in the hospital. Infection within the surgical wound will slow approximation of the wound edges, delaying wound healing.

Hallmark Signs and Symptoms

- Increase in pain at surgical wound due to inflammatory process early in infection
- Redness at wound edges which spreads if untreated
- Drainage from wound site owing to body's response to bacterial presence (change in color and odor of drainage)
- Fever because of infection
- Elevated WBC count

Common Test Results

- Elevated WBC due to body's response to bacterial presence.
- Elevated erythrocyte sedimentation rate due to inflammation.
- Culture of wound area will identify organism.
- Sensitivity test will identify appropriate antibiotic treatment.

Treatment

- Obtain culture and sensitivity test of wound.
- Administer appropriate antibiotics intravenously.
- Keep wound site clean and dry.

Nursing Diagnoses

- Risk for infection
- Impaired skin integrity
- Impaired tissue integrity
- Delayed surgical recovery

NURSING INTERVENTIONS

- Monitor vital signs; look for fever.
- Assess surgical wound for redness and drainage.
- Ask patient about pain at the surgical site.
- When obtaining wound culture, remove surface drainage with gauze, then obtain the specimen from within wound edge (this will ensure that the organism is actually from the wound and not from the skin).

8. Gastrointestinal Complications

Following administration of anesthesia or pain medication, patients may experience nausea, vomiting, constipation, or paralytic ileus.

What Went Wrong?

Nausea is a common side effect of both anesthesia and pain medications. A patient's reaction to anesthetic agents varies. Some patients have a lot of nausea after anesthesia that may last for several hours. Abdominal surgery may cause direct visceral afferent stimulation, resulting in nausea and vomiting. Medications may act upon the chemoreceptor trigger zone, located within the medulla outside the blood-brain barrier. Once the patient begins vomiting, antiemetic medication may be necessary to break the cycle. Opioid-based medications and decreased activity can both cause slowing of peristaltic activity, leading to constipation. Patients having abdominal procedures are at greater risk for paralytic ileus as a postoperative complication.

Hallmark Signs and Symptoms

- Nausea as a side effect of medication
- Vomiting due to visceral afferent stimulation or activation of chemoreceptor trigger zone
- Mild, generalized abdominal discomfort and distention with paralytic ileus owing to decreased intestinal motility
- Slow bowel sounds with constipation; absent bowel sounds with paralytic ileus because of changes in intestinal motility

Common Test Results

- Electrolyte abnormality due to vomiting.
- Abdominal flat and upright x-ray shows stool in constipation, gas-filled intestinal loops in paralytic ileus.

Treatment

- Monitor abdomen for distention; listen for bowel sounds.
- Assess for dehydration as a result of prolonged vomiting.
- Restrict oral intake in paralytic ileus or if nausea and vomiting are present.

- Nasogastric (NG) tube connected to suction to prevent vomiting in paralytic ileus.
- Progress diet as tolerated once bowel sounds return and patient is passing flatus rectally.
- Administer intravenous fluids.
- Administer total parenteral nutrition.
- Administer antiemetics as required.

Nursing Diagnoses

- Risk for imbalanced nutrition: less than what body requires
- Risk for imbalanced fluid volume
- Risk for delayed surgical recovery
- Risk for constipation
- Altered bowel elimination

NURSING INTERVENTIONS

- Ask the patient about the presence of nausea.
- Monitor vital signs for changes.
- Listen to bowel sounds; assess abdomen for distention.
- Monitor intravenous site for signs of infiltration, pain, and redness.
- Monitor intake and output.
- Monitor color and the amount of fluid drained from the NG tube.
- Ask patient if he or she is passing any flatus rectally or having bowel movement.

REVIEW QUESTIONS

1. **Donna is a healthy, 38-year-old woman scheduled for elective surgery next week. During the preoperative clearance, the physician, nurse practitioner, or physician assistant would include which of the following in her preoperative preparation?**

   A. Pulmonary function test and chest x-ray.

   B. Complete blood count, metabolic panel, and pregnancy test.

   C. Urine culture, thyroid panel, and cortisol level.

   D. Glucose tolerance test, ankle-brachial index, and electrocardiogram (EKG).

2. Lucinda is a 27-year-old woman with a history of asthma who is scheduled for an appendectomy later today. Due to her asthma, her preoperative teaching would include the need for postoperative:

   A. coughing and deep breathing exercises.
   B. leg exercises.
   C. wound dressing changes.
   D. all of the above.

3. Josie is the mother of a healthy 19-year-old woman having surgery tomorrow. After the surgeon discusses the surgery, risks, and benefits with the patient and her mother, the mother wants to sign the consent form. The most appropriate response to this would be:

   A. of course, she can sign the consent form; after all the patient is her daughter.
   B. no, she cannot sign the form.
   C. while you appreciate her concern for her daughter, the patient is a consenting adult and legally needs to sign her own consent form.
   D. encourage both the patient and her mother to sign the form.

4. Which member of the surgical team does not scrub into the operating room?

   A. The surgeon.
   B. The circulating nurse.
   C. The scrub nurse or surgical tech.
   D. The holding area nurse.

5. Suzette is having a minor surgical procedure performed in same-day surgical setting. Which type of anesthesia is most likely to be used?

   A. General.
   B. Epidural.
   C. Regional.
   D. Conscious sedation.

6. 65-year-old Dominic is being transferred into the PACU from the OR. Once there, initial assessment will focus on:

   A. Airway, breathing, circulation, and wound site.
   B. Intake, output, and intravenous access.
   C. Abdominal sounds, oxygen setting, and level of consciousness.
   D. Pulse oximeter, pupil responses, and deep tendon reflexes.

7. Denise is recovering from an open cholecystectomy. You know that because of the location of the surgery, she has an increased risk of postoperative:

   A. Myocardial infarction.
   B. Respiratory complications.

C. Deep vein thrombosis.

D. Wound infection.

8. **Three days after surgery, Mark notices that the wound site is more painful now than it was the day before. When you inspect the surgical site you are looking for redness or inflammation. Other indicators of infection would include:**

A. Elevated RBC and elevated respiratory rate.

B. Elevated WBC and elevated temperature.

C. Elevated erythrocyte sedimentation rate and decreased pulse.

D. Decreased platelets and decreased blood pressure.

9. **Paralytic ileus may occur as a postoperative complication. Which of the following patients would you be most concerned about the development of paralytic ileus?**

A. Kim, a 27-year-old postlaparoscopic appendectomy.

B. Joyce, a 39-year-old post–open right hemicolectomy.

C. Nancy, a 56-year-old postmediastinoscopy.

D. John, a 47-year-old post–total joint replacement.

10. **Steve has developed pneumonia following intrathoracic surgery performed last week. He has no comorbidities and the hospital does not have a high rate of MRSA infections. Treatment for postoperative pneumonia would most likely include a:**

A. Cephalosporin, such as cefazolin.

B. Penicillin, such as amoxicillin.

C. Fluoroquinolone, such as levofloxacin.

D. Tetracycline, such as doxycycline.

Chapter 14

Women's Health

LEARNING OBJECTIVES

At the end of this chapter, the student will be able to:

- Identify normal anatomy and physiology related to the female reproductive system
- Discuss the diseases-causing pathologic changes within the female reproductive system
- List four signs or symptoms of specific female reproductive disease or injury
- Recognize expected nursing and medical management of conditions or diseases specific to women's health

KEY CONCEPTS

1. Breast cancer
2. Cervical cancer
3. Dysmenorrhea
4. Ectopic pregnancy
5. Endometrial cancer
6. Fibroids (leiomyomas)
7. Infertility
8. Labor and delivery
9. Menopause
10. Ovarian cancer
11. Ovarian masses, benign
12. Pelvic inflammatory disease
13. Postpartum
14. Preeclampsia and eclampsia
15. Pregnancy
16. Rh incompatibility
17. Trophoblastic disease

KEY TERMS

Anovulation
Beta hCG serum levels
BRCA1
BRCA2
Cervical intraepithelial neoplasia (CIN)
Chemotherapy
Cone biopsy
Corpus luteum
Cryotherapy
Egg follicle
Endometrium
Estrogen
Follicle-stimulating hormone (FSH)
Human papillomavirus (HPV)
Leiomyomas
Luteal phase
Luteinizing hormone (LH)
Mastectomy
Menarche
Menstrual cycle
Menstruation
Oocyte
Papanicolaou (Pap) smear

The Female Body

The menstrual cycle is the series of changes a woman's body goes through monthly to prepare for conception and a growing fetus. If fertilization does not occur, the uterus will remove the prepared lining, termed menstrual bleeding. Figure 14–1 shows the anatomy of the female reproductive system. Menstruation begins in the early teens (menarche) and ends around the age of 50 years (menopause). The average age of menarche for African-Americans is 9 to 11 years while for Caucasians it is from 10 to 12 years. The cycle is controlled by hormones from the hypothalamus, pituitary, ovaries, and the uterus.

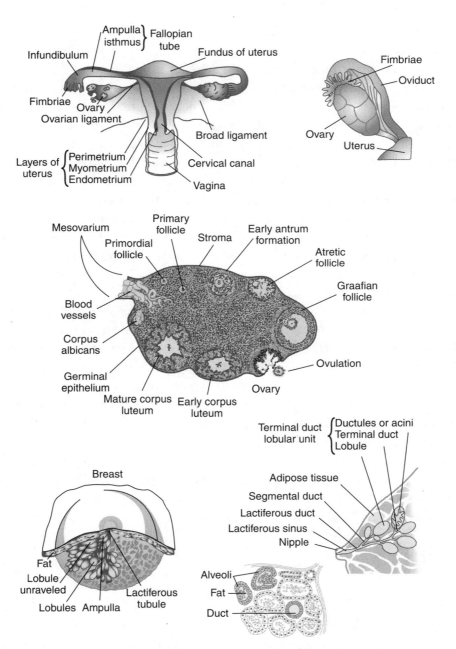

FIGURE 14–1 · Functional anatomy of the female reproductive tract. The female reproductive organs include the ovaries, the uterus, fallopian tubes, and the breasts or mammary glands.

Source: Reproduced with permission from: Molina PE: *Endocrine Physiology*, 3rd ed. New York, NY: McGraw-Hill; 2010, Fig. 9–1.

A normal menstrual cycle is 28 days, but only about 25% of women actually are on this schedule. The average can run from 21 to 35 days. The menstrual cycle is often divided into three phases, depending on the hormones.

The beginning of menstruation is the start of the follicular phase which lasts until day 14. As hormone levels are low, the thickened lining of the uterus begins to shed. The cramping that is felt is from small uterine contractions, helping to shed the lining. An egg follicle begins to mature due to growing levels of follicle-stimulating hormone (FSH), which also causes estrogen secretion. The increase in estrogen causes the endometrium to mature and thicken. The last 5 days of the follicular phase plus the day of ovulation are the most fertile days. Upon ovulation, on day 14, the oocyte, or egg, is released from the follicle due to a surge in luteinizing hormone (LH). The egg is expelled near the opening of one of the fallopian tubes (oviducts, uterine tubes), located laterally at the top of the uterus. Fertilization usually occurs in one of the tubes. The embryo now travels to the uterus, the primary job of which is to sustain development. A nonpregnant uterus measures about 7×5 cm. As it is a muscular organ, it is capable of great stretching. At the distal end of the uterus is the cervix which attaches to the superior portion of the vagina. The luteal phase starts next with LH causing the follicle to secrete progesterone instead of estrogen. Progesterone causes the endometrial lining to begin to thicken in preparation for implantation of a fertilized cell. Progesterone inhibits release of FSH and LH. If fertilization does not occur, the corpus luteum, containing the oocyte, dies, which lowers the level of progesterone. Sloughing of the lining begins about the 28th day of the cycle, resulting in a flow of blood and cellular debris through the vagina. The cycle will begin again. Primary amenorrhea is the absence of menses by the age of 16. Secondary amenorrhea is the absence of menses for more than 6 months in a woman who previously was menstruating regularly.

Just the Facts

1. Breast Cancer

Studies show that by the age of 80, about 1 in 8 women will have breast cancer. Ten percent of all breast cancers are inherited. Two major genes have been identified—BRCA1 and BRCA2.

What Went Wrong

Despite the research and advances in medicine, the cause of breast cancer is unknown. Some studies have implicated a higher-fat diet. Some medications, like estrogen, seem to increase the risk of breast cancer. Exposure to radiation also increases the risk. Childlessness and delayed childbirth also may be factors.

Prognosis

Breast cancer is the second leading cause of cancer death in women and the number one cancer in women. Prognosis depends on the stage at which the cancer is discovered. Those with no involved lymph nodes have the best expectations with a survival rate of 95% over 10 years. With lymph node involvement, survival ranges from 50% to 75% for 5 years.

Hallmark Signs and Symptoms

- Mass in breast, usually painless
- Nipple inversion, drainage
- Breast skin edema or "peau d' orange" leather-like appearance to the skin on the breast
- Dimpling in the skin of the breast
- Enlarged lymph glands, palpable in the axillary or supraclavicular areas
- Bone pain from metastasis
- Cough from lung metastasis

Common Test Results

- Mammography may show mass or abnormality
- Ultrasonography to further delineate the mass
- MRI of breast
- Biopsy is confirmative for cancer
- CT scan to check for metastasis

Treatments

Treatment for breast cancer is either curative or palliative, depending on the staging of the tumor and involvement of lymph nodes.

- Lumpectomy for small tumors and breast conservation.
- Mastectomy for larger tumors or more than two tumors in the same breast.
- Chemotherapy before surgery to shrink some tumors, or after surgery

- First-line regimes
  - Adriamycin and cytoxan
  - cytoxan, methotrexate and 5-fluorouracil
  - paclitaxel
  - docetaxel
- Hormonal therapy
  - For all estrogen receptor positive cancers
  - tamoxifen
- Use of nonsteroidal aromatase inhibitors
  - anastrozole used in postmenopausal women with early stage breast cancer, or in patients who have not responded to tamoxifen
- Radiation therapy
- Prophylactic bilateral mastectomy for women with BRCA1 or BRCA2 genes

Nursing Diagnoses
- Body image disturbance
- Anticipatory grieving
- Altered sexuality patterns

NURSING INTERVENTIONS

- Allow patient to voice concerns and questions over treatment plans.
- Monitor incision site, dressing, and drainage.
- Check for signs and symptoms of infection.
- **Explain to the patient:**
  - Disease process.
  - Use of affected arm.
  - Use of pain medication, timing, and side effects.
  - Urge follow-up mammography and treatment plan.
  - Discuss low-fat diet.
  - Encourage participation in support groups.

2. Fibroadenoma

This is a benign tumor that develops from breast tissue.

What Went Wrong

Fibroadenomas are composed of glandular tissue found within the breast. The cause of fibroadenomas is unknown.

Prognosis

This is a benign condition that will have a minimal effect on patient's overall health but may cause anxiety when a breast lump is first discovered.

Hallmark Signs and Symptoms

Nontender firm, rubbery, and breast mass that is encapsulated and well defined. Usually, 1 to 2 cm in diameter but may become larger, mass is painless. Mass is easily movable under the skin and there is no nipple discharge.

Common Test Results

- Ultrasound of breast
- Biopsy—may be open, guided by ultrasound or stereotaxic
- Mammogram

Treatment

- Observation and reevaluation of mass to assess growth
- Surgical excision

Nursing Diagnoses

- Body image disturbance
- Anxiety

NURSING INTERVENTIONS

- **Teach the patient:**
  - Disease process.
  - Follow-up examinations.
  - Importance of follow-up mammography.

---

2. Cervical Cancer

The Papanicolaou (Pap) smear has markedly increased early detection of cervical cancer and thus decreased the mortality.

What Went Wrong

Abnormal cells, cervical intraepithelial neoplasia (CIN), are the initial indication on a Pap smear, and they are more common in women with HIV and those infected with human *Papillomavirus* (HPV), subtypes 16, 18, 31, 33, 35, 39, 45, 51, 52, 58 (see Fig. 14–2). HPV is more common in women with multiple sexual partners, those having sex at an early age, and those with HIV or other immunosuppressive disorders. Smoking is also a risk factor.

Prognosis

Prognosis depends on the stage at which the cancer is discovered. The 5-year survival rate ranges as follows:

Stage I—85%
Stage II—65%
Stage III—35%
Stage IV—10%

Hallmark Signs and Symptoms

- Abnormal vaginal bleeding due to abnormal cells and ulceration of the cervix

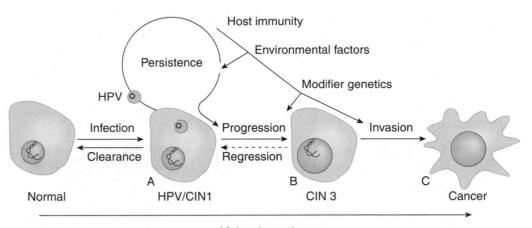

FIGURE 14–2 • Diagram illustrating genesis of cervical cancers. There are two critical endpoints on the spectrum of cervical dysplasia. A. This initial point represents the cell at risk due to active HPV infection. The HPV genome exists as a plasmid, separate from the host DNA. B. The clinically relevant preinvasive lesion, cervical intraepithelial neoplasia 3 (CIN 3) or carcinoma in situ (CIS), represents an intermediate stage in cervical cancer development. The HPV genome (red DNA strand) has become integrated into the host DNA, resulting in increased proliferative ability. C. Interactive effects between environmental insults, host immunity, and somatic cell genomic variations lead to invasive cervical cancer.

Source: Reproduced with permission from: Hoffman BL, Schorge JO, Schaffer JI, Halvorson LM, Bradshaw KD, Cunningham FG: *Williams Gynecology*, 2nd ed. New York, NY: McGraw-Hill; 2012. Fig. 30–1.

- Postcoital bleeding
- Pelvic or abdominal pain

Common Test Results

- Pap smear
- Colposcopy
- Biopsy to confirm disease and determine staging
- Cone biopsy which provides a sample of tissue of the lateral margins of the cervix

Treatment

- Cone biopsy may remove enough of the dysplasia.
- Ablation of the lesion with cryotherapy, which freezes the cells.
- Hysterectomy with lymph node biopsy for women with late-stage cancer or those with early-stage cancer who have completed childbearing.
- Radiation.
- Chemotherapy.
  - cisplatin
  - 5-fluorouracil

Nursing Diagnoses

- Altered sexuality patterns
- Personal identity disturbance
- Disturbance in self-esteem

NURSING INTERVENTIONS

- HPV vaccine as ordered.
- Offer pain and antiemetic medications.
- Abdominal assessment—distention, bowel sounds.
- Evaluate for vaginal bleeding.
- Assess urinary retention.

- Intake and output.
- Assess vital signs; check for fever.
- Remove vaginal packing when directed.
- Emotional reassurances.
- **Explain to the patient:**
  - Need for Pap tests as recommended.
  - All procedures.
  - Support through cancer treatments.
  - Use of pain relieving and antiemetic medications.
  - Benefit of early ambulation.
  - Safer sex practices.

3. Dysmenorrhea

Pain during menses that is not caused by any other pathologic condition is called primary dysmenorrhea. Pain during menses related to an underlying pelvic condition is called secondary dysmenorrhea.

What Went Wrong

Primary dysmenorrhea is caused by the changing hormones in the reproductive cycle. Uterine contractions from prostaglandins and blood vessel constriction in the uterine lining cause the discomfort as the enriched lining prepares to be sloughed off.

Secondary dysmenorrhea is caused by pelvic pathology such as tumors, sexually transmitted disease, or endometriosis.

Prognosis

Dysmenorrhea usually begins 1 to 2 years after menarche and becomes more acute with age. Pregnancy often diminishes the severity of dysmenorrhea, as does age. Some women are debilitated for several days per month. A large majority of women experience some degree of discomfort.

Hallmark Signs and Symptoms

- Cramps from small uterine contractions
- Lower abdominal pain and low back pain

- Nausea from fluctuating hormone levels
- Headache from declining hormone levels

Common Diagnostic Tests

- Pelvic examination is normal.
- Hemoglobin and hematocrit may be slightly low from excessive blood loss.
- Transvaginal ultrasound.

Treatment

- Over-the-counter preparations such as
  - Hot water bottles
- Home remedies
  - Herbal preparations
- Nonsteroidal anti-inflammatory drugs (NSAIDs) have antiprostaglandin activities, which decrease the discomfort.
  - ibuprofen
  - naproxen
  - nabumetone
- Oral contraceptives which inhibit ovulation as well as diminish the amount of menstrual flow and dysmenorrhea.

Nursing Diagnoses

- Intolerance for activity
- Pain, discomfort

NURSING INTERVENTIONS

- **Explain to the patient:**
  - The disease.
  - Benefit of exercise.
  - Medication use, timing, and side effects.

---

4. Ectopic Pregnancy

Ectopic pregnancy occurs when the fertilized ovum implants in an area other than the uterus. Most ectopic pregnancies occur in the fallopian tubes;

however, other possible sites for ectopic pregnancy include the ovary, cervix, and peritoneum.

What Went Wrong
When the fertilized ovum is unable to get to the uterus, it may settle in the fallopian tube. Any blockage, stricture, previous surgery on the tube, infection, or inflammation may impede the ovum from its final, proper destination.

Prognosis
Ectopic pregnancy is the greatest cause of maternal death early in the pregnancy if diagnosis cannot be made. Rupture of the involved organ and excessive bleeding into the peritoneum may occur.

Hallmark Signs and Symptoms
- Severe, lancinating (stabbing) lower pelvic pain from the growing embryo stretching the fallopian tube or other structure
- Backache from pressure on these structures
- Vaginal spotting; bleeding; amenorrhea

Common Test Results
- Beta hCG serum levels will be elevated but not as high as during an intrauterine pregnancy.
- Ultrasound will show an empty uterus.
- Urine pregnancy test will be positive.

Treatment
Surgery is planned to remove the fertilized egg. Often the egg can be retrieved laparoscopically if the pregnancy is early. Surgery will involve removal of the egg and may involve partial or complete removal of the fallopian tube (called salpingectomy—partial or complete).

Medical management of an ectopic pregnancy may be ordered for small ectopic pregnancies that have not ruptured. The most common treatment is methotrexate given for several doses.

Nursing Diagnoses
- Body image disturbance

- Anticipatory grieving
- Pain, discomfort

NURSING INTERVENTIONS

- **For surgical intervention:**
  - Check vaginal bleeding.
  - Check incision site.
  - Assess abdomen—bowel sounds, distention.
  - Assess voiding patterns.
  - Administer pain medication.
  - Check vital signs, temperature.
- **Explain to the patient:**
  - Use of pain medication.
  - Benefit of early ambulation.
  - Increased chance of future ectopic pregnancies.
- **For medical intervention:**
  - Pain and vaginal bleeding may occur, if severe bleeding occurs notify physician.
  - Avoid alcoholic beverages.

5. Endometrial Cancer

Endometrial cancer is one of the most common gynecologic cancers in women, and it is most often diagnosed in postmenopausal women.

What Went Wrong

Abnormal tissue grows rapidly, affected most often by estrogen. Eventually, this abnormal tissue, hyperplasia, turns into a cancer. Some causes of elevated estrogen levels are exogenous estrogen, polycystic ovarian disease, and estrogen-producing tumors. Risk factors for endometrial cancer include endometrial hyperplasia, tamoxifen, diabetes type II, nulliparity, and obesity (estrogen is stored in adipose tissue).

Prognosis

Prognosis depends on the stage and grade of the cancer upon diagnosis. Staging of the tumor (I–IV) can only be done via surgery, and grading is based on the histology of the tumor (GI, GII, GIII). In patients with stage IV, the 5-year survival rate is 26%.

Hallmark Signs and Symptoms

- Abnormal bleeding
- Postmenopausal bleeding
- Abnormal Pap test that contains endometrial cells

Common Test Results

- Pap test
- Endometrial biopsy
- Endocervical curettage
- Ca-125 (more commonly used to monitor ovarian cancer patient's response to treatment
- Transvaginal ultrasound
- CT scan
- MRI

Treatment

- Surgery initially for staging and to remove the tumor—usually hysterectomy, bilateral salpingo-oophorectomy, biopsy of nodes.
- Radiation.
- Hormone therapy.
  - progestins
- Chemotherapy used for cancers that recur outside the pelvis.
  - doxorubicin
  - cisplatin
  - ifosfamide

Nursing Diagnoses

- Anticipatory grieving
- Body image disturbance
- Sexual dysfunction

NURSING INTERVENTIONS

- Check vaginal bleeding.
- Check incision site.
- Assess abdomen for bowel sounds, distention.
- Check urinary output.
- Administer pain medication.
- Check vital signs, temperature.
- Emotional reassurance.
- **Explain to the patient:**
  - Use of pain medication.
  - Benefit of early ambulation.
  - Increased chance of future ectopic pregnancies.

6. Fibroids (Leiomyomas)

Leiomyomas are benign, smooth muscle tumors of the uterus. Since they are hormone-receptive, the tumors will change in size with the menses.

What Went Wrong

It is unknown what causes the proliferation of these smooth muscle tumors. Fibroids are more common in African-American women.

Prognosis

Since the tumors are hormone-responsive, they will shrink with menopause. However, in patients with large tumors, pain, and excessive bleeding, treatment is necessary.

Hallmark Signs and Symptoms

- Heavy menstrual bleeding
- Anemia
- Pelvic pain, from a large tumor
- Pelvic pressure

Common Test Results

- Laboratory work will show a declining Hgb and Hct.
- Ultrasound, MRI, CT scan, and hysteroscopy will all show a tumor.

Treatment

- Watchful waiting.
- Surgery—myomectomy if childbearing is to be preserved, or hysterectomy if childbearing is completed.
- Hormones may help to shrink the tumor.
  - Uterine artery embolization.

Nursing Diagnoses

- Pain, discomfort
- Fatigue
- Disturbed body image

NURSING INTERVENTIONS

- Monitor CBC to check anemia.
- Check vaginal bleeding.
- Check incision site.
- Administer pain medication.
- Check vital signs, temperature.
- **Explain to the patient:**
  - Use of pain medication.
  - Increased chance of future ectopic pregnancies.
  - Encourage early ambulation.

---

7. Infertility

Infertility is the inability of a reproductive-age couple to conceive after 12 months of unprotected sexual intercourse. More than 50% of the time the reproductive tract of the woman is at issue. Primary infertility is when a woman has never had a pregnancy; secondary is when it occurs in a woman who has had one or more pregnancies.

What Went Wrong

At fault may be decreased secretion of hormones from the anterior pituitary, failure to ovulate, endometriosis, or past infections causing blockage of the reproductive tract. Structural problems (blocked fallopian tubes, or anovulation), poor sperm motility and/or count, or multifactorial problems can cause infertility. Prior exposure to radiation, medications, exercise frequency, and menstrual cycle and length need to be evaluated. The male partner may have been exposed to conditions or illness that may have affected his sperm production. As a woman ages the ability to conceive decreases.

Prognosis

Infertility affects about 15% or more of couples. Ability to conceive depends on exact cause of the infertility.

Hallmark Signs and Symptoms

- Inability to achieve conception

Common Test Results

- Semen analysis
  - Ovulation tests
- Menstrual diary
- Sonogram to view endometrial anatomy
- Endometrial biopsy to check on hormone status and to determine if the lining is able to support a fertilized ovum, and if leiomyomas are present
- Laboratory work: hormone levels—progesterone, LH, FSH, and TSH to check on normal uterine, ovarian, pituitary, and thyroid function
- Hysterosalpingogram to view uterus, fallopian tubes
- Postcoital test—cervix is checked for patency and whether the mucous is thin enough for sperm to penetrate

Treatment

- Treatments depend on the cause of the infertility.
- For abnormal sperm findings:
  - Urology referral for the male partner
  - Check medications—calcium channel blockers can impair sperm function
  - Artificial insemination
- For anovulation:
  - LH/FSH to stimulate ovulation

- bromocriptine for hypothalamic dysfunction
- clomiphene to stimulate ovulation
- For structural aberrations:
  - Surgery to repair tube
  - Myomectomy to remove leiomyomas
  - Surgery to lysis adhesions
  - In vitro fertilization

Nursing Diagnoses

- Body image disturbance
- Defensive coping
- Risk for parenting

NURSING INTERVENTIONS

- **Explain to the patient:**
  - Suggest support groups.
  - Encourage questions.
  - Discuss tests.

8. Menopause

Menopause is defined as 12 months without menses. Few follicles are left to mature, levels of hormones decline, ovulation no longer occurs, and the uterine lining no longer needs to thicken in preparation for a fertilized egg.

What Went Wrong

- Natural progression of life

Prognosis

The average age of menopause in the United States is 51. About 50% of American women experience some symptoms of menopause.

Hallmark Signs and Symptoms

- Lack of menstrual cycle
- Breasts, vagina, and uterus shrink in response to decreased estrogen and progesterone

- Vasomotor flushing due to estrogen levels falling
- Moodiness because of changing hormone levels
- Cardiovascular risks increase as a result of less estrogen
- Osteoporosis is a risk factor due to less estrogen
- Vaginal mucous dryness from decreased levels of hormones

Common Test Results

- Increase in FSH during menopause
- Decrease in LH during menopause
- Estrogen levels decline

Treatment

Some women elect to begin hormone replacement therapy (HRT) (in women with a uterus) or estrogen replacement therapy (ERT) (in women without a uterus), to ameliorate the vasomotor flushing and menopausal signs and symptoms, and to decrease the risk of osteoporosis.

Nursing Diagnoses

- Effective management of individual therapeutic regimen
- Decisional conflict
- Personal identity disturbance

NURSING INTERVENTIONS

- **Explain to the patient:**
  - Bodily changes.
  - Effects of HRT and ERT.

---

9. Ovarian Cancer

Ovarian cancer is the deadliest gynecologic cancer because it is usually advanced before it is detected. There is no proven screening test for ovarian cancer. There are no definitive early signs. Some women experience vague abdominal discomfort and bloating.

What Went Wrong

A woman, who has never had a child or who has had only one or two children, is at higher risk for ovarian cancer. Women with a history of breast cancer, colon cancer, or a family history of these are at a higher risk of ovarian cancer. There is an association between endometriosis and ovarian cancer. A gene mutation (ARID1A) appears to be shared by endometriosis and two types of ovarian cancer.

Prognosis

Unfortunately, prognosis for ovarian cancer is poor. Over 75% of women are diagnosed at an advanced stage. The prognosis is more grim if the CA-125 level is elevated, and if the disease has spread. The prognosis for ovarian cancer depends on the stage at which it was diagnosed. The scale for staging ranges from I to VI. The higher the staging, the worse the prognosis. Stage I has a 5-year survival rate of 80% to 90%, Stage IV has a 5-year survival rate of 20% to 30%.

Hallmark Signs and Symptoms

- Many women affected by the early stages of the disease are asymptomatic. As the disease progresses symptoms develop.
- Bloating from the enlarging tumor.
  - Increased abdominal girth.
  - Constipation.
  - Abnormal vaginal bleeding.
  - Satiety after eating a small amount of food.
- Pelvic mass.
- Dyspnea due to pressure from the diaphragm from an enlarging tumor.
- Ascites—abnormal abdominal fluid.

Common Test Results

- An elevated CA-125 indicates a tumor may be malignant.
- Transvaginal ultrasound for detection of disease.
- CT scan

Treatment

- Treatment depends on the staging at diagnosis.
- Surgical staging is necessary.
- Complete abdominal hysterectomy, with bilateral salpingo-oophorectomy, omentectomy, and node dissection.

- Complete removal of all visible tumor and metastasis-debulking.
- Chemotherapy.
  - cisplatin
  - carboplatin
  - paclitaxel
- Radiation.

Nursing Diagnoses

- Ineffective breathing pattern
- Hopelessness
- Anxiety

NURSING INTERVENTIONS

- Monitor CBC to check anemia.
- Check vaginal bleeding.
- Check incision site.
- Abdominal assessment—check for bowel sounds, distention.
- Check vital signs, temperature.
- Administer pain medication.
- Emotional reassurance.
- **Explain to the patient:**
  - Benefit of early ambulation.
  - Use of pain medication.
  - Treatments promoted by the oncologist.

---

10. Ovarian Masses, Benign

The most common ovarian cysts are follicular. Other types of ovarian masses include endometriomas and dermoid cysts.

What Went Wrong

In follicular ovarian cyst, the cause is a disruption in normal ovulation. Usually, the egg is enclosed in a follicle as it waits to be expelled monthly from the ovary. When the follicle does not open to allow the egg out or the follicle is not reabsorbed, a benign cyst, a fluid-filled sac, may result.

An endometrioma is caused by endometrial tissue forming a cyst on the ovary. Dermoid cysts are benign germ cell tumors commonly found in adolescents.

Prognosis

Most follicular cysts resolve in several months. However, a small percentage of patients experience discomfort or pain when the cyst does not resolve.

Endometriomas and dermoid cysts require examination by a pathologist. If examination is benign, surgical excision will treat the condition.

Hallmark Signs and Symptoms

- Asymptomatic
- Changes in menstruation
- Unilateral pelvic pain (usually one ovary is involved)
- Sharp pelvic pain, which indicates rupture
- Dyspareunia

Common Test Results

- Pregnancy test
- Pelvic examination
- Ultrasound

Treatment

- Watchful waiting since most cysts resolve
- Oral contraceptives
- Surgery to remove the cyst

Nursing Diagnoses

- Pain, discomfort
- Anxiety

NURSING INTERVENTIONS

- Reassure her that a large majority of cysts resolve.
- **Explain to the patient:**
  - Cause of her pain.
  - The menstrual cycle, pain may be worse during ovulation.
  - Medication use.

11. Pelvic Inflammatory Disease

Pelvic inflammatory disease (PID) is a variety of inflammation and infection of the upper genital tract, which includes the uterus, fallopian tubes, ovaries, and other structures. It includes endometritis, salpingitis, oophoritis, tubo-ovarian abscess, and pelvic peritonitis.

What Went Wrong

Bacteria from the cervix and vagina migrate to the upper genital tract. Usual organisms include *Chlamydia trachomatis, Neisseria gonorrhoeae, Escherichia coli*, and *Bacteroides*. Most infections are due to a mix of bacteria. PID occurs most often in sexually active women, and it is more common in adolescents. PID is more common with multiple sexual partners, a young age, unprotected sex, and a history of sexually transmitted disease.

Prognosis

About one in ten sexually active women will experience PID in her lifetime and 25% of those will experience a major complication such as infertility, ectopic pregnancy, abscess, or chronic pain.

Hallmark Signs and Symptoms

- Abdominal tenderness
- Adnexal tenderness (ovaries and fallopian tubes)
- Cervical motion tenderness (pain on movement of the cervix) due to an infection
- Fever
- Vaginal discharge
- Dyspareunia (pain during intercourse)
- Elevated WBC count

Common Test Results

- CBC will show an elevated WBC.
- Pregnancy test—beta hCG.
- Chlamydia test.
- Gonorrhea test.
- Rapid plasma reagin (RPR) test for syphilis.

- Fluorescent treponemal antibody (FTA–ABS) test used to confirm syphilis.
- Chandelier sign—a great amount of pain is elicited when the cervix is touched (the woman will jump to the chandelier).

Treatment

- Most patients are able to be managed in an outpatient setting with antibiotics.
  - ofloxacin and metronidazole
  - ceftriaxone and doxycycline
  - azithromycin and metronidazole
- Those who are pregnant, who present with an abscess or peritonitis, or with GI symptoms require inpatient treatment.
  - cefotetan and doxycycline
  - clindamycin and gentamycin
  - azithromycin and metronidazole
- Sexual partners must also be treated.

Nursing Diagnoses

- Pain, discomfort
- Sexual dysfunction
- Risk of infection

NURSING INTERVENTIONS

- **Teach patient about:**
  - Spread of the disease.
  - Practicing safe sex.
  - Medication use and side effects.
  - Necessity of treating all partners.

12. Trophoblastic Disease

Trophoblastic neoplasias are abnormal cells that have resulted from an abnormal fertilization. There are four types of trophoblastic disease, hydatidiform mole (partial or complete), invasive mole, choriocarcinoma, and placental site trophoblastic tumor. A complete mole is formed when an egg that has no DNA is fertilized by a sperm. A partial mole has DNA from both parents and usually fetal parts. An invasive mole is a hydatidiform mole that has invaded the endometrium. Placental site trophoblastic tumors are trophoblasts which intrude the myometrium. If untreated, trophoblastic disease may develop into choriocarcinoma, a malignant disease. All of the trophoblastic diseases require a full metastatic workup, including CT scan of brain, kidneys, liver, and lung. Serial monitoring of human chorionic gonadotropin (hCG) levels is required to assess progression of disease.

What Went Wrong

There is thought to be a problem with the genetic material of the zygotes. The chances are increased with very young women or older women, prior molar pregnancy, and a history of miscarriage.

Prognosis

Prognosis is the best for a woman diagnosed with a hydatidiform mole. Approximately 20% of complete mole pregnancies result in further trophoblastic disease. The remaining three diagnoses may develop into malignancy. Most nonmetastatic malignancies have a good remission rate after treatment.

Hallmark Signs and Symptoms

- Usual pregnancy signs during the first trimester
- Vaginal passing of a grapelike cluster of vesicles
- Vaginal bleeding
- Abnormally elevated hCG
- Abnormally large uterus
- Absence of fetal heart tones
- Elevated blood pressure
  - Absence of fetus on ultrasound

Common Test Results

- Pelvic examination
- hCG higher than expected serum levels in blood pregnancy test
- Ultrasound

Treatment

- Dilation and curettage (D&C) to remove all trophoblastic cells
- Frequent testing of hCG levels to ensure no further cells remain
- Chest x-ray to assess for lung metastasis
- Liver function tests to assess for liver metastasis
- Contraception for a full year
- Chemotherapy till hCG levels return to normal
  - methotrexate
  - actinomycin-D
- Total abdominal hysterectomy and chemotherapy

Nursing Diagnoses

- Risk of altered parenting
- Anticipatory grieving
- Powerlessness

NURSING INTERVENTIONS

- **Explain to the patient:**
  - Trophoblastic disease.
  - Discuss further testing.
  - Allow for grieving.
  - Provide referrals to counselors, clergy.
  - Discuss need for year-long birth control.

13. Pregnancy

Gestational age is measured from the first day of the last menstrual period (LMP). Forty weeks from the LMP is the estimated due date.

Pregnancy is usually divided into trimesters. At each prenatal visit, the fundus (the top of the uterus) will be measured as to its location in the abdomen. This information is used to assess the growth of the fetus. After 20 weeks fundal height is measured in centimeters. Normal fundal height is equal in centimeters to the week of gestation.

The first trimester is from 0 to 14 weeks, and it starts at implantation. During this time, it is not uncommon to feel more fatigue, nausea, and morning sickness. At 2 months, the uterus is the size of a grapefruit. At 9 weeks, the embryo is called a fetus and is about 1 inch in length. During the first trimester, most major organs have developed.

The second trimester is from 14 to 28 weeks, and it is characterized by less breast tenderness, less fatigue, and a diminishing of morning sickness. However, some back pain may begin, as well as stretch marks, heartburn, and hemorrhoids. At 16 weeks, the fundus is halfway between the pubic bone and the umbilicus. At 16 to 18 weeks, fetal movement may be felt.

At 27 weeks, the fundus is 2 inches above the umbilicus or 27 cm. The third trimester is from 28 weeks to birth. Due to the limited space the fetus will not be able to change position as easily but the mother should still perceive fetal movement. The mother may feel some respiratory difficulty as the uterus is directly underneath the diaphragm, pushing up the lungs. She may experience some edema, have difficulty sleeping, and an increased urge to urinate due to pressure on the bladder. She may feel Braxton-Hicks contractions, which are mild abdominal cramping.

What Went Wrong
Normal complaints of pregnancy

Prognosis
Healthy baby after 9 months of gestation.

Hallmark Signs and Symptoms
Symptoms and signs are usually due to pregnancy, but none are diagnostic.

- Symptoms:
  - Nausea, vomiting
  - Breast enlargement and tenderness
  - Quickening (feeling fetal movements) at approximately 20 weeks
  - Weight gain
  - Absence of menses
- Signs:
  - Abdominal enlargement
  - Breast enlargement
  - Softening of cervix
  - Increased pigmentation and enlargement of areolae

- Chadwick's sign—vagina and cervix show a blue hue from increased vasculature
- Definitive signs:
  - Fetal heart sounds
  - Fetal appearance on ultrasound

Common Test Results

- Human chorionic gonadotropin
  - Plasma hCG—positive 3 to 4 weeks after LMP
  - Urine hCG—positive 1 week after first missed menses
  - Serum hCG—will also be elevated in ectopic pregnancy, trophoblastic tumors
  - Fetal heart tones—a positive test of pregnancy
  - Ultrasound—confirms pregnancy

Treatment

- Regular visits to healthcare provider
- Prenatal vitamins
- Routine laboratory work
- Ultrasound

Nursing Diagnoses

- Altered nutrition
- Body image disturbance

NURSING INTERVENTIONS

- Discuss bodily changes.
- Stress importance of prenatal vitamins.
- Reinforce diet, exercise.
- Remind of obstetrician appointments.
- Advise patient when to call the obstetrician.
  - Vaginal bleeding, discharge
  - Several-hour duration of cramping, pain

- Fever
- Diminished fetal movements
- Sustained vomiting
- **Explain to the patient:**
- Benefit of continued exercise.
- Observe for signs of dehydration.
- Eat small, frequent meals.
- Prenatal vitamins daily.
- Support hose for varicose veins.
- Stool softeners to aid in hemorrhoid pain.
- Avoid high heels if backache persists.
- Avoid prolonged sitting.
- Avoid MMR vaccine in pregnancy.
- Suggest Lamaze or other labor support groups.

14. Labor and Delivery

Labor is defined as the progressive dilatation and effacement of the cervix with eventual expulsion of the products of conception.

Labor is usually shorter in women who have previously had children than in first-time mothers. The average labor is anywhere from 12 to 24 hours. Labor is typically divided into three stages, with the first stage having two phases. The first stage starts with the beginning of labor, which is uterine contractions, which result in thinning (effacement) and dilation of the cervix. The first stage of labor ends with full dilation, at 10 cm, and complete effacement. This is the longest part of labor. First stage of labor is divided into the latent phase and the active phase. In the latent phase, contractions are milder, last 60 to 90 seconds, and are 15 to 20 minutes apart. The active phase occurs when the cervix dilates from 4 to 10 cm, contractions become stronger, last about 30 to 60 seconds, and are closer together. This is often when the membranes rupture, releasing amniotic fluid. A backache is common, as is some vaginal bleeding. When the cervix is fully dilated at 10 cm, the second stage of labor has started. This phase is fetal expulsion. Contractions continue, but feel different. There is pressure on the rectum, and a strong urge to push. The second stage of labor ends with the birth of the baby. Delivery of the placenta, or afterbirth, is the third stage of labor. Contractions will continue, but will be milder, as the uterus contracts, which helps to expel the placenta and slow the bleeding.

What Went Wrong
Normal labor and delivery.

Prognosis
Normal delivery of a healthy baby.

Hallmark Signs and Symptoms
- Bloody show which is the mucous plug, expelled from the vagina
- Rupture of membranes, which releases amniotic fluid (commonly referred to as water breaking)
- Regular uterine contractions

Common Test Results
- CBC to assess any anemia
- Blood typing
- Rh factor
- Urinalysis to look for protein and glucose
- Ultrasound

Treatment
- Some medications may be administered to stimulate uterine contractions.
  - oxytocin
  - prostaglandins
- Pain medications may be administered, but always with the safety of the fetus in mind. The risk versus the benefit must be weighed.
- Analgesia and sedation.
  - Stadol
  - butorphanol
  - meperidine
  - fentanyl
  - nalbuphine
- Regional anesthesia.
  - pudendal block
  - paracervical block
  - spinal block

- Epidural analgesia.
- Local infiltration.

Nursing Diagnoses

- Anxiety
- Pain, discomfort

NURSING INTERVENTIONS

- **Explain to the patient:**
- Observe for signs of dehydration.
- Eat small, frequent meals.
- Monitor vital signs.
- Monitor fetal heart rate.
- Suggest Lamaze or other labor support groups.

15. Postpartum

The time from birth to 6 weeks when involutionary changes occur.

What Went Wrong

Normal part of pregnancy.

Prognosis

- Return to prepregnant state.

Hallmark Signs and Symptoms

- Vaginal drainage (lochia) lessens, becomes lighter in color
- Uterus shrinks in size
- Abdomen shrinks
- Breasts enlarge and fill with milk
- Body weight decreases

Common Tests Results

- CBC to assess blood loss

Treatment

- Iron supplementation if indicated

Nursing Diagnoses

- Fatigue
- Disturbance in body image
- Effective breastfeeding

NURSING INTERVENTIONS

- Explain lochia (postpartum vaginal discharge)—color and amount.
- Answer breast-feeding questions.
- Remind patient to call obstetrician if fever develops, or if there is excessive vaginal bleeding, chest pain, or dyspnea.
- Discuss contraception—ovulation may occur before menses resume.
- Discuss signs of postpartum depression and to call provider if they occur.

---

16. Rh Incompatibility

What Went Wrong

Rh incompatibility is assessed on each mother during pregnancy. An antigen, Rh, may or may not be on the surface of the red blood cell (RBC). If a mother is Rh positive, she carried the rhesus antigen on the RBC. A fetus has antigens from its mother and father. The Rh is problematic when the mother is Rh– and the father is Rh+. When the mother is Rh– and the fetus is Rh+, she may develop antibodies that will cross the placenta and attack the fetal RBCs, which are recognized as foreign.

Prognosis

Prognosis is good as all mothers are tested during prenatal care.

Hallmark Signs and Symptoms

- Incompatibility with Rh of mother and baby

Common Test Results

- Blood type and Rh, antibody screen

Treatment

- RhoGAM is Rh IgG (immunoglobulin) to prevent an immune response by the mother.

Nursing Diagnoses

- Safety
- Risk for injury

> **NURSING INTERVENTIONS**
>
> - Retest if unsure of antibody titer.
> - Administer RhoGAM.
> - Explain Rh status to the mother, need for testing and possible RhoGAM with every pregnancy.

17. Preeclampsia and Eclampsia

Preeclampsia is a condition that women may get in the latter half of pregnancy. It is pregnancy-induced hypertension and more often occurs in a first pregnancy. If preeclampsia is left untreated, eclampsia (which is severe) will result.

What Went Wrong

The etiology of preeclampsia and eclampsia is unknown. Prepregnant hypertension, obesity, and poor nutrition may be contributing factors. First-time mothers have a greater risk of preeclampsia, as do women with a family history of the condition.

Prognosis

Preeclampsia can cause a small baby, premature birth, and learning disabilities. Untreated eclampsia can lead to seizures, coma, and even death of the mother and baby.

Hallmark Signs and Symptoms

- Preeclampsia (may be asymptomatic):
  - BP more than 140/90 mmHg
  - Proteinuria (presence of excess serum protein in the urine) more than 300 mg/24 hours
  - Elevated creatinine
  - Headache

- Edema
- Pulmonary edema
- Hemolysis
- Rapid weight gain
- Abdominal pain
- Diminished urine output
- Excessive vomiting and nausea
- Eclampsia:
  - As above
  - Seizures

Common Test Results

- Chemistry panel to assess hydration status as well as kidney and liver function
- CBC to asses anemia and platelet count
- Urinalysis to look for protein and creatinine in the urine
- Fetal ultrasound

Treatment

Birth of the baby is the only cure for eclampsia and preeclampsia. Mild preeclampsia with mild hypertension and a small amount of protein in the urine can be managed at home with rest and frequent healthcare provider checks, depending on the status and gestational age of the baby. All other preeclampsia and eclampsia patients are hospitalized.

- Bed rest
- Low-salt diet
- Medications to control blood pressure:
  - hydralazine
  - labetalol
  - methyldopa
  - nifedipine
- To control seizures:
  - magnesium sulfate

Nursing Diagnoses

- Safety
- Risk for altered parenting
- Altered growth and development

NURSING INTERVENTIONS

- Monitor blood pressure.
- Monitor protein in the urine.
- Assist during bed rest.
- **Explain to the patient:**
  - The disease
  - Necessity of low-salt diet
  - All tests

REVIEW QUESTIONS

1. The start of the luteal phase of the menstrual cycle is marked by:

   A. Menstruation.

   B. Pelvic pain.

   C. Ovulation.

   D. Cramping.

2. Symptoms of an ectopic pregnancy include:

   A. Hematuria, pelvic pain, and dizziness.

   B. Amenorrhea, pelvic pain, and vaginal spotting.

   C. Constipation, nausea, and fainting.

   D. Fallopian pain, nausea, and breast enlargement.

3. Symptoms indicative of cervical cancer include:

   A. Irregular vaginal bleeding.

   B. Bloating.

   C. Weight gain and nausea.

   D. Dyspareunia.

4. Which of the following is a definitive sign of pregnancy?

   A. Amenorrhea.

   B. Positive hCG.

C. Morning sickness.

D. Fetal heart sounds.

5. **Which of the following is a finding that is most often associated with endometrial cancer?**

   A. Thickened endometrial lining on ultrasound.

   B. Irregular periods.

   C. Young age.

   D. Dyspareunia.

6. **The main action of luteinizing hormone is:**

   A. Beginning of menses.

   B. Menopause.

   C. Ovulation.

   D. Pregnancy.

7. **Your patient is a 25-year-old woman just diagnosed with hydatidiform mole. You would expect:**

   A. A positive hCG.

   B. Weight loss and wasting as with other malignancies.

   C. Braxton-Hicks contractions.

   D. A cough.

8. **The most important laboratory value to monitor in a patient with heavy bleeding due to fibroids is:**

   A. Hemoglobin.

   B. Luteinizing hormone.

   C. White blood cell count.

   D. Potassium.

9. **The third stage of labor is when:**

   A. Contractions reach their peak.

   B. The head is visible.

   C. The water breaks.

   D. The placenta is delivered.

10. **One risk factor that increases a woman's chances of getting breast cancer includes:**

    A. Family history.

    B. Young age at first birth.

    C. Multiple births.

    D. Underwire bras.

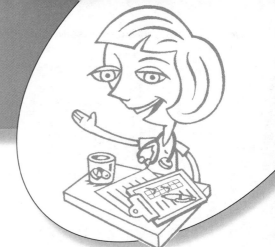

Chapter **15**

Pain Management

At the end of this chapter, the student will be able to:

- Identify the neuroanatomic and physiologic aspects of pain
- List four signs or symptoms of acute and chronic pain
- Discuss the treatments commonly used in pain management
- Recognize expected nursing and medical treatment of pain treatment

KEY CONCEPTS

1. Acute pain
2. Chronic pain
3. Drug addiction
4. Peripheral neuropathy
5. Phantom limb pain
6. Substance use disorders

KEY TERMS

Adjuvant modalities
Biofeedback
Breakthrough pain
Electromyography
Endorphins

Enkephalins
Likert scale
Neuroleptics
Serotonin
Serum levels

Pain

Pain is sensed through nerve endings, which are generously spread throughout the internal tissues and the skin. The brain is the only structure without pain receptors. Internal organs and skin have nerve fibers (nociceptors) that sense painful stimuli (see Fig. 15–1). When pain receptors are stimulated, the perception of discomfort or pain results, prompting that action be taken to remove the cause of the pain. The pain impulse travels along sensory fibers of the spinal nerves to the spinal cord and then to the brain, which interprets the degree and source of the pain. The brain can then signal nerve fibers to release chemicals to inhibit pain signals. Some of the chemicals—enkephalins, serotonin, and endorphins—are able to suppress pain signals and provide endogenous pain control. Visceral pain is pain from an organ and may be secondary to surgery, cramping, ischemia, stretching, or spasms. Visceral pain tends to be diffuse or difficult to localize. Referred pain is the sensation of pain coming from another part of the body than where it actually originates. It is common for heart pain to be felt in the arm, jaw, or back. The pain impulses from the heart travel the same circuit as the receptors in these areas, confusing the interpretation in the brain.

Various individuals can experience different levels of pain with the same injury. Researchers have sought to explain this phenomenon. The gate control theory postulates that there is a "gate" in the spine which controls the impulses

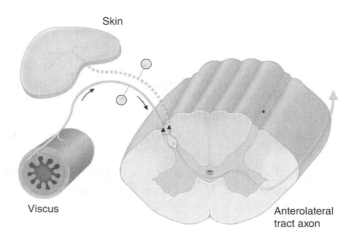

Skin

Viscus

Anterolateral
tract axon

FIGURE 15−1 · Convergence-projection hypothesis of referred pain. According to this hypothesis, visceral afferent nociceptors converge on the same pain-projection neurons as the afferents from the somatic structures in which the pain is perceived. The brain has no way of knowing the actual source of input and mistakenly "projects" the sensation to the somatic structure.

Source: Reproduced with permission from: Longo DL, Fauci AS, Kasper DL, Hauser SL, Jameson JL, Loscalzo J: *Harrison's Principles of Internal Medicine,* 19th ed. New York, NY: McGraw-Hill; 2012. Fig. 11–3.

from the finger on the hot stove to the brain. The brain controls this gate to allow total or partial signals through. However, the interpretation is based on current emotions, memories, expectations, ideals, and cultural biases. If your mind is busy elsewhere, the pain may be somehow lessened, for example, the Lamaze experience through labor and childbirth. Emotional pain can produce many symptoms, as varied in their presentation as the etiology of the pain. Psychogenic pain is the result of emotional or mental influences.

Pain is subjective. You must elicit information from the patient about the quality, location, and duration of pain. Pain scales are useful tools to assess the severity of pain and quality of life. They will help the patient to accurately assess the pain and the impact it is having. Pain scales often are measured on a Likert scale from 0 (no pain) to 10 (the worst pain ever). The Wong pain scale for children uses a happy smiling face to a sad, tearful one. Another useful tool is a pain diary, in which the patient records severity, location, activity at the time, precipitating factors, and what, if anything, relieved the pain. It is a helpful tool to assess worsening or alleviating pain and also reactions to pain medications.

Patients need different amounts of noxious stimulus (perception threshold) to cause pain, and varied points that will cause the patient to react (tolerance threshold) to stop the pain. Age, gender, ethnicity, and past experience may all contribute to these thresholds. Pain may be controlled with medication, biofeedback, electrical stimulation, acupuncture, hypnosis, and other complementary therapies.

Just the Facts

1. Acute Pain

Acute pain usually points to an aberration or an illness. It is differentiated from chronic pain by the duration, usually less than 4 to 6 months.

What Went Wrong

Pain nerves are stimulated by pressure, cuts, heat, cold, stabs, surgery, and so on. Other causes include fractures, burns, and bruises.

Prognosis

Acute pain is usually managed and terminated in less than 4 to 6 months.

Hallmark Signs and Symptoms

- Intense sharp pain (moderate to severe)
- Fleeting, momentary, or ongoing
- Cramping, spasmodic

Common Test Results

- Ultrasound
- X-rays
- CT scans
- MRI

Treatments

- Surgery
- Delivery of child for labor pain
- Anesthesia
- Analgesics
  - acetaminophen
  - aspirin
  - COX-2 inhibitors
  - NSAIDs
    - celecoxib
    - diclofenac

- flurbiprofen
- ibuprofen
- indomethacin
- ketorolac
- nabumetone
- naproxen
- Opioids
  - codeine
  - hydrocodone
  - hydromorphone
  - levorphanol
  - meperidine
  - methadone
  - morphine
  - oxycodone
- Antispasmodics
- Muscle relaxers
- Neuropathic pain relievers
  - Tricyclic antidepressants
    - amitriptyline
    - desipramine
  - Nontricyclic antidepressants
    - bupropion
  - Neuroleptic medication
    - carbamazepine
    - clonazepam
    - gabapentin
    - pregabalin
  - Anxiolytics
  - Steroids
  - Heat/cold
  - Transcutaneous electrical nerve stimulation (TENS) unit
  - Epidural injection

- Physical therapy
- Acupuncture
- Biofeedback
- Chiropractic

Nursing Diagnoses

- Acute pain
- Powerlessness

NURSING INTERVENTIONS

- Assess the level of pain.
- Monitor for effectiveness of pain medication.
- Cold or hot packs.
- Massage.
- Meditation.
- Support groups.
- Prayer.
- **Explain to the patient:**
  - Diagnoses.
  - Tests and treatments.
  - Use of pain medication, timing, and side effects.
  - Use of alternative therapies.

2. Chronic Pain

Chronic pain is lingering pain after identification of etiology of the initial onset. It may be less intense after 4 to 6 months or may be the same degree of pain.

What Went Wrong

- Arthritis
- Backaches
- Cancer
- Headaches
- Neurogenic pain
- Psychogenic pain

Prognosis

Prognosis for chronic pain is poor. The longer the pain has been present without adequate intervention, the more difficult it is to treat. Adjuvant modalities may help ease the long-term effects of chronic pain.

Hallmark Signs and Symptoms

In addition to the presentation of acute pain, other manifestations may include

- Anger
- Decreased mobility
- Decreased energy
- Depression
- Restlessness or anxiety
- Tense muscles

Common Test Results

- Heart rate, blood pressure, and respiratory rate may be elevated.
- Pain scales.

Treatment

- Anxiolytics
- Antidepressants
- Neuroleptics

Nursing Diagnoses

- Chronic pain
- Hopelessness
- Self-esteem, situational low

NURSING INTERVENTIONS

- Recommend counseling or joining a support group.
- Daily exercise.
- Physical therapy.

- Massage.
- Deep breathing and meditation.
- Biofeedback.
- Monitor use and effectiveness of medications.
- Monitor for breakthrough pain—pain that presents even with the regular use of pain medication at times when the medication should still be effective.

3. Peripheral Neuropathy

This is the degeneration or disease of the peripheral nerves that affect motor and/or sensory nerves. The peripheral nerves include all but the brain and spinal cord. Neuropathic pain is often described as "pins and needles" or tingling, burning, electric, or stabbing in nature.

What Went Wrong

The neuropathies are poorly understood. When peripheral nerves are damaged, the brain becomes confused when processing communication from the damaged nerves. Pain or numbness may be out of proportion to the damage or may be present where skin and tissue are intact. Peripheral neuropathy may affect motor nerves, sensory nerves, or both. It is often a sequela (secondary result) of poorly controlled diabetes, autoimmune diseases, hypothyroidism, toxic substances, HIV/AIDS, vitamin deficiencies, alcohol abuse, or some infections.

Prognosis

Treating the underlying disease state may help to relieve the pain. Often, treating the pain is the best option.

Hallmark Signs and Symptoms

Symptoms result from pressure on the nerve or damage to the nerve, either sensory or motor.

- Pain
- Numbness
- Tingling
- Muscle weakness

- Loss of sensation
- Burning

Common Test Results

- Comprehensive history and physical
- Reflexes and sensation may be abnormal
- Muscle strength
- EMG—electromyography
- Nerve conduction studies
- Low serum level of vitamin B_{12}, which may be the cause of nerve disturbances

Treatment

Treatment options include management of the underlying disease to ameliorate the neuropathy and treatment of the pain or symptoms caused by the neuropathy.

- Pain relief
  - acetaminophen
  - NSAIDs
- Neuroleptic medication
  - gabapentin
  - pregabalin
  - carbamazepine—helps neuropathic pain for unknown reasons
- Tricyclic antidepressants
  - amitriptyline
  - desipramine
  - imipramine—works by blocking the signals sent to the brain
- Lidocaine patch—a topical anesthetic applied directly to the site
- Biofeedback
- Acupuncture

Nursing Diagnoses

- Risk for peripheral neurosensory dysfunction
- Alterations of tactile sensory perception

> ## NURSING INTERVENTIONS
>
> - Relaxation
> - Protect feet—loss of sensations will make injuries undetectable
> - Exercise
> - Remove pressure from affected limbs
> - Heat/cold application

4. Phantom Limb Pain

Pain, mild to severe, felt in the area where an extremity has been amputated, is called phantom limb pain. It occurs more commonly in upper extremity amputation. The sensation may decrease as time passes.

What Went Wrong

The nerve endings at the surgical site continue to relay pain signals to the brain. The missing limb could be the result of surgical amputation or trauma.

Prognosis

Some patients experience little or no phantom pain. Other patients' pain diminishes with time. Poor prognosis is associated with ongoing pain for 4 to 6 months.

Hallmark Signs and Symptoms

- Pain distal or proximal to the amputation
- Itch
- Cramps
- Tingling

Treatment

- Physical therapy
- Analgesics
- Pain relievers
- Neuroleptics
  - gabapentin
  - pregabalin

Nursing Diagnoses
- Pain, discomfort
- Powerlessness
- Grieving

NURSING INTERVENTIONS

- Heat.
- Massage.
- **Explain to the patient:**
  - Nerve conduction.
  - Medications, timing, and side effects.

---

5. Substance Use Disorders

Substance abuse is defined as an irresistible urge for drugs, alcohol, or other substances, including physical, physiologic, and psychological longings, and a need for more and greater dosages to satisfy the cravings. Abused substances produce euphoria and intoxication, which include changes in mental status, decreased coordination, and slurred speech. Seizures and loss of consciousness are late signs. Usual abused substances include alcohol, club or illegal drugs, and cigarettes. However, food, caffeine, and sex may be included in some definitions.

What Went Wrong

Research shows a varied set of internal and external circumstances leading to drug abuse. There seems to be a genetic factor involved, as well as environmental and social elements. Individuals may slowly begin a habit for pleasure, depression, hunger issues, weight reduction, societal pressures, or to escape from pressure. Teen use often begins early.

Prognosis

Prognosis depends on the drug, its potency, the duration of usage, and genetic factors of the user. Research shows that a history of prolonged abuse changes some brain functions, leading to increased cravings. Substance use disorders may start with one substance and may progress to others; for example, it is not uncommon to begin with marijuana and progress to cocaine or heroin.

Hallmark Signs and Symptoms

- Removing oneself from sports, work, and friends
- Decrease in grades, interest in school
- Irritability, depression
- Stealing money to support habit
- Hangovers
- Forgetfulness from effects of drug on the brain
- Fever
- Epistaxis from nasal administration, snorting
- Pain at injection sites
- Tremors
- Chest pain
- Abdominal pain
- Discolored, dark urine
- Tobacco
  - Heart disease
  - Lung cancer
  - Emphysema
  - Peptic ulcers
  - Stroke
- Alcohol
  - Depression
  - Slurred speech
  - Diminished coordination
  - Decreased inhibitions
  - Irregular heartbeat
  - Anxiety
  - Seizures
  - Liver failure
- Cannabis (marijuana)
  - Diminished memory and coordination
  - Progression to harsher drugs

- Stimulants/amphetamines (cocaine, methedrine, ecstasy, methylphenidate, phenmetrazine, methamphetamines)
- Change in pupil size
  - Paranoia
  - Heart damage
  - Hyperactivity
  - Tachycardia
  - Hypertension
  - Stroke
  - Psychoses
  - Coma
- Opioids/narcotics (heroin, opium)
  - Change in pupil size
  - Vomiting, diarrhea
  - Confusion
  - Bradypnea
  - Increased risk for HIV/AIDS
- Designer/club drugs
  - Respiratory depression
  - Euphoria
  - Tremors
  - Hallucinations
  - Paranoia
  - Tachycardia
- Benzodiazepines/barbiturates (Rohypnol, hydroxybutyrate G [GHB])
  - Hypotension
  - Sedation
  - Confusion
  - Cramps
- Dissociative anesthetics (phencyclidine [PCP], ketamine)
  - Impairs memory
  - Aggression

- Depression
- Dyspnea
- Hallucinogens (LSD, mescaline)
  - Hallucinations
  - Tachycardia
  - Delusions
  - Paranoia
- Inhalants (aerosols, solvents, gasoline, lighter fluid, paint thinners, cleaning fluids)
  - Euphoria
  - Confusion
  - Hallucinations
  - Memory loss
  - Vomiting

Common Test Results

For alcoholism, several screening tests are available to assess for dependency. The CAGE screening test is commonly used for the following:

- Have you ever felt you should **C**ut down on your drinking?
- Have you ever felt **A**nnoyed by others questioning your drinking?
- Has your drinking ever made you feel **G**uilty?
- Do you need a drink first thing in morning for an **E**ye-opener?

In addition, the following tests may be performed.

- Blood alcohol levels
- Screening tests for drug use
  - Blood work
  - Urinalysis

Treatment

Those treatments for alcohol abuse that include behavior modification seem to be the most effective. Often, a combination of behavior modification, support group, and/or medication may be needed.

- ABCs of emergency support—airway, breathing, and circulation
- Inpatient facilities

- Outpatient settings
- Counseling
- Support groups
- Abstinence
- Behavior modification
- Activated charcoal
- Toxicity medications
  - For opioids
    - naloxone
    - nalmefene
  - For benzodiazepines
    - flumazenil
  - For alcohol
    - acamprosate
    - disulfiram
  - For acetaminophen
    - acetylcysteine
  - For ethylene glycol
    - fomepizole

Nursing Diagnoses

- Ineffective denial
- Hopelessness
- Altered family processes: alcoholism
- Ineffective individual coping

NURSING INTERVENTIONS

- Prevent relapse.
- **Explain to the patient:**
  - Adopt strategies to cope with cravings.
  - Use of medication.
  - Physical symptoms of withdrawal.
  - Benefit of attendance at group sessions.

6. Drug Addiction

Drug addiction is the chronic overuse and abuse of legal or illegal substances causing interpersonal, social, and family problems. Addiction occurs when the use of the substance causes an abnormal physical or psychological dependence in which the sudden discontinuance will cause severe trauma. This differs from tolerance in which the desired effectiveness of the drug diminishes over time. Larger quantities of the drug must be used to achieve the same effect. Severe addiction is usually characterized by the inability to carry out work requirements, school responsibilities, or family obligations and duties.

What Went Wrong

Some patients who take pain medications other than directed or to achieve a sensation different than pain relief are more at risk for addiction. Addiction is a multifaceted problem caused by peer pressure, genetic factors, social non-conformity, stress, depression, and mental anxiety. Those who have a family member with an addiction or who have themselves had an addiction in the past are at an increased risk. Societal pressures and environmental pressures can influence the probability of becoming addicted. Research has determined that long-term drug use results in changes in brain function, which increases the compulsion to abuse drugs.

Prognosis

People of all ages, young ones in particular, are dying in unprecedented numbers because of their addictions. Most of the deaths are due to addiction to diverted prescription analgesics, alcohol, and benzodiazepines. Since addiction is such a multifaceted problem, treatment prognosis varies greatly. Relapses, unfortunately, are frequent. Studies have shown that women and older patients respond better to treatment programs and have fewer relapses. The greatest incidence of drug addiction occurs in men between the ages of 18 and 25. Active participation in a treatment program increases the chances of success.

Hallmark Signs and Symptoms

- Tachycardia
- Dilated pupils
- Restlessness
- Weight loss due to poor appetite
- Hypervigilance

- Euphoria
- Death because of overdose

Common Test Results

- Urinalysis for initial diagnoses and to monitor compliance; it will determine substance and toxicity.
- Blood tests will identify the drug used up to 12 hours before testing.

Treatment

- ABCs of emergency support—airway, breathing, and circulation
- Referral to a specialist in substance abuse
- Behavioral therapy (counseling, cognitive therapy, and/or psychotherapy)
- Avoidance of situations detrimental to well-being
- Residential programs
- Outpatient programs
- Medications—methadone, naltrexone, and bupropion
- Antidepressants—paroxetine, fluoxetine, sertraline, amitriptyline, and trazodone
- Mood stabilizers—olanzapine and risperidone
- Acupuncture
- Biofeedback

Nursing Diagnoses

- Altered family process
- Social isolation
- Risk for loneliness

NURSING INTERVENTIONS

- Assess for HIV/AIDS, tuberculosis, and hepatitis.
- Different approaches work for different people.
- Drug abuse is a result of multiple issues and treatment must address all of these issues.

> - **Explain to the patient:**
>   - Disease process.
>   - Long-term treatment is more effective.
>   - Benefit of continued counseling.
>   - Treatment, medications, and side effects.
>   - Detoxification.
>   - Benefit of avoidance of high-risk behaviors.
>   - Recovery process is a long-term commitment.
>   - Strategies for coping.
>   - Prevention strategies.

REVIEW QUESTIONS

1. **A mother is concerned about her teenaged son who is depressed and irritable. His school teachers have called, concerned about his declining grades. You would ask:**

   A. If you can recommend a psychiatrist.
   B. If he has a fever.
   C. About any family history of substance use disorders.
   D. About any allergies.

2. **A 2-day postoperative right-below-the-knee amputation patient complains of severe right foot pain. Your appropriate nursing response would be to:**

   A. Refer the patient to psychiatry.
   B. Explain to the patient that the pain is not real because the foot is not there.
   C. Medicate the patient for pain.
   D. Encourage guided imagery or another diversion technique.

3. **Prior to giving a requested pain medication, you would:**

   A. Wait longer; the patient did not appear to be uncomfortable.
   B. Administer after the family left.
   C. Assess the vital signs.
   D. Call the doctor.

4. **You are caring for a patient who borrowed pain medication from a friend at a beauty salon. She seems to be experiencing side effects of the medication. Your most appropriate response would be:**

   A. Stop the medication and call the friend's practitioner.
   B. Continue the medication if pain relief is adequate.

C. Instruct the patient as to the dangers of using a medication prescribed for someone else.

D. Take the medication with milk.

5. **Your postdischarge instructions for a 65-year-old man with peripheral neuropathy from diabetes would include:**

A. Walk barefoot to increase the stimulation.

B. Wear socks and shoes.

C. Check feet weekly for wounds.

D. Soak feet in hot water daily.

6. **An elderly patient with chronic arthritis asks you for suggestions for pain relief. You advise:**

A. Increasing caffeine.

B. Marijuana.

C. Decreasing caffeine.

D. Guided imagery.

7. **It would not be unusual for a patient with chronic pain to be taking:**

A. Tricyclic antidepressants.

B. Antibiotics.

C. Antidiabetic medications.

D. Hypertensive medications.

8. **On the first postoperative day after a fractured femur, the patient is resting quietly, watching TV. Your nursing interventions would include:**

A. Asking the patient what their pain level is on a scale of 1 to 10.

B. Administering an ordered dose of opioid.

C. Encouraging ambulation.

D. Telling the next shift nurse not to give any pain medication.

9. **The most appropriate assessment of the efficacy of administered pain medication would be:**

A. The nurse's visual assessment.

B. Changes in blood pressure, pulse, and respiratory rate.

C. The nurse's verbal assessment.

D. The patient's perception measured on a pain scale.

10. **An elderly patient has a 2-year history of back pain from arthritis. You would encourage:**

A. Lifestyle modification and NSAIDs.

B. Use of narcotics for pain management.

C. Diagnostic tests.

D. Vigorous physical therapy.

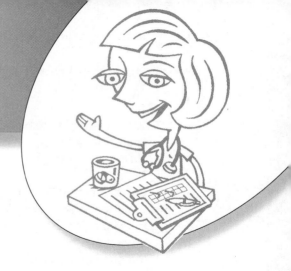

Chapter **16**

Geriatrics

At the end of this chapter, the student will be able to:

- Identify physiologic changes related to the aging process
- Discuss diseases and disorders that present atypically in the geriatric patient populations
- List four signs or symptoms of specific disease or injury common to geriatric patients including geriatric syndromes
- Recognize expected nursing and medical management of geriatric patients

KEY CONCEPTS

1. Cardiovascular system
2. Endocrine system
3. Fluids and electrolytes
4. Frailty
5. Gastrointestinal system
6. Genitourinary system
7. Hematologic system
8. Immune system
9. Integumentary system
10. Mental health
11. Musculoskeletal system
12. Nervous system
13. Pain management
14. Perioperative care
15. Postoperative care
16. Respiratory system
17. Women's health

KEY TERMS

Bradykinesia
Dysphagia
Dyspnea
Essential tremor
Hypernatremia
Immune senescence
Myelofibrosis
Myelopathy
Normal decline

Parkinsonism
Polypharmacy
Pharmacokinetics
Pharmacodynamics
Polycythemia vera
Pressure ulcers
Pulmonary thromboembolism
Thrombocythemia

Why the Elderly Are Different?

Older patients ($\geq$ 65 years) represent an increasing proportion of the US population. Starting in 2011, the first of the baby boomers will become eligible for Medicare at the rate of 10,000 per day. Between 2010 and 2030, the US population over the age of 65 years is projected to increase from 13.1% (about 35 million people) to about 25% of the population (> 70 million people). There will be three to four times greater increase in those over the age of 85. This tidal wave of the elderly will have a significant impact on the healthcare system. For increasing numbers of healthcare providers working in the United States, the likelihood of caring for an older patient is fast becoming a certainty that will challenge and change the way in which healthcare is delivered.

Individuals age very differently. While some suffer from a variety of impairments, others may age more successfully, largely avoiding disease and disability. The concept of successful aging stresses that the process of growing old is not necessarily accompanied by illness and dysfunction. Normal decline—a process by which the capacity for cell division, growth, and function is reduced over time—differs from disease.

Both normal aging and disease can cause significant changes in all systems of the body, often affecting more than one at the same time. As a result, older adults typically present with multiple medical problems that reflect multiple underlying physiologic causes. Older adults may have an exaggerated response to change or present with atypical symptoms. It may also take the older patient longer to return to a normal state than younger patients.

Atypical presentations of disease can vary widely among the elderly, depending upon their specific situations. For example, myocardial infarction may present without chest pain, and acute appendicitis may not produce typical signs and symptoms. Additional factors that complicate diagnosis of older patients may include the following:

- Cognitive impairment
- Differing, "non-normal" values for some diagnostic tests
- Decreased functional reserves
- Inadequate social support
- Unclear or unknown baseline functional status
- Psychosocial status

Treatment of multiple problems among older patients often involves multiple healthcare providers in different specialties. Such fragmented care frequently results in polypharmacy. The combination of prescription medication (which may have been ordered by multiple healthcare providers), over-the-counter (OTC) medications and supplements may interact with each other causing symptoms or making diagnosis and appropriate treatment difficult. Furthermore, pharmacokinetics—what the body does to drugs—and pharmacodynamics—what drugs do to the body—frequently change with age. Therefore, extra attention must be paid not only to which medications are administered to older patients, but also to their dosage and titration. The cardinal rule, "start low, go slow," should always apply.

As people age, physical assessment can be more difficult as the various body systems may not have a "normal" presentation. Each older patient, by virtue of age and life experience, is unique in almost every way. This makes the rendering of sensitive care to the elderly distinctively rewarding.

Geriatric Syndromes

The term geriatric syndromes is used to highlight the unique features of common health conditions in the elderly. Geriatric syndromes include delirium, dementia, falls, gait impairment, osteoporosis, dizziness, syncope, malnutrition, eating and feeding problems, pressure ulcers and wound care, sleep problems, incontinence, frailty, and visual and hearing impairments. The syndromes are widespread, multifactorial, and associated with substantial morbidity and poor outcomes.

1. Cardiovascular System

More than 30% of individuals aged 65 years or older have clinical manifestations of coronary artery disease; it is the most common cause of death in this age group. There are well-documented differences between cardiovascular performance in older and younger individuals; however, the effects of interactions among disease, lifestyle, and age are still frequently disregarded. Whether such disorders as hypertension, coronary artery disease, and heart failure result from an aging process or, simply, longer exposure to risk has yet to be established.

Certain elements of age-related change in cardiovascular *structure*, cardiovascular *function*, and *lifestyle* have been associated with cardiovascular disease. Structural changes in the cardiovascular system can include an increase in the intimal thickness of blood vessels systemically which may lead to loss of compliance. Increased vascular stiffness related to structural change may lead to systolic hypertension and stroke. As the vessel walls become less pliable, the vascular system has greater difficulty responding to change which can lead to increased pressure within the vessels. A buildup of plaque on the inner layer of the vessel walls also contributes to loss of compliance as well as narrowing of the vascular lumen. This buildup increases the risk of cardiovascular disease, such as myocardial infarction or stroke. An increase in left ventricular wall thickness can result in slowed cardiac filling, increased cardiac filling pressure, and a lower threshold for dyspnea. Increased left atrial size may lead to atrial fibrillation.

Functional changes in the cardiovascular system may affect the regulation of vascular tone leading to a stiffening of the vasculature and hypertension, similar to the damage that results from structural changes. Functional changes may also lead to decreased cardiovascular reserve which may lower the threshold for heart failure and increase its severity.

An older person's lifestyle may include certain risk factors that are modifiable and can improve health, such as cessation of cigarette smoking, reduction of dietary fat and cholesterol, and weight loss. Common lifestyle changes in the elderly frequently involve significant reduction of physical activity, which can have widespread and potentially devastating effect. Insufficient physical activity can exacerbate age-associated structural and functional cardiovascular change, dramatically increasing the risk of vascular disease, hypertension, and heart failure.

Presentation of cardiovascular problems in older adults may differ from those more commonly manifested in younger individuals. Myocardial ischemia (MI) may be evidenced more by dyspnea on exertion than by the chest pain typical of angina pectoris. The pain of angina pectoris in older adults may be described as less severe and of shorter duration than is the case with younger individuals, and may manifest in the back and shoulders or in burning epigastric pain. Among older patients, acute MI may also be evidenced by neurologic or gastrointestinal (GI) symptoms.

Syncope is defined as a transient loss of consciousness (T-LOC). The incidence increases with advancing age. Cardiac causes such as bradyarrhythmias, neurocardiogenic syncope, carotid hypersensitivity syndrome, and orthostatic hypotension are more common as people age. Syncope has an estimated 1-year mortality rate of 18% to 33%, and it is strongly associated with falls, a potentially devastating contributor to morbidity and mortality among the elderly. It is difficult to determine the cause of syncope. Good history-taking and physical examination is important for formulating the diagnosis and testing strategy. Comorbidities and medications must be considered since they can exacerbate syncopal symptoms.

Dizziness is similarly associated with poor outcomes in the elderly, overlapping substantially with syncope and falls through commonly shared pathophysiologic mechanisms. Dizziness has many possible causes, including inner ear disturbance, motion sickness, and medication effects. It can also be caused by an underlying health condition, such as poor circulation, infection, or injury. To provide the best care for this vulnerable patient population, it is very important to recognize the causes and associated risk factors, as well as appreciate their influence on diagnosis and management.

2. Respiratory System

Pure age-related pulmonary changes should not result in clinically significant airway obstruction or shortness of breath among people who have not smoked. However, pulmonary function does decline with aging. At about the age of

55 years, respiratory muscles begin to weaken. Among older individuals, changes in connective tissue reduce the size of airways and cause alveolar sacs to become smaller. Calcifications and arthritic changes may affect chest wall flexibility, and muscle atrophy may reduce strength of the diaphragm by 25%.

The most common respiratory symptoms and complaints among older patients include dyspnea (subjective shortness of breath), chronic cough, and wheezing. Dyspnea commonly occurs with end-stage lung diseases such as chronic obstructive pulmonary disease (COPD) and can be a good predictor of quality of life. Over 90% of chronic cough is caused by postnasal drip, asthma, and gastroesophageal reflux. However, other important diagnostic considerations of cough include drug effects, heart failure, infection, aspiration, or respiratory tract abnormalities. Wheezing may be associated with asthma, postnasal drip, heart failure, pulmonary edema, and, especially among current or prior smokers, bronchitis.

Among older patients, major respiratory disease includes asthma, COPD, obstructive sleep apnea (OSA), pulmonary embolism, and pneumonia. After childhood, the prevalence of asthma peaks after the age of 65, with 5% to 10% of older adults experiencing symptoms. Mortality attributable to asthma has increased most significantly among those aged 65 or older, who account for up to 45% of all deaths caused by the disease. This is likely due to reduced awareness and under treatment of symptoms among both patients and clinicians. Inhaled corticosteroids and bronchodilating drugs are mainstay asthma therapies in both the elderly and the young. However, neurologic, muscular, arthritic, and other problems among older people can lead to improper use of inhaler devices used to treat asthma. Lower doses of medication are typically used to treat older patients than is the case with their younger counterparts.

COPD affects approximately 15 million people in the United States. It is the fourth most common cause of death after heart disease, cancer, and stroke. This disease continues to affect more people each year, especially the elderly. COPD also continues to have a significant mortality rate. In people aged between 55 and 85, 1 in 10 may have COPD. COPD is actually a group of diseases, usually including chronic bronchitis and emphysema in the presence of chronic airflow obstruction. Common signs of COPD include cough, increased sputum production, dyspnea, and wheezing. The disease may be accompanied by bronchospasm, pulmonary infection, pulmonary hypertension, hypercapnia, and hypoxemia. Risk factors for COPD include genetic predisposition, environmental exposure, cigarette smoking, and other inhaled substances. Chest x-rays, spirometry, and arterial blood gas (ABG) levels are typically used to diagnose the disease. Treatment for COPD is palliative; there is no cure.

Sleep-related breathing disorders are very common in older people, and OSA is the most common type of sleep-related breathing disorder. It is caused by temporary collapse of the oropharyngeal wall, typically occurring in people who are moderately or severely obese, especially those who sleep supine. The disorder is more common in men than in women and is precipitated or exacerbated by use of alcohol or hypnotics. Obstructive sleep apnea is characterized by episodes of partial or complete interruption of respiration during sleep, for periods that may last for 10 seconds or more, which may occur hundreds of times during a night. To resume normal breathing, patients unknowingly awake, spending excessive time in lighter stages of sleep, leaving them feeling restless and unrefreshed during the day. Obstructive sleep apnea may cause serious health problems, including systemic and pulmonary hypertension, cardiac arrhythmias, exacerbated angina, renal dysfunction, stroke, heart attack, cognitive impairment, and depression. Diagnosis of OSA is confirmed by overnight monitoring of apneic episodes. Treatment for the disease may be complex and include weight loss, use of nasal continuous positive airway pressure (CPAP) or dental devices, laser surgery, and tracheostomy, which are reserved for the most severe cases.

Incidence of pulmonary thromboembolism triples between the ages of 65 and 90 years. Up to 10% of patients will have a recurrence within a year. Hypercoagulability is an age-specific risk factor for pulmonary thromboembolism, and anticoagulants are a principal therapy. Warfarin (Coumadin) is frequently the therapy of choice. It is very important to note that warfarin interacts with many drugs that are commonly used among older patients; these drugs may increase or decrease the international normalized ratio (INR) level when used with warfarin. Risk of bleeding must also be considered with implementation of anticoagulant therapy, especially among older patients who may be at risk for falls.

Pneumonia is one of the most common and significant health problems in the elderly. It is often the terminal event after prolonged serious illness and has been called "the old man's friend." The annual incidence of community-acquired pneumonia ranges from 20 to 40 people per thousand; in long-term care facilities, the annual incidence of pneumonia is 100 to 250 per thousand. Hospital-acquired pneumonia is common among older patients who have undergone thoracic or abdominal surgery, mechanical ventilation, or tube feeding. Major risk for developing the disease is the presence of other serious illness. The mortality rate associated with pneumonia is directly related to the number of such comorbidities, increasing from 9/100,000 without comorbidity to 217/100,000 with one high-risk condition and 979/100,000 with two or more high-risk conditions. In up to 50% of pneumonia cases among older patients, no specific pathogen is detected. It is important to note that fever, cough, and production of sputum—the characteristic clinical features of pneumonia—may present subtly or incompletely among older patients. Only 33% to 60% of older patients with pneumonia may have a high fever. Rather, the elderly may present with acute confusion, delirium, or general deterioration of baseline functions. Diagnosis of pneumonia is usually by x-ray, though this does not indicate cause. As leukocytosis (an elevated white blood cell [WBC] count) with immature WBCs (typically released from the bone marrow to help fight off significant infections) develops less frequently in older patients, blood cultures are frequently performed. Treatment for pneumonia includes antimicrobial drug therapy, respiratory, and other types of supportive care, as well as drainage of fluids resulting from chest infection.

3. Immune System

Infection is the major cause of mortality in 40% of people over the age of 65, and contributes to death in many others. Hospitalization may result from the infection itself or because the infection has exacerbated other preexisting conditions. Pneumonia, urinary tract infections (UTIs), septicemia, and respiratory infections are among the top diagnostic groups paid by Medicare.

Fundamental changes occur in the immune response of elderly patients; this is called immune senescence, which can cause inappropriate, inefficient, and sometimes harmful immune response. With age, both adaptive (acquired) immunity and natural (innate) immunity may be adversely affected, and the latter particularly in frail elderly patients. Adaptive immunity relies on the proper functioning of T- and B-lymphocytes. Changes in the creation and function of these cells contribute to compromised immune response. The specialized cellular components of natural immunity—dendritic cells, macrophages, and natural killer cells—as well as the complement system also change with age, adversely affecting immunity. A third type of immunity—mucosal immunity—also provides resistance to infection and is adversely affected as the body ages. Age-related declines in the effectiveness of these types of immunity occur in response to exogenous, or outside, antibodies. It should be noted, however, that the autoimmune reactivity of some elements of the immune system may increase with age; there appears to be an age-related tendency to lose tolerance to self (Merck Manual).

A major influence on immune function among older people is nutritional status. Undernutrition is present in 30% to 60% of people (65 years of age or older) on admission to the hospital. Outside the hospital, 11% of older adults suffer from undernutrition. Ninety percent of these older adults outside the hospital can attribute the undernutrition to reversible underlying conditions, including depression, poorly controlled diabetes mellitus (DM), and side effects of medicine. Undernutrition may be associated with delayed wound healing, extended lengths of hospital stay, hospital-acquired infection, and increased mortality.

Older persons are at greatly increased risk for epidemic diseases such as influenza. Seasonal influenza vaccination can decrease the likelihood of contracting influenza. Broad use of antibiotics has also increased the risk of the elderly for acquiring diseases caused by organisms that are increasingly resistant to antibiotic therapy.

It is important to note that typical signs and symptoms of disease may be absent among older patients, even those with very significant infection. Fever, for example, may be absent in 30% to 50% of frail older adults with serious infections, including pneumonia and endocarditis. The absence of fever is but a single instance of atypical presentation of infectious disease in older persons. Infections may manifest in confusion, falling, and decreased eating and drinking. Exacerbation of underlying illness(es) may become the most salient indication of infection. Also, cognitive impairment may contribute to atypical presentation of infection in older patients, as they may be unable to communicate key symptoms effectively.

4. Hematologic System

Changes to the hematologic system among older persons are usually due to changes in the bone marrow. In the presence of a disease in the elderly, there is a reduced capacity of marrow to quickly make new blood cells. This can cause a problem among older patients. Age-related changes that occur in marrow function include reduction in the number of stem cells (which go on to mature to different types of blood cells), reduced incorporation of iron into RBCs, and decreased production of new RBCs in response to hemorrhage, hypoxemia, or severe infection ("decreased marrow reserve"). Among both men and women, average hemoglobin and hematocrit values decrease with age, but remain within the normal range for adults. The lifespan of RBCs, total blood volume, the volume of RBCs, and the morphology of platelets are essentially unchanged with age, though platelet counts may be reduced. The lymphoid system sustains age-related change that affects immunity, possibly contributing to the increased susceptibility of older persons to infections and malignancy.

While the annual incidence of anemia in the general population is estimated to be 1% to 2%, it is reported to be four- to sixfold higher in people of 65 years of age or older. In those 65 years of age or older, the incidence of anemia appears to be higher in men than in women. Anemia is never normal. It is a sign rather than a diagnosis, and proper identification of its underlying cause is almost always warranted. Anemia may be caused by benign disease and may be a marker of chronic illness, or it may be a sign of serious disease, including cancer. Vitamin B_{12} deficiency anemia accounts for up to 9% of all anemias in the elderly, and 3% to 12% of all older persons have low serum vitamin B_{12} levels. Neurologic damage and dementia may occur before anemia or any hematologic changes are found.

Hypercoagulable states among older patients may be either inherited or acquired. The predisposition to intravascular thrombosis among older patients is likely due to multiple processes that can present in a variety of clinical manifestations. Incidence of both venous and arterial thromboembolism increases with age, especially after the age of 55 years. Arterial thromboembolism can lead to MI and stroke. Venous thromboembolism includes deep vein thrombosis (DVT) and pulmonary embolism, and it remains a major cause of death and disability among hospitalized older patients. It is estimated that more than 250,000 cases are diagnosed annually in acute care hospitals, with as many, if not more, cases going unrecognized. It is believed that the incidence of venous thromboembolism may be twice as high in rehabilitation centers and nursing homes because these patients are less active.

There are a variety of anticoagulants available for use in treating hypercoagulable states. Especially among older patients, these must be monitored carefully and continuously. It is very important to remember that some disorders, some medications (either prescription or OTC), and herbal remedies may influence the action of anticoagulants, either increasing or decreasing their effects.

Chronic myeloproliferative disorders constitute a group of diseases of the bone marrow in which excess blood cells are produced. Among these, the classic-chronic disorders include primary thrombocythemia (overproduction of platelets), polycythemia vera (an abnormal increase in blood cells, primarily RBCs), and myelofibrosis (bone marrow is replaced by fibrous, scar tissue, disrupting normal production of blood cells).

5. Nervous System

The brain and nervous system sustain natural changes as people age. With normal aging, there is a decrease in the number of nerve cells in the brain, with some areas sustaining more cell loss than others. From about the age of 20 to 90 years, brain weight declines about 10%. Intellectual performance is typically maintained until at least the age of 80, and tasks may take longer to perform due to slowing in central processing. Cognitive changes (memory problems, confusion, disorientation, etc.) are not a normal part of aging. Verbal skills remain largely unimpaired until the age of 70, after which some healthy individuals may sustain a reduction in vocabulary, acquire a tendency to make semantic errors and evidence changes in various features of speech. It should be remembered that mild forgetfulness in noncritical areas is different from dementia in that it does not affect recall of important memories or affect function.

With normal aging, senile plaques and neurofibrillary tangles do occur among older persons, but without clinical evidence of dementia. Free radicals, a normal byproduct of metabolism, accumulate over time and may have a toxic effect on some nerve cells. Normal aging brings changes in the enzymes and receptors of neurotransmitter systems; increases in some and decreases in others may be an omen of the onset of ailments such as Alzheimer's and Parkinson's diseases.

Cerebral blood flow decreases by about 20% with normal aging; illnesses like diabetes and hypertension may cause even greater decreases, resulting in small-vessel cerebrovascular disease. The number of cells in the spinal cord also decreases with age, but does not appear to adversely affect its normal function. Decreased muscle strength likely results from lost muscle fibers (sarcopenia) rather than from loss of nerves.

Dementia is a broad term used with reference to a series of disorders that cause significant decline in two or more areas of cognitive functioning, one of which must be sufficiently severe to cause functional decline. Dementia is progressive, disabling and not reversible; it is distinct from normal aging and not an inherent part of the normal aging process.

Alzheimer's disease (AD) is a type of dementia afflicting an estimated 4 million people in the United States, typically beginning in late life. Beyond its major impact on society, with associated costs approaching $100 billion annually, AD can cause an immense emotional toll on both patients and their families. Almost half of primary caregivers of dementia patients experience psychological distress, especially depression. The two greatest risk factors for AD are family history and age; by the age of 90, almost half of individuals with parents or siblings with AD develop the disease themselves. Other types of dementia syndrome include mild cognitive impairment, vascular dementia, Lewy body dementia, and frontotemporal dementia. Each of these is distinct in onset, cognitive domain, cognitive symptoms, and progression and has its own set of appropriate laboratory tests and diagnostic imaging.

Primary treatment goals for patients with dementia include enhanced quality of life and maximized functional performance. Both pharmacologic and non-pharmacologic treatment is available to improve cognition, mood, and behavior of patients diagnosed with dementia. While the elderly patients are particularly sensitive to the effects of drugs, those with some degree of neurologic disease are often even more sensitive. In patients with underlying neurologic disorders, hypnotics may cause confusion or delirium in older persons. Stress and depression can also worsen brain disease and produce pseudodementia, a dementia-like syndrome in older patients.

Essential tremor is a very common form of abnormal action tremor, present when the limbs are in active use—for example, while writing or holding a cup. The tremor usually involves the arms, but the head and voice are commonly involved. A notable feature of essential tremor is its variable amplitude, such that it may be mild or even absent at times, severe at others. The tremor typically disappears when the body is at rest. Stress or anxiety can exacerbate essential tremor. Its prevalence increases with age, affecting as many as 1% to 5% of people aged 60 years or older.

Parkinsonism is a syndrome characterized by tremor, muscular rigidity, bradykinesia, and loss of postural reflexes. Most cases of parkinsonism are Parkinson's disease, the incidence of which increases dramatically with age. Among all age groups in the United States, the prevalence of Parkinson's disease is about 100 cases per 100,000 but is approximately 50% lower among blacks than among whites. The incidence among all age groups is 10 to 20 cases per 100,000. Among people in their seventies and eighties, the incidence of Parkinson's disease is about 200 cases per 100,000 in the United States and about 1000 to 2000 cases per 100,000 in other countries (Iceland, India, Scotland, Australia). The disease most commonly appears between the ages of 50 and 79 years, affecting both sexes and all races.

Symptoms and signs of parkinsonism may appear alone or in combination. Tremor, usually involving the fingers in a pill-rolling motion, is one of the most common initial symptoms, usually in one hand but sometimes in both. It is present at rest, usually decreasing with voluntary movement and disappearing during sleep. Muscular rigidity is usually evident with passive movement of a limb—either a smooth resistance or one manifesting as a ratchet-like jerk (cogwheel phenomenon). Bradykinesia is a lack of spontaneous movement or movement that is slow. Patients with parkinsonism may also experience a freezing, or sudden interruption, of movement that renders them incapable of completing an action. Gait becomes shuffled, sometimes with quick, short steps breaking into a run (festination) as the patient's arms fail to swing. With parkinsonism, postural abnormalities are evident; erect posture is not assumed or maintained and the head tends to fall forward onto the trunk. Postural reflexes become diminished, causing the body to fall forward or backward unless supported. Beyond these classic symptoms of parkinsonism, patients may experience rapid speech degenerating into a mumble, altered handwriting, a masklike face lacking expression, diminished eye blinking, difficulty swallowing, drooling, oily skin, mood abnormalities (usually depression or anxiety), cognitive impairment, and dementia.

Parkinsonism is progressive, sometimes developing rapidly but, more often, with a course that is slow and protracted, as patients may remain functional for many years. Diagnosis of the disease is clinical and no cure exists for parkinsonism due to any cause other than drugs (side effects or adverse effects of medication that has been taken). Nondrug treatment consists of regular exercise, physical therapy, and occupational therapy. Drug treatment includes the use of carbidopa-levodopa, bromocriptine, pergolide, pramipexole, ropinirole, selegiline, and amantadine.

Other common dysfunctions of the aging nervous system include myelopathy or spinal cord dysfunction, most often the result of compression of the spinal cord, typically in the cervical region; radiculopathy or pain, numbness, weakness, or tingling which appears to radiate from the spine outward to cause symptoms away from the source of the spinal nerve, typically in the limbs; and peripheral neuropathy or damage to the nerves of the peripheral nervous system. The presence of peripheral neuropathy in older patients is estimated to be as high as 20%. It may be particularly devastating among the elderly, as the resulting sensory and motor deficits cause gait impairment and falls. Among developed countries, diabetes is the most common cause of peripheral neuropathy; up to 60% of patients with DM who are over 60 years of age have some form of peripheral neuropathy. Medications, alcohol abuse, nutritional deficiencies, renal disease, and cancer may also cause peripheral neuropathies. Treatment depends upon the cause.

Stroke is a cerebrovascular accident and a leading cause of death and disability among older persons. Its incidence increases with advancing age, about doubling with each decade of life. About 72% of people who have a stroke in a given year are aged 65 or older. Of the approximately 750,000 Americans who have strokes each year, about 150,000 of them die. Among persons who die of stroke, 88% are aged 65 or older. Stroke is the third leading cause of death in the United States and most other industrialized countries. In addition to high mortality rates, stroke may significantly alter survivors' quality of life, adversely affecting activities of daily living.

There are two types of stroke, each reflecting a different etiology. Ischemic stroke is a cerebrovascular disorder caused by insufficient blood flow in an area of the brain. Ischemia accounts for about 80% of strokes. Risk factors for this type of stroke include hypertension, heart disease, arrhythmias, hyperlipidemia, and the effects of age on cerebral vessels. Ischemia that engenders stroke may occur in many different arteries and may have several causes. Transient ischemic attacks (TIAs) are focal neurologic abnormalities that occur suddenly, are of brief duration, and are due to a temporary blockage of blood flow to the brain. By definition, they last 24 hours or less; 75% last less than 5 minutes, but some may last for several hours. About a third of patients who have had at least one TIA will have a stroke; having had a TIA increases the risk of stroke by 9.5 times. Hemorrhagic stroke is caused by bleeding into brain tissue or meningeal spaces, and accounts for about 20% of strokes. Intracranial hemorrhage is most often a result of aneurysms, vascular malformations, bleeding disorders, head trauma, and use of illicit drugs. Vascular malformations are less likely to be life-threatening among persons older than 60 years. Head trauma, however—especially common among older patients, who tend to fall—is often undiagnosed. After a fall, older patients may be confused or unable to remember what happened to them, raising the possibility of delayed or missed diagnosis of a hemorrhagic event.

Among older patients, there are many strategies to prevent and treat the causes, the neurologic and functional results, and the complications of stroke. The symptoms and signs of stroke are varied, reflecting many possible etiologies as well as the presence or absence of prior ischemic or hemorrhagic events. Rapid diagnosis and treatment of stroke is, in all circumstances, imperative.

Delirium is common and associated with substantial morbidity. Under recognition of delirium is a major problem. Delirious patients must be evaluated for reversible causes. A formal mental status examination that includes testing of attention should be administered. It is important to reduce the risk factors for delirium. Medications are the most common reversible causes.

6. Musculoskeletal System

Musculoskeletal complaints are among the most common reason that older adults seek medical attention and are responsible for about 25% of their visits to primary care providers. From about the age of 50 years, bone density decreases progressively in both sexes, but does so more rapidly in women. This process, along with deterioration of the microarchitecture of the skeleton, results in bone fragility with increased risk of fractures. This state is diagnosed as osteoporosis when bone density is at least 2.5 standard deviations (SD) below the young adult mean. Osteopenia is diagnosed when bone density lies between 1 and 2.5 SD below the young adult mean.

Between the ages of 30 and 75, lean body mass decreases as skeletal mass is lost and the number and size of muscle fibers decrease in a process called sarcopenia; by the age of 75, half of muscle mass has disappeared.

Osteoarthritis (OA) is a degenerative disease of cartilage, present in anywhere from 50% to 90% of older adults. While strongly correlating with age, the pathologic change in osteoarthritic cartilage differs from changes present in normal aging cartilage. OA subsumes a group of related joint disorders with varying causes which may be genetic, associated with diseases of metabolism, due to joint malformation or joint trauma, or to damage from other joint disease. Repetitive mild joint trauma (which is often work related) causes the pain and associated tissue damage to joints in a predictable manner. Joints in the lower body (knees, hips, ankles) are often affected earlier in people who carry heavy weights or are overweight themselves. Underlying pathology of OA does not feature inflammation and is notable for pain and reduced joint motion with associated ligamental instability and muscle atrophy. These changes put affected joints at biomechanical disadvantage, further increasing pain and causing even more rapid joint deterioration. Pain control and efforts to strengthen atrophied muscles constitute basic management of OA. Weight loss may help improve function as well as joint injection with corticosteroids. Steroid injections into joint spaces cannot be a frequent therapeutic management. In some cases, total joint replacement surgery is the ultimate solution.

Gout most often appears in middle-aged men and postmenopausal women. It results from a metabolic disorder where the body does not properly metabolize purines (the end product of metabolism of certain proteins). It is characterized by acute onset of inflammatory arthritis, usually in a joint of the big toe. This joint inflammation of the metatarsal joint of the big toe is called podagra. Resulting tenderness is so intense that the weight of bedclothes results in exquisite pain. In some cases, inflammation may extend beyond the affected joint, suggesting cellulitis. Patients may also develop subcutaneous deposits of uric acid crystals (often seen along the outer ear) or uric acid crystallization within the kidney (nephrolithiasis or kidney stones). Acute treatment starts with nonsteroidal anti-inflammatory drugs (NSAIDs); xanthine oxidase inhibitors (eg, allopurinol or febuxostat) or uricosuric drugs (eg, probenecid) are used to treat chronic states.

Rheumatoid arthritis (RA) is a chronic autoimmune syndrome causing inflammation of peripheral joints, which results in progressive damage and destruction of the affected joint structures. It typically occurs symmetrically. Its prevalence increases up to the age of 80 and constitutes an important cause of disability among older persons. The cause is not known. RA occurs principally in the joints of the hands and feet and in the larger joints (elbows, shoulders, knees). Symptoms include pain, swelling, and stiffness in the affected areas, particularly in the morning and lasting an hour or more. The long-term prognosis for RA is poor, as many patients endure progressive disability despite treatment. Physical modalities of treatment are essential, with rest when symptoms are severe. However, prolonged bed rest among older patients may serve to accelerate age-related loss of exercise tolerance and muscle strength, and may lead to irreversible immobility. It is vital to note that older patients may easily cross the threshold at which functional ability is so severely compromised that it cannot be restored. Pharmacologic treatment includes NSAIDs to relieve pain and swelling. Corticosteroids may also help reduce pain and disability, while their long-term adverse effects (osteoporosis, cataracts, poor wound healing, hyperglycemia, hypertension, hyperlipidemia, risk of increased infection) must be balanced against their benefits. Disease-modifying antirheumatic drugs (DMARDs) slow the disease process, improve function, and reduce mortality. Used early in the course of the disease, these prevent joint destruction and disability, and may even improve survival. These medications include methotrexate, hydroxychloroquine, sulfasalazine, minocycline, and leflunomide. Immunosuppressant medications are used to directly affect the autoimmune cause of the disease and include azathioprine, cyclosporine, and cyclophosphamide. Patients taking immunosuppressants may have an increased risk of infection. Tumor necrosis factor alpha (THN-alpha) inhibitor medications can ease symptoms due to inhibiting an inflammatory substance (TNF-alpha) within the body. Examples of these medications include etanercept, infliximab, adalimumab, golimumab, and certolizumab. There is increased risk for infection, heart failure, and certain cancers with these medications. These treatment options are sometimes used as combination therapy, which has been demonstrated to be more effective than monotherapy. Both individually and together, however, these medications frequently have significant and irreversible adverse effects which must be very closely monitored.

Polymyalgia rheumatica (PMR) is a syndrome occurring in older adults as early as the age of 50 but, mostly, after age 60. The classic symptom of PMR is extreme stiffness and pain in muscles of the limb girdles. Usually the hips and shoulders are affected, less often affected are the knees and sternoclavicular joints. Giant cell (temporal) arteritis (GCA) is a chronic inflammatory process involving the extracranial arteries. The classic symptom of giant cell arteritis is a continuous, throbbing temporal headache. Fatigue, weight loss, and fever are hallmarks of both disorders. Although PMR and GCA may occur separately, 40% to 60% of patients with GCA have clinical features of PMR; 10% to 25% of patients with PMR have clinical or pathologic features of GCA. These disorders are 10 times more common in patients more than 80 years old than among those aged between 50 and 59 years. They are twice as common in women as in men and are found more commonly in whites than in blacks. The causes of PMR and GCA are unknown. A key symptom of both disorders is a high erythrocyte sedimentation rate (ESR); with GCA, this is often combined with elevated C-reactive protein. Standard treatment for both GCA and PMR is oral prednisone.

Gait Impairment

Gait and balance disorders are common in older adults and are the most common causes of falls. They often lead to injury, disability, loss of independence, and reduced quality of life. Gait and balance disorders are usually multifactorial in origin and require a detailed physical examination and a functional performance evaluation to determine contributing factors. Generally effective options for patients with gait and balance disorders include surgery, exercise, medical, and physical therapy.

Falls

Falls are the leading cause of injury deaths and the most common cause of nonfatal injuries and hospital admissions for trauma. All falls in long-term care facilities must be reported to the Centers for Medicare and Medicaid Services (CMS). According to the Centers for Disease Control and Prevention, one out of five falls causes a serious injury such as broken bones or a head injury, more than 95% of hip fractures are caused by falling. Falls are the most common cause of traumatic brain injuries. The etiology of falls is multifactorial. A comprehensive assessment is essential in assessing fall risks. A variety of fall risk instruments are available.

7. Gastrointestinal System

Most of the GI tract has considerable functional reserve capacity, so aging has relatively little direct effect on GI function. However, advancing age may be associated with accumulating disorders involving many body systems that do affect the structure and function of the GI tract. Consequently, clinically significant abnormalities related to GI function need to be evaluated. Changes in connective tissue can limit the elasticity of the gut, and changes in nerves and muscles can impair motility. Increased use of medications associated with disorders and diseases common among older patients may have direct effects on intestinal mucosa and motility. Atherosclerosis and DM can compromise gastrointestinal function. GI problems may rapidly compromise an older person's ability to maintain nutrition, leading to fatigue, weight loss, and inability to effectively recover from disease.

Taste sensation decreases with age, impairing ability to enjoy foods or identify them by taste, and may adversely affect appetite. The ability to sense sweetness is one of the last taste sensations to be lost. Many drugs and diseases can also affect taste, while poor dentition may also contribute to reduced caloric intake.

Dysphagia—inability to swallow or difficulty in swallowing—is a common problem among older adults. Patients with oropharyngeal dysphagia experience food getting stuck after swallowing, inability to initiate a swallow, difficulty transferring food from mouth to esophagus, nasal regurgitation, or coughing. Dysphagia may be progressive or intermittent, depending upon the cause, which may include cerebrovascular accidents (CVAs), neuromuscular disorders, esophageal strictures, mechanical obstruction, or oropharyngeal tumors. It is especially important to review medications, as anticholinergics, antihistamines, and some antihypertensives can reduce salivary flow. Decrease in saliva causes dryness in the mouth and may impair the ability to swallow. Treatment of dysphagia depends upon the cause and may include swallowing rehabilitation; dietary modification; careful feeding with a cup, straw or spoon, or surgery.

Gastroesophageal reflux disease (GERD) is defined as the presence of chronic symptoms or mucosal damage produced by abnormal reflux of gastric content into the esophagus. It is fairly common among patients 65 years of age or older, with symptoms of heartburn or acid regurgitation occurring weekly in at least 20% of this population and at least monthly in 59%. Sliding hiatal hernia is found in about 30% of patients 50 years of age or older, which may contribute to acid reflux and regurgitation. Anticholinergic drugs can have the effect of reducing salivary secretions, compromising the ability of the esophagus to buffer the effects of refluxed acid and aggravating mucosal injury. Uncomplicated GERD is treated with acid-suppressing drugs. Proton pump inhibitors are the preferred choice of treatment, as they eliminate heartburn and regurgitation in 80% of cases. Less expensive H_2 antagonists relieve symptoms in 60% of cases. Symptoms of GERD commonly reoccur after therapy is stopped and lifelong therapy is often needed. It is important to note that gastric acidity protects the body against ingested pathogens; one concern regarding gastric acid inhibition in an increased risk of intestinal infection. GERD complicated by the presence of anemia, dysphagia, GI bleeding, vomiting, and weight loss should be referred for endoscopy.

A decrease in esophageal peristalsis is common among older patients. This can reduce clearance of ingested materials, including pills; esophageal injury may occur as a result of prolonged contact of caustic medications with the mucosa of the esophagus. Salivation and swallowing are significantly reduced during sleep, so pill intake just before lying down without adequate fluids can result in pill retention and injury. Tetracyclines, aspirin, NSAIDs, potassium chloride, quinidine, iron, and alendronate are among the most common offenders.

Use of NSAIDs by those over 60 can be problematic, as risk of ulcers and their complications among this group is five times greater than among nonusers. Older patients with NSAID-related ulcers usually present with anemia, bleeding, or perforation without warning symptoms; they commonly require emergency surgery for serious complications.

Helicobacter pylori infection causes about 80% of duodenal ulcers and approximately 60% of gastric ulcers. Most older patients with ulcers will complain of dyspepsia, though anemia and acute abdominal pain may occur as well. Among those diagnosed with dyspepsia who also test positive for *H pylori*, 30% with underlying peptic ulcer will benefit from antibiotic therapy.

Gallstones, formed mostly in the gallbladder, may obstruct the common bile duct, and cause inflammation (cholangitis) and biliary pain. When stones obstruct the ampulla, pancreatitis may result. Biliary pain is acute, intense upper abdominal pain that may last for more than an hour and may radiate to the back or scapula. Biliary pain is frequently associated with restlessness, nausea, or vomiting. Isolated alkaline phosphatase elevation without jaundice may reflect biliary obstruction in older patients and always warrants evaluation. In any older person presenting with gallstones, the possibility of cancer should be considered.

Constipation, defined as a stool frequency of less than 3 per week, occurs in about 30% of adults 65 years of age or older, more commonly in women. It may occur as a side effect of drugs or a manifestation of metabolic of neurologic abnormality. Colonic obstruction must always be excluded. Fluids, dietary fiber, and bulk laxatives are effective in increasing the frequency and softening the consistency of stool with minimal adverse effect. Chronic use of stimulant laxatives, including bisacodyl and senna, may cause hypokalemia, loss of protein, and impaired bowel motility. Patients with fecal impaction should have their colons evacuated with enemas or polyethylene glycol electrolyte solution until cleansing is complete.

Diverticulosis is prevalent among 30% of persons by the age of 60, and among 65% by the age of 85. Most patients remain asymptomatic, 20% develop symptomatic diverticulitis, and 10% may develop diverticular bleeding. Symptoms of diverticulitis include left lower quadrant pain and, sometimes, nausea, vomiting, constipation, and diarrhea. Older, immunosuppressed patients with comorbidities may present atypically, from minimal symptoms to frank peritonitis. Treatment ranges from outpatient to hospitalization for surgical relief.

It is not uncommon for older patients to have a positive stool test for occult blood or to be diagnosed with iron deficiency anemia. Causes of a positive stool test include esophagitis, peptic ulcers, esophageal and gastric malignancies, benign colon polyps, inflammatory bowel disease, or hemorrhoids. Among older persons, a high prevalence exists of colorectal cancer as well as benign polyps with a positive fecal occult blood test.

About 40% of the US population aged 50 years and more have one or more colonic polyps. These are usually asymptomatic, though they may bleed or predispose a patient to cancer. Detection and removal of these adenomas can substantially reduce morbidity and mortality associated with colorectal cancer. Old age and male gender are major risk factors. First-degree relatives of patients with adenomas are at increased risk for colorectal cancer and should undergo screening. Colorectal cancer is the third leading cause of cancer in the United States and the second leading cause of cancer death. Advancing age brings a dramatic increase in the risk of colorectal cancer; over 90% of cases occur in people older than 50 years. Risk of colorectal cancer in patients with rectal bleeding relates to age, reaching 25% among patients aged 80 years and more. Fewer than 10% of colorectal cancers are within the reach of digital rectal examination.

The American Cancer Society recommends that, beginning at age 50, both men and women should undergo flexible sigmoidoscopy every 5 years with a colonoscopy if the test is positive; or colonoscopy every 10 years; or double-contrast barium enema every 5 years with a colonoscopy if the test is positive; or CT colonography (virtual colonoscopy) every 5 years with a colonoscopy if the test is positive.

8. Endocrine System

The two major areas of importance are thyroid disorders and diabetes. Thyroid disorders are common in the older population and are more common as people get older. In general, the thyroid gland does not change significantly with aging in healthy adults. The gland undergoes moderate atrophy and fibrosis occurs. There are increasing numbers of colloid nodules and lymphocytic infiltration within the gland. Subclinical disorders of thyroid function are more prevalent than overt dysfunction. Production of thyroxin (T4) decreases with age. Triiodothyronine (T3) levels stay the same. The decrease in T4 is considered a compensatory mechanism for the decreased use of the hormone by peripheral tissues and is not a symptom of thyroid disease. The body's decreased use of T4 is thought to be caused by the age-related decline in lean body mass, such as metabolically active, protein-rich tissue (ie, muscle, skin, bone, and viscera).

The causes of overt and subclinical hypothyroidism in elderly individuals are similar to those in younger people. The term subclinical hypothyroidism is defined by a normal serum-free T4 level and an elevation of the thyroid-stimulating hormone (TSH) level. The patient has no symptoms attributable to hypothyroidism. Signs and symptoms in the older patient are often vague and subtle. Symptoms common to geriatric syndromes (confusion, anorexia, weight loss, falling, incontinence, decreased mobility, arthralgias) are seen in the elderly with an underactive thyroid. There will be an elevated serum TSH level.

Hyperthyroidism in elderly patients is more often due to multinodular and uninodular toxic goiter than to Graves' disease. A common iatrogenic cause of hyperthyroidism is from the use of amiodarone, a cardiac drug containing iodine, or from ingesting too much T4 and T3. Signs and symptoms include tachycardia, weight loss, fatigue (or weakness or apathy), and atrial fibrillation. There will be a subnormal serum TSH level.

Glucose intolerance and type 2 DM increases with age and is much more common than type 1. Adults from age 50 to 80 have no significant change in fasting glucose but the postprandial (after eating) blood glucose rises with age. Up to 30% of diabetic older adults do not present with polyphagia, polydipsia, and polyuria. Signs and symptoms include dry eyes, dry mouth, confusion, and incontinence. Some patients will be asymptomatic and diagnosis is made incidentally by blood test done for some other reason.

9. Genitourinary System

Renal function declines substantially with age but is usually sufficient for removing bodily wastes and regulating the volume and composition of extracellular fluid. The most important functional decline is a decrease in glomerular filtration. Creatinine clearance declines at a rate of 10 mL per decade. Many drugs excreted primarily by the kidneys require adjustment to compensate for decreases in renal function. The renal threshold for glucosuria increases with age. The older kidney exhibits decreased ability to regulate sodium (excretion and conservation) and reduced ability to concentrate urine. Age-related reduction in renin and aldosterone levels contributes to the development of various fluid and electrolyte abnormalities. The most common renal disorders in the elderly are nephrotic syndrome; glomerulonephritis; renal artery stenosis, thrombosis, or embolism; and acute or chronic renal failure.

The important types of glomerulonephritis in the elderly are acute (postinfectious) glomerulonephritis and glomerulonephritis associated with systemic disease or an unknown cause. Signs and symptoms in elderly patients are often nonspecific. Symptoms may include nausea, malaise, arthralgias, pulmonary infiltrates, and worsening of a preexisting illness, especially heart failure. About 75% of elderly persons with glomerulonephritis have renal failure at presentation, with 20% requiring dialysis.

Acute renal failure (ARF) is more common in the elderly. The prognosis is nearly as favorable in the elderly as in younger patients; therefore, treatment need not be denied because of age. Chronic renal failure is much more common in the elderly. Some chronic illnesses common in the elderly (eg, DM, hypertension, urinary tract obstruction, and hydronephrosis secondary to prostatic hypertrophy or cancer, arterial obstruction secondary to atherosclerosis) can cause chronic renal failure. Long-term use of drugs such as NSAIDs and certain analgesics (especially in combination) can cause chronic interstitial nephritis and papillary necrosis, resulting in chronic renal failure.

Urinary tract infection is a common problem in the elderly. Diagnosis, prevention, and treatment can often be complex because clinical manifestations can be atypical and host defenses diminish with age. Asymptomatic bacteriuria is a common finding in the elderly, especially in women. Only about 70% of asymptomatic patients with high colony counts in a single urine sample have true bacteriuria.

In women, asymptomatic bacteriuria should not be treated unless coexisting conditions increase the risk of symptomatic invasive disease. In men, asymptomatic bacteriuria should be investigated to exclude complicating factors such as residual urine, calculi, or tumors. While the diagnosis is being determined and causative factors are eliminated, treatment should usually be given.

Urinary Incontinence

Urinary incontinence (UI) is involuntary leakage of any amount of urine. It affects 15% to 30% of all adults 65 years old or older and 60% to 70% of nursing home residents. It is a stigmatized, underreported, underdiagnosed, and undertreated condition that is mistakenly thought to be part of normal aging. UI affects quality of life and is associated with falls, skin irritations, infections, UTIs, and pressure ulcers. Treatment includes bladder training, bladder relaxants, bladder outlet stimulants, surgery, and mechanical and electrical devices.

10. Integumentary System

The incidence of skin disease increases with aging and sun exposure. The skin of older individuals is characterized by a number of changes including increased fragility. Each of the skin layers changes with aging. The epidermis becomes flattened with reduced keratinocytes and melanocytes, contributing in part to the increased time needed for wound healing. Epidermal-dermal separation occurs more readily in elderly skin, causing skin to tear or blister. In aging skin, there is a decrease in the number of immune antigen-presenting cells, which may lead to increased skin infections. Vitamin D production declines with age. One common reason is insufficient sun exposure (especially in the institutionalized elderly) and poor intake of dairy products (the dietary source of vitamin D).

The thickness, shape, color, and growth rate of the nails change with age, reflecting changes in the supporting nail bed. Nails become dry and brittle and flat or concave instead of convex, often with longitudinal ridging. Nail color may vary from yellow to gray. Occasionally, the nails become grossly thickened and distorted (onychogryphosis). Yellow thickened nails with distal separation of the nail plate from the nail bed (onycholysis) may indicate a fungal infection (onychomycosis). No effective treatment exists for age-related nail changes. Brittle fingernails can be protected by wearing gloves while doing housework and laundry. Nails should be kept short, and use of nail polish remover, which dehydrates the nail, should be minimized.

Pressure ulcers are a serious and common problem for older adults, affecting approximately 1 million adults in the United States. The CMS has designated pressure ulcers as one of the three primary markers of quality of care in the long-term care setting. In 2008, Medicare made the decision to stop paying for hospital-acquired stages III and IV pressure ulcers. Thus, it is critical for clinicians to be aggressive in both pressure ulcer prevention and treatment programs.

11. Fluids and Electrolytes

Normal aging leads to impaired water conservation and sodium balance. Older adults have a delayed and less intense thirst response. The older body tends to secrete antidiuretic hormone (ADH) despite decreased blood tonicity (the syndrome of inappropriate ADH secretion [SIADH]), especially if the individual suffers from chronic cardiac, hepatic, or renal disease. A rise in ADH concentration and secretion greatly adds to the risk of hyponatremia when fluid intake increases. This situation commonly occurs with IV hydration during hospitalization or surgery.

Renal filtration of sodium and water at the glomerulus, renal tubular conservation of sodium, and renal tubular natriuretic substances (eg, atrial natriuretic peptide, renal prostaglandins) are all altered with aging (all but atrial natriuretic peptide decrease). Other factors that affect sodium balance include cardiac output, blood pressure, renal blood flow, glomerular filtration rate, and renal sympathetic nerve activity. Many of these parameters are severely altered in elderly people who have coexisting cardiovascular or renal disease.

With age, total body water decreases because of an increase in fat and a decrease in lean body mass (from about 60% of body weight in healthy young adults to about 45% of body weight in the elderly). Therefore, the margin of error is reduced for maintaining normal electrolyte balance when water losses occur during acute illness due to fever, because of increased moisture loss with respiration in tachypnea, or as a result of renal and GI losses.

Serum sodium concentration is determined primarily by body water balance; thus, hyponatremia usually results from excessive water retention and hypernatremia from water loss. With total body sodium and water excess, edema may result. With pure water excess, edema is not present. With a sodium and water deficit, the presentation often includes orthostatic hypotension. With a pure water deficit, vital signs do not change.

The ability to concentrate urine decreases with age in part because of tubular senescence. Many elderly persons also have resistance to the renal action of ADH, that is, a form of acquired partial nephrogenic diabetes insipidus.

The ability to decrease renal sodium excretion is impaired with age and may result partly from an age-related nephron loss, a decrease in circulating renin and aldosterone, and partly from decreased responsiveness to acute stimuli. Elderly persons with an acute illness who are not ingesting sodium develop a negative sodium balance quicker than do younger persons. In the elderly, basal blood levels of atrial natriuretic peptide are increased; atrial natriuretic peptide inhibits aldosterone secretion and may decrease aldosterone blood levels.

In most cases of hyponatremia in the elderly, the concentration of sodium or any other osmotic substance in the plasma is low relative to water content (ie, is hypo-osmolar). Dilutional hyponatremia is probably the most common type of hyponatremia in the elderly; it is often the most severe hyponatremia, resulting in the greatest morbidity and mortality in the elderly. A common cause of dilutional hyponatremia in elderly patients is the use of nutritional supplements such as Isocal, Ensure, and Osmolite, which are low in sodium. IV fluid administration of hypotonic fluids may also cause dilutional hyponatremia, especially in patients with elevated ADH levels. Primary polydipsia (excessive fluid intake in association with a neuropsychiatric disorder) occurs rarely in the elderly.

Lower body weight is a risk factor for hypernatremia in the elderly. Mortality rate is about 40% in the elderly hospitalized patient and is highest in patients with a rapid onset and in those with serum sodium concentrations greater than 160 mEq/L.

Hypokalemia is common in the elderly. Common causes include decreased intake of potassium during acute illness, nausea and vomiting, and treatment with thiazide or loop diuretics.

Hyperkalemia can be caused by a number of disorders or drugs. A relatively small shift of potassium from the intracellular to the extracellular compartment can result in marked hyperkalemia in patients with metabolic acidosis, especially diabetic ketoacidosis.

In the elderly, serum calcium tends to decrease for many reasons, including decreased intake of dairy products, lower serum albumin levels, and decreased vitamin D intake or activation resulting in hypocalcemia. Impaired vitamin D activation is due in part to decreased exposure to sunlight and decreased vitamin D synthesis of the skin. Drugs may reduce body stores of calcium by increasing elimination (eg, the loop diuretics are calciuric) or reduced absorption (eg, anticonvulsants stimulate hydroxylation pathways that produce metabolites of vitamin D that are less effective at absorbing calcium from the gastrointestinal tract).

In the elderly, hypercalcemia most often results from malignancy such as metastatic breast cancer and multiple myeloma. It can also result from primary hyperparathyroidism.

Hypomagnesemia is common in elderly patients. Causes of magnesium depletion include dietary deprivation, renal loss, and GI disorders, including vomiting, diarrhea, malabsorption syndrome, and alcoholism.

Hypermagnesemia is rare except in renal failure or after parenteral magnesium administration. It can depress central nervous system and cardiac functions.

Mild hypophosphatemia is common in the elderly and most likely results from decreased intake and impaired intestinal absorption of phosphate. The age-related increase in parathyroid function might also lower the renal threshold for tubular reabsorption of phosphate. Severe hypophosphatemia usually results from prolonged, severe decreased dietary intake, and impaired absorption or from renal tubular dysfunction. Vomiting, acidosis, and alcoholic keto-acidosis may also contribute to hypophosphatemia. Aluminum hydroxide antacids, renal dialysis, and a rapid recovery of renal function after acute renal failure or transplantation are other causes of phosphate loss.

Hyperphosphatemia occurs most commonly in patients with chronic renal failure. In rare cases, severe hyperphosphatemia occurs in patients who undergo rapid cell lysis with release of phosphate. This condition can occur in patients with leukemia or other tumors who receive chemotherapy. Excessive intake of phosphate rarely causes hyperphosphatemia, partly because a high phosphate concentration leads to diarrhea and partly because renal excretion is efficient.

Dehydration is the most common fluid and electrolyte disturbance of the elderly. A history of decreased food or fluid intake, febrile illness, polyuria, vomiting, diarrhea, chronic renal disease, DM, use of diuretics, or nasogastric suction is common. Other factors include impaired renal concentrating ability, reduced thirst, and impaired access to water due to neurologic or orthopedic problems or to deconditioning from medical or surgical conditions. Hot weather is a common contributing factor. Nurses can help prevent dehydration by closely monitoring fluid balance in elderly patients.

12. Mental Health

Many changes in mental function in the elderly are the result of underlying disease. Decreases in cognition, memory, intelligence, personality, and behavior may be due to depression, hypothyroidism, or other illnesses and socioenvironmental factors including the care setting. A rapid decrease in cognition is almost always due to physiologic disease and requires investigation by the nurse. Psychiatric disorders have the highest occurrence among individuals aged 65 years or older residing in nursing homes. It is important to rule out a physical cause in elderly patients, especially when there is a rapid onset of symptoms.

In the elderly, several medical disorders (eg, hyperthyroidism, cardiac arrhythmias, hypoglycemia, dementia, delirium) and drugs (anticholinergics, caffeine, drug withdrawal, OTC sympathomimetics) may cause anxiety or similar symptoms that can be easily mistaken for an anxiety disorder.

Treatment is aimed at correction of all potential organic causes including evaluation of medications that may be contributing to the anxiety. These medications should be stopped if possible, after consulting with the prescribing healthcare provider. Dosage of benzodiazepines for elderly patients is usually lower (eg, alprazolam 0.125 mg po bid or tid) than that for younger patients.

Depression is one of the most common psychiatric disorders among the elderly and one of the most common risk factors for suicide. Elderly patients who have suffered a major loss (such as death of a longtime spouse) have an increased risk for suicide. Major depression occurs less often in later life. A thorough history and physical examination, including complete neurologic and mental status assessment, are necessary. A complete review of drug use (including illicit drugs) and alcohol use is also critical. The geriatric depression scale and the Hamilton depression rating scale are useful assessment instruments. Some medical conditions common in the elderly may cause depressive symptoms, eg. vitamin B_{12} and B_6 deficiency, thyroid conditions, deficiencies in folic acid, thiamine, zinc, magnesium, vitamin D, protein, electrolyte imbalances, and dehydration. Usual starting doses of antidepressants in otherwise healthy elderly patients are typically one-half the usual adult doses. Antidepressants must be closely monitored for adverse reactions. Elderly persons who have been treated for schizophrenia for many years are likely to have adverse effects of antipsychotic drugs (eg, tardive dyskinesia).

13. Perioperative Care

Many of the changes of normal aging affect the perioperative management of the older surgical patient. For example, cardiac and vascular stiffening complicate fluid management and optimization of intravascular volume. Volume overload and volume depletion occur commonly and are poorly tolerated by many older adults. Stiffening of the thoracic cage and decreases in ciliary function contribute to a reduction in pulmonary reserve and heightened risk of postoperative pneumonia. Diminished thermoregulation places the older surgical patient at particular risk of perioperative hypothermia. Changes in the brain that occur with normal aging make older individuals exquisitely susceptible to postoperative cognitive changes. Older patients benefit from a multidisciplinary approach to perioperative care and recovery.

14. Postoperative Care

The most common cardiovascular problems that arise in older adults after surgery are hypertension, rhythm disturbances, and heart failure. Postoperative pulmonary complications, most commonly atelectasis and pneumonia, occur more often in older adults than in younger age groups. Impaired preoperative kidney function increases the risk of postoperative kidney failure. Many drugs administered during the perioperative period may require dosage adjustments in patients with diminished renal function.

Untoward effects of well-intentioned interventions are common among older hospitalized adults. Some of the more common pitfalls to be avoided include mobility restriction, excessive use of catheters, inattention to nutrition and hydration status, and inappropriate use of medications.

Surgery in older adults often results in destabilization of chronic, coexistent medical conditions. Additionally, because of the diminished physiologic reserve common in older adults, new medical problems can arise in the post-operative period.

Constipation is quite common postoperatively, as a consequence of the combined effects of altered diet, immobility, and usually use of narcotics and other constipating medications.

Postoperative diarrhea should raise concern for fecal impaction and antibiotic-associated or *Clostridium difficile* diarrhea in the setting of recent antibiotic use.

Perioperative hyperglycemia among diabetic and nondiabetic patients is associated with morbidity and mortality in medical and surgical intensive-care-unit (ICU) patients (SOE=B) and in patients undergoing coronary artery bypass grafting (SOE=C) or carotid endarterectomy (SOE=B).

Delirium is one of the most common postoperative complications. The oldest-old and cognitively impaired patients appear to be at highest risk for undertreatment of pain, so they deserve particular attention. Undertreatment of pain, at least in nondemented individuals, appears to be a more powerful predictor for development of postoperative delirium than narcotic use.

15. Women's Health

Aging and Sexual Function

Sex and sexuality after the age of 60 years may be affected by both individual physical changes of aging and the physical changes of aging in her partner. Therefore, with age comes a decrease in sexual activity. The incidence of sexual dysfunction in postmenopausal women is well over 80%. Hormonal changes associated with menopause can lead to dyspareunia due to decreased elasticity and lubrication of the vaginal walls and increased fragility of the vaginal mucosa. One-third of sexually active women over 65 years old complain of painful intercourse. Testosterone influences female sexual behavior with low levels leading to impaired sexual desire, arousal, responsiveness, genital sensation, and orgasm. However, there is minimal decline in circulating androgen levels in the postmenopausal period.

A major issue for the aged female is the availability of a partner who is also capable of sexual activity. According to statistics there are approximately four single elderly women for every single elderly man. Another important factor for older women who live with their adult children or who are institutionalized is loss of privacy. Several chronic illnesses may impair sexual functioning. There are many medications that can interfere with sexuality such as antipsychotics, antiepileptics, antihypertensives, antidepressants, neuroleptic medications, diuretics, alcohol, and illicit drugs.

Although sexuality remains an important component of emotional and physical intimacy that most men and women desire to experience throughout their lives, it is unfortunately a topic many healthcare professionals have difficulty raising with their patients.

Depression can play an important role in the reduction of sexual interest as well as antidepressant medications that may interfere with sexual functioning. The practitioner must integrate all such data into a comprehensive sexual dysfunction treatment plan. Identified physiological conditions should be treated, and any drugs likely to interfere with sexual function should be withdrawn and replaced. If the dysfunction is thought to have a psychological component, the use of medications to improve desire or arousal should be considered. Appropriate referrals for counseling may prove beneficial for specific sexual problems.

Pelvic Organ Prolapse

Pelvic support disorders are hernia-like protrusions into the vagina by the bladder, rectum, or uterus, caused by weakness of pelvic ligaments, connective tissue, and muscles. The more common pelvic support disorders include rectoceles, enteroceles, cystoceles, or a combination of these defects. Progressive weakening of the connective tissue and muscular supports of the genital organs through childbearing, constipation, chronic coughing, estrogen deficiency, and heavy lifting are activities that increase intra-abdominal pressure. This often leads to genital prolapse. The success rate for surgical interventions is high. Nonsurgical interventions also have an excellent prognosis. Signs and symptoms include heaviness or pressure in the vaginal area, protrusion of a mass at the introitus, difficulty passing stool, lower back or sacral pain, and stress or overflow urinary incontinence. Tests will only be taken if complications are present, that is, infections, or the patient decides to have surgery. Treatments include Kegel exercises to strengthen the pelvic floor muscles, the use of pessaries, and possibly surgery.

16. Pain Management

Pain is one of the most common complaints of the elderly. Pain is undertreated in acute care, long-term care, and home care settings. It can lead to depression, sleep disorders, decreased socialization, and impaired mobility. Culture, ethnicity, family, and individual characteristics all influence one's tolerance and expression of pain. Coexisting medical conditions and the potential risk for adverse effects play a large role in treatment choices for older adults. Pain management and interventions often differ from those of other age groups because of concerns regarding cognitive function and the use of such therapies as TENS, antidepressants, or relaxation techniques. Another issue in pain management of the elderly is their fear of losing self-control and fear of addiction. The cognitively impaired elderly may demonstrate pain by increased levels of confusion, restlessness, or withdrawal. Nurses should not assume that patients who cannot verbalize their pain clearly because of cognitive impairment do not have pain or as much pain as others who are cognitively intact, but must be alert to the cues that suggest that pain and discomfort are present.

Generally, pain relief is achieved by medication that blocks or alters pain impulses as they travel to the higher brain centers. It is recommended that an initial dose is one-half to two-thirds of the usual dose given to a younger person and increased in increments of 25% as needed. Opioids are usually reserved for moderate to severe pain. Opiates produce a greater analgesic effect, a higher peak, and a longer duration of effect in the older adult as a result of altered absorption, distribution, metabolism, and excretion. Opioids that can safely be used with older adults are morphine (safest), oxycodone, hydrocodone, hydromorphone, and transdermal fentanyl. The use of meperidine (Demerol) should be avoided because of the toxic metabolite accumulation, as well as the long half-life of drugs such as methadone. Nonnarcotic agents (adjuvants) are usually effective for mild to moderate pain but may be combined with opioids if necessary. It is necessary to be aware of equianalgesic doses so that when parenteral pain medications are replaced with oral medications, or one oral medication is replaced with another, the dosage has pain relief power equivalent to the previous drug.

Mild and moderate pain relief may be achieved with adjuvant medications such as the NSAIDs or acetaminophen. The NSAIDs bind with proteins and may induce toxic responses in elders if serum albumin levels are low. Other drugs that older people routinely take may compete for the same protein receptor sites and may be displaced by the NSAID, creating unstable therapeutic effects. NSAIDs should be used with extreme caution because of increased risk of adverse effects, especially gastrointestinal bleeding and renal impairment.

Aspirin and acetaminophen use should be monitored because of reduced renal and hepatic function with aging.

Pain that is not responsive to NSAIDs or narcotics may respond to adjuvant drug therapy. Adjuvant drugs are anticonvulsants or antidepressants that can alter pain responses at either the transmission, pain perception, or modulation phase of the pain process. When used in combination with analgesics, they may potentiate or enhance the overall analgesic effects.

Although older persons frequently respond well to adjuvant pain management, it is important to remember that many adjuvant drugs have a very long half-life, which increases plasma concentration in elders. Drugs that cause central nervous system (CNS) effects should be used with caution in older people who are sensitive to CNS effects.

17. Frailty

Frailty is a chronic, progressive condition. The most severely frail older adults appear to be in an irreversible, pre-death phase with high mortality over 6 to 12 months. There are two types of frailty: primary frailty, which results from intrinsic aging processes, and secondary frailty, which is associated with the end stages of several chronic diseases, such as cancer associated with inflammation and wasting, heart failure, COPD, and HIV/AIDS.

Sarcopenia (loss of lean body mass) is a central component of frailty. Comprehensive geriatric assessment and management is designed to optimize outcomes for frail older adults, particularly to prevent loss of independence.

REVIEW QUESTIONS

1. **It is estimated that the population of people aged 65 or older in United States will increase to:**
   A. 13%.
   B. 20%.
   C. 25%.
   D. 38%.

2. **Medications are given to older adults for many different conditions. A good rule to follow for medication use in older adults is to:**
   A. Use once daily dosing.
   B. Take all medications at the same time.
   C. Request brand name medications.
   D. Use the lowest possible effective dose.

3. **The most common cause of death in patients age 65 or older is:**

   A. Chronic obstructive pulmonary disease.

   B. Breast cancer.

   C. Coronary artery disease.

   D. Alzheimer's disease.

4. **Systolic hypertension and stroke are due to:**

   A. Increased vascular stiffness related to structural changes.

   B. Loss of peripheral vascular tone.

   C. Buildup of soft plaque within the veins.

   D. Changes within the basement membrane.

5. **Expected age-related changes of the pulmonary system include:**

   A. Significant airway obstruction.

   B. Shortness of breath.

   C. Development of emphysema.

   D. A modest, gradual decline in pulmonary function.

6. **Lack of adequate nutrition in older adults may lead to:**

   A. Delayed wound healing.

   B. Shorter hospital stays.

   C. Improved immune status.

   D. Decreased mortality rates.

7. **You are reviewing lab findings on an 88-year-old patient and note that her vitamin B_{12} level is low. A decrease in B_{12} among older adults frequently results in:**

   A. Aplastic anemia.

   B. Pernicious anemia.

   C. Folate anemia.

   D. Wernicke's anemia.

8. **Cognitive changes include memory problems, confusion, and disorientation. These changes:**

   A. Occur in 75% of patients over age 65.

   B. Are not a normal part of aging.

   C. Are due to enhanced cerebral blood flow.

   D. Cause senile plaques and neurofibrillary tangles.

9. Which of the following statements about sexual function in older people is true?

   A. Impotence is an inevitable consequence of aging.
   B. Slower arousal and reaction times are normal signs of aging.
   C. Moderate alcohol consumption can improve sexual dysfunction.
   D. Hormonal replacements are necessary for sexual satisfaction.

10. The World Health Organization (WHO) recommends the use of three-step analgesic ladder when deciding on pain management. In order of first choice to second choice to third choice, the following drug categories are used:

   A. NSAIDs, nonopioids, and opioids.
   B. Nonopioids, opioid antagonists, and opioids.
   C. Nonopioids, opioids, and adjuvant agents.
   D. NSAIDs, opioids, and adjuvant agent.

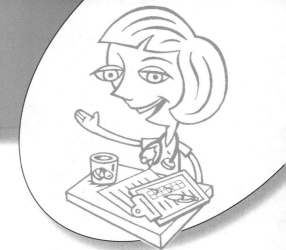

Chapter 17

Substance Abuse

At the end of this chapter, the student will be able to:

- Identify normal anatomy and physiology related to substance abuse
- Discuss the disease-causing pathologic changes associated with substance abuse
- List four signs or symptoms of specific substance abuse disorders
- Recognize expected nursing and medical management of substance abuse disorder.

KEY CONCEPTS

1. Alcohol dependence disorder
2. Amphetamine abuse disorder
3. Anxiolytic, hypnotic, sedative-dependent disorder
4. Cannabis abuse disorder
5. Cocaine abuse disorder
6. Hallucinogen abuse disorder
7. Inhalant abuse disorder
8. Nicotine-dependent disorder
9. Opioid-dependent disorder

KEY TERMS

Abuse
Addiction
Alcohol metabolism
BAL
Blood alcohol level
Cravings
Delirium tremens (DT)
Dependency
Detoxification
Hallucinogen

Narcotics Anonymous (NA)
Neural transmission
Physical dependency
Psychological dependency
Recovery
Substance dependency
THC
Tolerance
Triggers
Withdrawal

How the Substance Abuse Works

Substance abuse occurs when a person continues to use a substance knowing that the substance will have an adverse effect on their health and activities of daily living. For example, a person may use the substance to "relax" on Friday and Saturday and then abstains on Sunday with hopes to return to normal and fully functional for work on Monday.

Substance dependency occurs when a person uses a substance to feel normal. Initially, the person uses the substance to "relax." However, the person goes through withdrawal symptoms as the level of the substance in the bloodstream decreases and the body attempts to compensate for the missing substance. Withdrawal symptoms are uncomfortable and may cause serious health problems such as seizures depending on the substance. The person reuses the substance in order to elevate the withdrawal symptoms. In addition, the person builds a tolerance for the substance requiring a higher dose to achieve "relaxation" and to prevent withdrawal symptoms.

There are two types of substance dependency. These are physical dependency and psychological dependency. Physical dependency occurs when the person experiences withdrawal symptoms when abstaining from the substance. Psychological dependency occurs when the person exhibits drug-seeking behaviors after the physical dependency has dissipated.

Addiction is a psychiatric disorder that occurs when a person is psychologically dependent on a substance. A person who is addicted to a substance will spend most of the person's waking hours focused on obtaining and using the substance with total disregard for activities of daily including family and employment responsibilities.

Dependency and Medication

Some medications such as opioids for pain and benzodiazepine for anxiety have shown a high risk for dependency. Practitioners balance the therapeutic needs of a patient with the risk of dependency when prescribing medication and are careful to reduce the dose or change to a different class of medication at the first sign of the patient becoming dependent on the medication.

Patients who are in severe pain will become dependent on opioids if prescribed opioids for a relatively long period of time. However, the practitioner will employ pain management protocols to reduce the dependency on a particular medication and alter medication to ensure that the patient does not build a tolerance to the medication. The patient will then be detoxed from opioids after the underlying cause of the pain is resolved. Proper pain management prevents a patient from becoming addicted to the medication.

Detoxification

Detoxification is a process of removing the substance from the patient's body. Once the substance is removed and the patient's body stabilized, the patient is no longer physically dependent on the substance. Detoxification begins when the patient stops taking the substance and ends when all traces of the substance are removed from the body.

The patient experiences withdrawal symptoms once the patient stops taking the substance. The time when withdrawal symptoms begin depends on many factors that include the nature of the substance, the amount of substance taken, and patient's health.

Typically, the practitioner lets the patient's body naturally remove the substance. The liver is the major organ that detoxifies substances from the bloodstream. The liver neutralizes the substance, which is then excreted through the kidneys or during a bowel movement.

The body then gradually returns to the normal neural transmission as the nervous system is no longer influenced by the substance. During this adjustment, the patient's neural transmission continues to malfunction until the body's adjustment is completed. It is during this period when the patient feels uncomfortable and shows signs of withdrawal. Alcohol and anxiolytic withdrawal place the patient at risk for seizures and other serious medical conditions in addition to making the patient feel uncomfortable.

During the detoxification process, the practitioner will order medications to ease withdrawal symptoms and to reduce the risk of medical complications. For example, the practitioner will likely order anxiolytic medication for a patient who is dependent on anxiolytic and then tapper the dose over several days to prevent the patient from having a seizure.

The practitioner may order extraordinary measures to detox a patient if the substance is at a critical level in the bloodstream caused by a high dose ingested by the patient or poor health preventing the body from naturally removing the substance from the body. For example, the practitioner may order kidney dialysis for a patient who has acute alcohol poisoning.

Triggers and Recovery

Recovery is the process of coping with life's challenges without the assistance of the substance. Recovery begins when detoxification ends. However, there is no end to recovery. The patient is in recovery for the rest of the patient's life. Although the patient is no longer physically depended on the substance because detoxification is completed, the patient remains psychologically dependent on the substance and will have ongoing cravings to use the substance.

The patient faces the same challenges as a patient who wants to lose weight. Both sincerely want to succeed and have a plan to prevent a relapse back to old habits. However, the craving to relapse is strong. Events called triggers can bring about craving. A trigger can be a song, memories of a place, or meeting certain people that the patient associates with using the substance or binging on junk food. For example, walking into a fast food place triggers the craving to go off a diet—the person relapsed. Patients in recovery call this people, places, and things.

A patient can expect to relapse many times during his or her life. The goal of recovery is to increase periods between relapses. Drug treatment programs are designed to help the patient avoid relapse. At the beginning of recovery, the patient is helped to identify triggers and to recognize cravings and how long cravings last. The patient is then helped to identify ways to cope with triggers and cravings. For example, the patient may realize that a craving lasts for 30 minutes. The patient must be distracted himself or herself for 30 minutes until the craving goes away. There are self-help groups most notably Alcoholics Anonymous (AA) and Narcotics Anonymous (NA) that are run by people in recovery and provide support 24/7 for those in recovery. Each member has a sponsor who provides one-on-one help and is available to help the patient deal with cravings.

Social Support

Dependency on a substance typically affects the patient's activities of daily living. The combination of withdrawal symptoms and cravings results in drug-seeking behavior where the patient's daily activities are focused around acquiring and using the substance. As a result, the patient forgoes family and employment obligations resulting in loss of income.

The lack of income leads to the patient stealing to pay for drugs and encounters with the law. Home life is ruined. The patient has burned bridges with family and friends. The patient's entire support system is destroyed, leaving the patient homeless and penniless. The patient has challenges reclaiming the his or her life. Finding employment becomes increasingly difficult even during recovery because many substance abuse patients have a criminal record. No employment. No support system. No home. These are factors that increase despair and depression leading the patient to relapse and continuing the cycle of substance abuse.

Common Signs of Substance Abuse

Substance abuse does not occur overnight but gradually develops beginning with social or recreational use of the substance occasionally. The periods between use narrows from occasionally to Friday and Saturday and then occasionally during weekday nights. Eventually, use of the substance prevents the patient from going to work on time and perform his work. As stress increases, the patient turns more to using drugs to cope with stress. The patient moves from abusing the substance to becoming dependent on the substance.

The followings are signs of substance abuse:

- Poor hygiene
- Secretive behavior
- Missing money
- Items missing from the home
- Stolen credit cards
- Eyes less responsive to changes in light
- Inappropriately wearing sunglasses
- Pupils fixed dilated or pinpoint
- Frequent unnecessary trips outside the house
- Change in weight
- Change in appetite
- Dress in long sleeves on hot days
- Sinus congestion
- Frequently missed days from school or work
- Not being able to function normally
- Agitated behavior when confronted with behavior change

Just the Facts

1. Alcohol Dependence Disorder

What Went Wrong

Alcohol dependence disorder occurs when the patient develops a physical dependency on alcohol. The patient has developed a tolerance for alcohol that requires the patient to increase alcohol intake to achieve the desired physiological effect. Furthermore, the absence of alcohol results in the patient becoming increasingly uncomfortable and displaying withdraws symptoms that are relieved by ingesting alcohol. A patient frequently reports needing an alcoholic drink in the morning to feel normal. The patient totally focuses on obtaining and ingesting alcohol during waking moments.

Alcohol alters inhibitions. Patients tend to exhibits behavior different from behavior when sober. For example, the patient may become overly friendly and the life of the party commonly referred to as a happy drunk. Other patients demonstrate violent controllable behavior commonly referred to as a nasty drunk.

Since the patient is always at some level of intoxication, the patient is unlikely to maintain activities of daily living including employment. It is not uncommon for a patient diagnosed with alcohol dependency disorder to be unemployed, homeless, and without family and friends who have distanced themselves from the patient's abnormal behavior. The patient continues ingesting alcohol regardless of the consequences of his actions.

The patient likely tried to stop drinking alcohol without success because of psychological dependency on alcohol. Psychological dependency occurs when the patient associates a pleasurable feeling with the use of alcohol. The patient may report that all his troubles go away when intoxicated.

When a patient seeks treatment for alcohol dependency disorder, the patient is likely unemployed, homeless, malnourished, and without a support system. Treatment is difficult because the patient experiences withdraw symptoms and a structured lifestyle that the patient does not control. Patients tend to report there are too many rules and they are not permitted to sleep beyond 8 hours. The psychological dependency is compulsive. The patient believes he or she can handle requirements of treatment if he or she has one drink. It is common for the patient to discontinue treatment and return to using alcohol. The patient typically has many attempts at treatment that results in relapse.

Characteristics of alcohol use are as follows:

- Current use: At least one drink in the past 30 days.

- Binge use: Five or more drinks on the same occasion within the same time or within a couple of hours of each other on at least 1 day in the past 30 days.

- Heavy use: Five or more drinks on the same occasions on each of 5 or more days in the past 30 days.

- Abuse: The patient uses alcohol frequently but does not experience withdrawal symptoms and does not have a physical or psychological dependency on alcohol.

- Physical dependency: The patient experiences withdrawal symptoms that subside when the patient ingests alcohol. The patient is unable to stop drinking alcohol regardless of consequences of drinking alcohol.

- Psychology dependency: The patient has compulsive thoughts about acquiring and ingesting alcohol. The patient views alcohol as a means to achieve a positive feeling and avoid negative feelings. The patient is preoccupied with acquiring alcohol.

Alcohol Metabolism

Alcohol passes from the stomach to the intestine where the alcohol is absorbed into the bloodstream. Blood vessels transport alcohol to the liver where liver enzymes convert alcohol into carbon dioxide and water. A small amount of alcohol is not metabolized and is excreted in urine and is exhaled by the lungs.

The rate of alcohol metabolism depends on the amount of alcohol dehydrogenase (ADH) enzymes available in the liver. Alcohol absorption is faster than alcohol metabolism. The following are the factors that influence alcohol absorption and metabolism:

Food: The higher the fat content of food recently ingested with alcohol, the longer time alcohol has to be absorbed into the bloodstream. The emptier the stomach, the shorter time alcohol has to be absorbed into the bloodstream.

The patient may ingest any form of alcohol including mouthwash, lighter fluid, and aftershave lotion. Ingestion of these forms of alcohol can lead to acute kidney failure and require kidney dialysis. As a general rule, a blood alcohol level (BAL) of 0.016 takes 1 hour to metabolize resulting in a BAL of zero; however, other factors can affect a person's metabolism of alcohol.

There is no known cause of alcohol dependence disorder; however, some researchers believe there is genetic predisposition to alcoholism although other factors influence whether or not the person develops alcohol dependency. Other researchers believe a person who is impulsive and use alcohol as self-medication for anxiety and to escape from responsibilities and facing life's challenges are at risk for alcoholism. Peer pressure combined with an active social life increases the risk for a person to become alcohol dependent.

Prognosis

Brain: Alcohol can have a long-term effect on communication pathways within the brain leading to disruption in coordination, clear thinking, and results in behavior and mood changes. The patient may experience alcoholic dementia, seizure disorders and Wernicke's encephalopathy.

Cardiovascular: The patient may experience esophageal varices and hypertension.

Cancer: Alcohol abuse and dependence is linked to breast, mouth, esophagus, throat, and liver cancer.

Heart: Over time alcohol abuse and dependency can lead to cardiomyopathy and arrhythmias related to hypertension. Cardiac arrhythmias can lead to blood clots and stroke.

Immune system: Alcohol decreases the ability of the body to absorb nutrients that are required to energize elements in the immune system. Alcohol also suppresses the growth of white blood cells. A material decrease in white blood cells decreases the body's ability to fight infection.

Liver: Alcohol is metabolized in the liver. Alcohol abuse and dependency over-works the liver resulting in an abnormal destruction of liver cells. Fat deposits develop in the liver and liver cells are replaced by scare tissue leading to liver fibrosis and liver cirrhosis. With decreased liver cells, metabolism of alcohol and other chemical decrease leading to an increase of those substances in the blood. Alcohol blood levels can reach critical levels leading to alcohol poisoning and death. When liver cells in the blood enter a lower than normal range, the patient is possibly in liver failure and requires a liver transplant to live. Alcohol can also cause inflammation of the liver called alcoholic hepatitis.

Pancreas: Alcohol abuse and dependence can cause inflammation of the pancreatic duct preventing unobstructed flow of active pancreatic enzymes from flowing into the duodenum. As a result, active pancreatic enzymes remain in the pancreatic duct and pancreatitis causing pancreatitis.

Fetal alcohol spectrum disorder (FASD): Drinking alcohol at any stage of pregnancy can have an adverse effect on the fetus and lead to fetal alcohol spectrum disorder. First trimester: alcohol may disrupt fetal brain cell formation. Second trimester: facial features may be affected by alcohol. Third trimester: hippocampus format may be affected resulting in problems with vision and hearing. FASD results in delayed intellectual development, visual problems, hearing problems, abnormal behavior, and neurological problems that can lead to an abnormal gait. The fetus can experience facial deformities such as thin upper lip, missing grove in the upper lip, flatten mid-face, or shortened eye openings.

Hallmark Signs and Symptoms

- Patient response when alcohol is discussed with the patient:
  - Denies having a problem
  - Blames others for the problem
  - Angry when confronted about alcohol use
  - Avoids discussion about alcohol use

- Blood alcohol level and related behavior/impairment
  - 0.01 to 0.029
    - Normal
  - 0.03 to 0.059
    - Talkativeness
    - Decreased inhibition
    - Relaxed
    - Impaired concentration
    - Mild euphoria
  - 0.06 to 0.09
    - Impaired reasoning
    - Impaired vision
    - Emotional
    - Assertive
    - Excitable
    - Disregard for social conventions
    - Tactless
    - Disregard of feelings of other
    - Impaired recovery when a light source is shined into the eyes
  - 0.1 to 0.19
    - Anger
    - Emotional swings
    - Sadness
    - Loud
    - Impaired reflexes
    - Staggering
    - Erectile dysfunction
    - Slurred speech
    - Decreased libido
  - 0.2 to 0.29
    - Blackout
    - Stupor

- Motor impairment
- Impaired sensations
- 0.3 to 0.39
  - Unconsciousness
  - Impaired breathing
  - Depressed central nervous system
  - Impaired heart rate
  - Impaired bladder function
  - Risk of death
- 0.4 to 0.5
  - Impaired breathing
  - Impaired heart rate
  - Unconsciousness
  - Visible jerkiness in eye movement (positional alcohol nystagmus)
  - Risk of death
- \> 0.5
  - Alcohol poisoning
  - Risk of death
- Withdrawal symptoms:
  - 0 to 6 hours since last drink
    - Slurred speech
    - Anxiety
    - Unsteady gait
    - Anorexia
    - Lack of coordination
    - Insomnia
    - Impaired judgment
    - Nausea
    - Impaired memory
    - Fever
    - Label mood

- 6 to 24 hours since last drink
  - Delusions
  - Restlessness
  - Vomiting
  - Hallucinations
  - Poor concentration
  - Tremors
  - Excessive sweating
  - Increase anxiety
  - Hypertension
  - Tachycardia
- 12 to 24 hours since last drink
  - Grand mal seizure
    - Loss of consciousness
    - Violent muscle contractions
- 24 to 72 hours since last drink
  - Delirium tremens (DT)
    - Tachycardia
    - Increase temperature
    - Severe agitation
    - Disorientation
    - Restlessness
    - Unable to recognize others and self
- Ingesting alcohol while taking Antabuse (disulfiram)
  - Respiratory distress
  - Hypotension
  - Palpitations
  - Blurred vision
  - Flush
  - Confusion
  - Sweating
  - Increase thirst
  - Nausea

- Vomiting
- Tachycardia
- Weakness
- Chest Pain

Common Test Results

- Blood alcohol level: Reported in a tenth of one percent of the person's blood volume is alcohol. For example, 0.1 is one-tenth of one percent of the tested blood volume is alcohol. A blood alcohol test is typically reported as a whole number such as 290. This means 0.29 or 0.29% of the tested blood volume is alcohol.
- Alcohol use disorder identification test (AUDIT): 10-item assessment scored by a range of 0 to 40.
- Alcohol use disorder identification test-consumption (AUDIT-C): 4-item assessment scored by a range of 0 to 12.
- Alcohol use disorder identification test-primary care (AUDIT-PC): 5-item assessment scored by a range of 0 to 20.
- CAGE test: 4-item assessment scored as yes or no.
- Michigan alcoholism screening test (MAST): 25-item assessment scored as yes or no.
- Brief Michigan alcoholism screening test (MAST): 10-item assessment scored as yes or no.
- Short Michigan alcoholism screening test (MAST): 13-item assessment scored as yes or no.
- The initial step is to rule out physiological and other mental disorders causing the symptoms before reaching a psychiatric diagnosis. The psychiatric diagnosis of alcohol dependence disorder requires the following:
  - A patient must exhibit a maladaptive pattern that has had significant impairment indicated by at least three of the following over the previous 1 month:
    - Require an increasing amount of alcohol to reach the desired effect or a decrease in the desired effect when using the same amount of alcohol.
    - Experienced withdrawal symptoms or use alcohol to relieve or prevent withdrawal symptoms.
    - Ingesting large amounts or over longer periods than intended.
    - Persistently tries to reduce the use of alcohol without success.

- Spending significant time acquiring alcohol, using alcohol or recovering from the effects of alcohol.
- Reducing or eliminating social or occupational activities due to alcohol use.
- Continually using alcohol despite physical or psychological problems caused by alcohol use.

Treatment

- Chronic:
  - Group therapy: The goal of group therapy is to focus on underlying psychiatric problems that may be present.
  - Alcoholics Anonymous (AA): Alcoholics Anonymous is a 12-step program that helps the patient stay in recovery. The 12-step program is facilitated by recovering alcoholics. In addition to the 12-step program, a member of AA volunteers to sponsor the patient. The sponsor provides one-on-one support and advice 24/7. AA has meeting 24/7 in practically every area of the country. An 800 number is available to the patient and is to be called whenever the patient feels the urge to relapse.
  - Al-Anon: Al-Anon is a family self-help group that focuses on encouraging family member not to blame themselves for the patient's addiction to alcohol.
  - Alateen: Alateen is a self-help group for children of patients who are addicted to alcohol and has the same focus as Al-Anon.
  - Administer:
    - For aversion: Antabuse (disulfiram)
    - For cravings: Vivitrol (naltrexone), Revia (naltrexone IM), and Campral (acamprosate)
- Withdrawal:
  - Administer:
    - Thiamin, B-complex vitamins to assist in glucose metabolism and nutritional deficiency.
    - Benzodiazepines: Librium (chlordiazepoxide), Ativan (lorazepam), Xanax (alprazolam), and Serax (oxazepam) to reduce the risk of seizures.
    - Barbiturates: phenobarbital for sedation.
    - Anticonvulsants: Neurontin (gabapentin), Tegretol (carbamazepine), and Trileptal (oxcarbazepine) to prevent psychosis and hyperactivity.

- Antipsychotics: Haldol (haloperidol) to prevent psychosis and hyperactivity.
- Beta blockers: Inderal (propranolol) and Tenormin (atenolol) to treat hypertension and tremors.
- Lasix (furosemide) for over hydration.
- Magnesium sulfate to reduce central nervous system irritability.

Nursing Diagnoses

- Risk for memory impairment related to increasing ingestion of alcohol
- Risk for altered nutrition less than body requirements related to decreasing food intake while intoxicated
- Risk for impaired social interaction related to intoxication.

NURSING INTERVENTION

- Patient is not withdrawing
  - Develop a therapeutic rapport with the patient.
  - Be emphatic to the patient.
  - Acknowledge that the patient's addiction to alcohol resulted in a breakdown in the patient's health, welfare, family, and support structure.
  - Help the patient rationalize that the patient's addiction is the root cause of the patient's problem. No one is to blame but himself or herself.
  - Explain the physiological of addiction.
  - Tell the patient that the patient will be in recovery for the rest of the patient's life.
  - Discuss options for AA, Al-Anon, Alateen, inpatient rehabs, outpatient rehabs, partial hospital programs, and treatment options.
  - Acknowledge that the patient has tried and failed at treatment options.
  - Tell the patient the goal is to extend the length of time between relapses.
  - Ask the patient how long is the urge to drink (ie, 20 minutes, 60 minutes, 2 hours). Devise a plan that the patient can enact when the patient has the urge to drink (ie, call a sponsor and friends who are in recovery).
- Patient is withdrawing
  - Focus on the physiological aspect of withdrawal.
  - Develop a therapeutic rapport.
  - Assess how much alcohol the patient ingested.
  - Determine the last time the patient ingested alcohol. This will give you an idea when the patient will begin withdrawing.

- Monitor the patient's vital signs.
- Place the patient in a quiet environment.
- Place the patient on seizure precaution.
- Be alert for signs of DT (see Hallmark signs and symptoms).
- Monitor the patient for safety. The patient may have an unsteady gait and be confused.
- Monitor the patient's blood pressure. The patient may be hypotensive related to medication and be unable walk without assistance.
- Place the patient on constant observation if the patient is violent. Some patient exhibit aggression when intoxicated and during withdrawal.
- **Explain to the patient:**
  - Do not attempt to confront the patient about the patient's denial being addicted to alcohol or addressing treatment and recovery until the patient is near the end or has finished detox.
  - The risk of abusing alcohol.
  - Treatment options.

2. Amphetamine Abuse Disorder

What Went Wrong

An amphetamine is a stimulus that increases alertness and decreases fatigue resulting in a temporary pleasurable rush. Amphetamines are prescribed for a number of disorders including Attention Deficit Hyperactive Disorder (ADHD), narcolepsy, and sleep disorder. Amphetamines are dextroamphetamine, methamphetamine, and amphetamine sulfate. Commonly prescribed amphetamines are Ritalin, Adderall, and Dexedrine. Street names for amphetamine are Bennies, Black beauties, Crank, Crystal, Glass, Ice, Krystal meth, Louee, Meth, Shabu, Speed, and Uppers.

Amphetamine abuse disorder occurs when a person self-medicates with amphetamine to experience a feeling of a pleasurable high and is seeking to improve performance and staying awake for long periods. The effects of amphetamines will vary based on the person's size, weight, health, and tolerance to the drug, and the route with which the drug is administered. Injection and smoking amphetamine produce an immediate effect. Snorting or swallowing takes upward of 30 minutes to produce the effect.

The patient increases stress on the body by combining amphetamines with cocaine, ecstasy, alcohol, cannabis, benzodiazepines, and heroin. Using amphetamines with cocaine and ecstasy can lead to a stroke. Patients typically will binge on amphetamines, which is called a run. For days, the patient injects or smokes amphetamines every 3 hours forgoing sleep and food. The run ends when the patient has exhausted money for amphetamines or is physically unable to continue.

Amphetamine releases dopamine, norepinephrine, and serotonin creating pleasurable high related to high levels of dopamine within the area of the brain that regulates pleasure. Feeling high lasts several minutes afterward there is a feeling of irritability, depression, and radical mood swings during the withdrawing from the drug. A combination of feeling uncomfortable during withdrawal and the desire to feel pleasurable high results in becoming physical dependent on amphetamines.

Prognosis

The effects of amphetamine abuse resolve several days after the patient stops using amphetamines. The patient can develop amphetamine psychosis resulting in delusions, hallucinations, and bizarre behavior, if the patient uses frequent high doses of amphetamines. Long-term effects of amphetamine use can lead to hypertension, cardiac disease, kidney failure, malnutrition, insomnia, dental disease, memory loss, depression, risk of stroke, paranoia, panic, decrease immune system, and short of breath. These symptoms can last years after the patient stops taking amphetamines.

Hallmark Signs and Symptoms

- Under the influence
  - Feeling of euphoria and sense of well-being
  - Alert
  - Need for less sleep
  - Sense of superiority
  - Talkativeness
  - Increased libido
  - Dilated pupils
  - Sweating
  - Increased temperature
  - Itching/scratching
  - Picking at skin thinking insects are crawling on their body (formication)
  - Palpitations

- Increase blood pressure
- Decrease appetite
- Overdose
  - Irregular breathing
  - Blurred vision
  - Seizures
  - Hallucinations
  - Aggressive behavior
  - Loss of coordination
  - Collapse
  - Stroke
  - Coma
  - Tachycardia
- Withdrawal
  - Irritable
  - Restless
  - Aggression
  - Mood swings
  - Exhaustion
  - Depression
  - Paranoia
  - Lethargy

Common Test Results

- Urine toxicology: Positive for amphetamine.
- The initial step is to rule out physiological and other mental disorders causing the symptoms before reaching a psychiatric diagnosis. The psychiatric diagnosis of amphetamine abuse disorder requires the following:
  - A patient must exhibit a maladaptive pattern that has had significant impairment indicated by at least three of the following over the previous 1 month:
    - Require an increasing amount of amphetamine to reach the desired effect or a decrease in the desired effect when using the same amount of amphetamine.

- Experienced withdrawal symptoms or use amphetamine to relieve or prevent withdrawal symptoms.
- Ingesting large amounts or over longer periods than intended.
- Persistently tries to reduce the use of amphetamine without success.
- Spending significant time acquiring amphetamine, using amphetamine or recovering from the effects of amphetamine.
- Reducing or eliminating social or occupational activities due to amphetamine use.
- Continually using amphetamine despite physical or psychological problems caused by amphetamine use.

Treatment

Chronic:

- Cognitive behavioral therapy: The goal is for the patient to change behavior and develop alternative coping mechanisms than self-medicating with amphetamine.
- Narcotics Anonymous (NA): Narcotics Anonymous is a 12-step program that helps the patient stay in recovery. The 12-step program is facilitated by recovering drug abuses. In addition to the 12-step program, a member of NA volunteers to sponsor the patient. The sponsor provides one-on-one support and advice 24/7. NA has meeting 24/7 in practically every area of the country. An 800 number is available to the patient and is to be called whenever the patient feels the urge to relapse.

Withdrawal:

- Amphetamine withdrawal is treated symptomatically.
- Monitor vital signs
- Gastric lavage is performed to remove amphetamines that were ingested, if needed.
- Apply a cooling blanket, if needed.
- Administer:
  - IV fluids restore fluids.
  - Nutritional supplements for malnutrition
  - Vitamins for malnutrition
  - Ativan (lorazepam), Klonopin (clonazepam), and Valium (diazepam) to prevent seizures and induce sleep.

- Imodium for diarrhea
- Osmitrol (mannitol) to increase urination related to acute kidney failure
- Benadryl (diphenhydramine) and Cogentin (Benztropine) for muscle relaxation

Nursing Diagnoses

- Risk for self-injury related to aggressive behavior
- Risk for confusion related to the effects of amphetamine
- Risk for malnutrition related to decreasing eating

NURSING INTERVENTION

- Patient is not withdrawing.
  - Develop a therapeutic rapport with the patient.
  - Be emphatic to the patient.
  - Help the patient rationalize that the patient's addiction is the root cause of the patient's problem. No one is to blame but himself or herself.
  - Explain the physiological of addiction.
  - Tell the patient that the patient will be in recovery for the rest of the patient's life.
  - Discuss options for NA, inpatient rehabs, outpatient rehabs, partial hospital programs, and treatment options.
  - Acknowledge that the patient has tried and failed at treatment options.
  - Tell the patient the goal is to extend the length of time between relapses.
  - Ask the patient how long is the urge to use amphetamine (ie, 20 minutes, 60 minutes, 2 hours). Devise a plan that the patient can enact when the patient has the urge to use amphetamine (ie, call a sponsor and friends who are in recovery).
- Patient is withdrawing
  - Focus on the physiological aspect of withdrawal.
  - Monitor the patient's vital signs. The patient may have tachycardia, hypertension, and increased temperature.
  - Place the patient in a quiet environment.
  - Place the patient on seizure precaution.
  - Be alert for signs of seizures
  - Monitor the patient for safety. The patient may be confused and agitated.
  - Monitor and treat symptoms of withdrawal.

> - **Explain to the patient:**
>   - Risks of continued substance abuse.
>   - Treatment options.

3. Anxiolytic, Hypnotic, Sedative-Dependent Disorder

What Went Wrong

Anxiolytic, hypnotic, sedative-dependent disorder occurs when the patient becomes dependent on anxiolytic, hypnotic, or sedative medication. Collective these classes of drugs reduce anxiety and induce sleep and can be taken orally or injected intramuscular or intravenously. Depending on the route, the effect can be immediate or take several minutes and lasts up to 8 hours.

Medication includes Librium (chlordiazepoxide), Ativan (lorazepam), Klonopin (clonazepam), Xanax (alprazolam), Valium (diazepam), Ambien (zolpidem), and Sonata (zaleplon). Street names for these drugs include yellow jackets, dolls, and roaches.

Anxiolytic, hypnotic, and sedatives decrease the potential of the gamma-aminobutyric acid (GABA) neurotransmitter resulting in slowing the actions of the central nervous system and a relaxing feeling. Over time, the patient develops a tolerance to the medication requiring a higher dose to achieve the calming effect. The patient experiences a jittery feeling and becomes irritable during withdrawal leading the patient to administer the drug to remove withdrawal symptoms. Withdrawal symptoms begin within 4 days after the last dose and may reoccur intermittently for a year after the last dose. The patient is treated with benzodiazepine in tapering doses to prevent seizures.

Prognosis

Long-term use may lead to irritability, depression, memory impairment, sleep disorder, and personality changes. The patient may become psychologically and physiologically dependent on the medication and unable to cope with stress without using the medication.

Hallmark Signs and Symptoms

Under the Influence:

- Slurred speech
- Increase appetite

- Aggression
- Personality changes
- Anxiety
- Decrease muscle coordination
- Drowsiness
- Hypotension
- Memory loss
- Insomnia

Overdose:

- Blurred vision
- Unresponsiveness
- Coma
- Decrease muscle tone
- Depressed respiration
- Hallucinations
- Uncontrolled body movement

Withdrawal:

- Confusion
- Seizures
- Hypertension
- Paranoia
- Panic attacks
- Headache
- Sweating
- Abdominal pain
- Insomnia
- Decrease appetite

Common Test Results

- Urine toxicology: Positive for anxiolytic, hypnotic, or sedative
- The initial step is to rule out physiological and other mental disorders causing the symptoms before reaching a psychiatric diagnosis. The psychiatric

diagnosis of anxiolytic, hypnotic, or sedative dependency disorder requires the following:

- A patient must exhibit a maladaptive pattern that has had significant impairment indicated by at least three of the following over the previous 1 month:
  - Require an increasing amount of alcohol to reach the desired effect or a decrease in the desired effect when using the same amount of anxiolytic, hypnotic, or sedative.
  - Experienced withdrawal symptoms or use anxiolytic, hypnotic, or sedative to relieve or prevent withdrawal symptoms.
  - Ingesting large amounts or over longer periods than intended.
  - Persistently tries to reduce the use of anxiolytic, hypnotic, or sedative without success.
  - Spending significant time acquiring anxiolytic, hypnotic, or sedative, using anxiolytic, hypnotic, or sedative or recovering from the effects of anxiolytic, hypnotic, or sedative.
  - Reducing or eliminating social or occupational activities due to anxiolytic, hypnotic, or sedative use.
  - Continually using alcohol despite physical or psychological problems caused by anxiolytic, hypnotic, or sedative use.

Treatment

- Chronic:
  - Group therapy: The goal of group therapy is to focus on underlying psychiatric problems that may be present.
  - Cognitive behavioral therapy: The goal is for the patient to change behavior and develop alternative coping mechanisms than self-medicating with anxiolytic, hypnotic, or sedative.
  - Narcotics Anonymous (NA): Narcotics Anonymous is a 12-step program that helps the patient stay in recovery. The 12-step program is facilitated by recovering drug users. In addition to the 12-step program, a member of NA volunteers to sponsor the patient. The sponsor provides one-on-one support and advice 24/7. NA has meeting 24/7 in practically every area of the country. An 800 number is available to the patient and is to be called whenever the patient feels the urge to relapse.

- Withdrawal:
  - Administer:
    - Benzodiazepines: Librium (chlordiazepoxide), Ativan (lorazepam), Xanax (alprazolam), and Serax (oxazepam) to reduce the risk of seizures

Nursing Diagnoses

- Risk for impaired social interaction related to the sedated effect of the medication.
- Ineffective coping related to self-administering medication to cope with stress.
- Ineffective denial related to denial that the patient is dependent on medication.

NURSING INTERVENTION

- Patient is not withdrawing.
  - Develop a therapeutic rapport with the patient.
  - Be emphatic to the patient.
  - Acknowledge that the patient's addiction to anxiolytic, hypnotic, or sedative resulted in a breakdown in the patient's health, welfare, family, and support structure.
  - Help the patient rationalize that the patient's addiction is the root cause of the patient's problem. No one is to blame but himself or herself.
  - Explain the physiological of addiction.
  - Tell the patient that the patient will be in recovery for the rest of the patient's life.
  - Discuss options for NA, inpatient rehabs, outpatient rehabs, partial hospital programs, and treatment options.
  - Acknowledge that the patient has tried and failed at treatment options.
  - Tell the patient the goal is to extend the length of time between relapses.
  - Ask the patient how long is the urge to use drugs (ie, 20 minutes, 60 minutes, 2 hours). Devise a plan that the patient can enact when the patient has the urge to use drugs (ie, call a sponsor and friends who are in recovery).
- Patient is withdrawing.
  - Focus on the physiological aspect of withdrawal.
  - Develop a therapeutic rapport.
  - Monitor the patient's vital signs.

- Place the patient in a quiet environment.
- Place the patient on seizure precaution.
- Monitor the patient for safety. The patient may have an unsteady gait and be confused.
- Monitor the patient's blood pressure. The patient may be hypotensive related to medication and be unable to walk without assistance.

4. Cannabis Abuse Disorder

What Went Wrong

A patient diagnosed with cannabis abuse disorder ingests cannabis for the recreational purpose to induce euphoria. Cannabis is a drug that is extracted from the hemp plant, in leaf form it is called marijuana and its resin form is called hashish. In leaf form, cannabis is smoked or ingested as tea. Leaves are rolled to form cigarettes. Alternatively, a cigar is opened and the tobacco is replaced with marijuana to form a blunt. In resin form, cannabis is smoked using water pipes called bongs. Street names for cannabis are 420, Acapulco gold, Aunt Mary, baby, bale, bomber, weed, joint, doobee, hooch, Jane, Jay smoke, loco, tea, roach, refer, and blunt. The onset effect of cannabis is within 2 hours of ingestion and can have a diminishing effect for up to 12 hours. Researchers believe that cannabis is psychologically addictive and some cannabis uses experience withdrawal symptoms.

Patients who use cannabis may combine cannabis with other drugs such as crack cocaine, PCP, and opioid to achieve a combined effect from both drugs. Medical cannabis is used as an antiemetic for patients undergoing chemotherapy to prevent nausea and vomiting.

The active ingredient in cannabis is tetrahydrocannabinol (THC). THC enters the bloodstream when cannabis is ingested by the patient and is carried to the brain. THC attaches to cannabinoid receptors in the brain leading to the sense of pleasure and effecting coordination, learning, perception, and memory.

Prognosis

Some researchers believe that the long-term use of cannabis can lead to anxiety, depression, decrease memory, and psychosis. Other researchers believe that cannabis is a gateway drug and use of cannabis may encourage a patient to experiment with other prescribed and street drugs. Regular use of cannabis may lead to disruptions of activities of daily living including employment resulting in financial hardship.

Hallmark Signs and Symptoms

Cannabis use:

- Dry mouth
- Hypertension
- Red eyes
- Decrease reaction time
- Increase heart rate
- Increase breathing
- Increase appetite
- Paranoia
- Short-term memory loss
- Depression
- Grandiose
- Euphoria
- Perceptual distortion
- Hyperalertness
- Poor coordination
- Time distortion
- Depression
- Magical thinking

Cannabis overdose:

- Aspiration pneumonia
- Respiratory distress
- Hypotension
- Pulmonary edema

Cannabis withdrawal:

- Mood swings
- Restlessness

- Craving for cannabis
- Insomnia
- Weight change (loss/gain)
- Increase appetite
- Headaches

Common Test Results

- Urine toxicology: Positive for THC
- The initial step is to rule out physiological and other mental disorders causing the symptoms before reaching a psychiatric diagnosis. The psychiatric diagnosis of cannabis abuse disorder requires the following:
  - A patient must exhibit a maladaptive pattern that has had significant impairment indicated by at least three of the following over the previous 1 month:
    - Require an increasing amount of cannabis to reach the desired effect or a decrease in the desired effect when using the same amount of cannabis.
    - Experienced withdrawal symptoms or use cannabis to relieve or prevent withdrawal symptoms.
    - Ingesting large amounts or over longer periods than intended.
    - Persistently tries to reduce the use of cannabis without success.
    - Spending significant time acquiring cannabis, using cannabis or recovering from the effects of cannabis.
    - Reducing or eliminating social or occupational activities due to cannabis use.
    - Continually using cannabis despite physical or psychological problems caused by cannabis use.

Treatment

Chronic:

- Cognitive behavioral therapy: The goal is for the patient to change behavior and develop alternative coping mechanisms than self-medicating with amphetamine.
- Narcotics Anonymous (NA): Narcotics Anonymous is a 12-step program that helps the patient stay in recovery. The 12-step program is facilitated

by recovering drug abuses. In addition to the 12-step program, a member of NA volunteers to sponsor the patient. The sponsor provides one-on-one support and advice 24/7. NA has meeting 24/7 in practically every area of the country. An 800 number is available to the patient and is to be called whenever the patient feels the urge to relapse.

Withdrawal:

- Cannabis withdrawal is treated symptomatically.
- Monitor vital signs
- Administer:
  - Ativan (lorazepam), Klonopin (clonazepam), and Valium (diazepam) reduce restlessness and insomnia.

Nursing Diagnoses

- Risk for self-injury related to poor coordination
- Ineffective individual coping related to the use of cannabis to cope with life's challenges
- Risk for disturbed personal identity related to grandiose behavior

NURSING INTERVENTION

- Patient is not withdrawing.
  - Develop a therapeutic rapport with the patient.
  - Be emphatic to the patient.
  - Help the patient rationalize that cannabis can be psychologically addicting.
  - Acknowledge that the patient has tried and failed at treatment options.
  - Tell the patient the goal is to extend the length of time between relapses.
  - Ask the patient how long is the urge to use cannabis (ie, 20 minutes, 60 minutes, 2 hours). Devise a plan that the patient can enact when the patient has the urge to use cannabis (ie, call a sponsor and friends who are in recovery).
- Patient is withdrawing
  - Focus on the physiological aspect of withdrawal.
  - Monitor the patient's vital signs.
  - Place the patient in a quiet environment
  - Monitor the patient for safety. The patient may be confused and agitated.
  - Monitor and treat symptoms of withdrawal.

- **Explain to the patient:**
  - Risk of substance abuse.
  - Treatment options.
    - Tell the patient that the patient will be in recovery for the rest of the patient's life.
    - Discuss options for NA, inpatient rehabs, outpatient rehabs, partial hospital programs, and treatment options.

5. Cocaine Abuse Disorder

What Went Wrong

Cocaine abuse disorder occurs when a patient takes cocaine to realize a feeling of hyper alertness, euphoria, and energy. Cocaine is contained in coca leaves. The effects of cocaine can be felt by chewing coca leave. Cocaine abusers use a purified form of cocaine called cocaine hydrochloride. Cocaine can be prescribed as an anesthetic for eye, ear, and throat surgeries. Cocaine is known on the street as coke, snow, blow, flake, or C, and it is usually dilute with cornstarch, sugar, talcum powder, or combined with amphetamine, procaine, or heroin. The combination of cocaine and heroin is called a speedball.

Two forms of cocaine are abused. These are water-soluble hydrochloride salt and water-insoluble cocaine base. Water-soluble hydrochloride salt cocaine is injected IV or snorted. Water-insoluble cocaine base, called freebase, is processed into a smokable substance called crack.

The effect of cocaine occurs immediately and can last up to an hour. During that period the patient decreases food intake and sleep. The patient experiences an immediate down feeling once the effect of cocaine wears off.

The most commonly used combined drug is cocaine and alcohol. The combination is converted into cocaethylene that increases the duration of the effects of the drugs and increases the toxic level of the drugs that can result in death.

Cocaine enters the bloodstream through nasal mucous when cocaine is sniffed. Cocaine that is smoked (crack) enters the lungs in vapor, and it is absorbed by lung tissue into the bloodstream. Cocaine travels through the bloodstream into the ventral tegmental area (VTA) of the brain where neurons are effected leading to an increase in dopamine in the pleasure centers of the brain.

Prognosis

The patient develops a tolerance for cocaine with prolong use that results in the patient increasing the amount of cocaine used to achieve the initial euphoric feels called chasing the high. The patient will become increasingly restless, irritable, and develop paranoid psychosis. In addition, the patient is at risk for cardiac disorders, stroke, seizures, and respiratory failure with long-term use of cocaine as cocaine over taxing the cardiorespiratory system. Prolong snorting cocaine may result in damage to the nasal septum.

Hallmark Signs and Symptoms

Cocaine use:

- Dilated pupils
- Euphoria
- Increase sociability
- Vertigo
- Runny nose
- Energetic
- Increase alertness
- Nasal congestion
- Decrease pain
- Abnormal EKG

Cocaine withdrawal:

- Restlessness
- Nausea and vomiting
- Agitation
- Craving for cocaine
- Pain
- Insomnia
- Fatigue

Common Test Results

- Urine toxicology: Positive for cocaine
- The initial step is to rule out physiological and other mental disorders causing the symptoms before reaching a psychiatric diagnosis. The psychiatric diagnosis of cocaine abuse disorder requires the following:
  - A patient must exhibit a maladaptive pattern that has had significant impairment indicated by at least three of the following over the previous 1 month:

- Require an increasing amount of cocaine to reach the desired effect or a decrease in the desired effect when using the same amount of cocaine.
- Experienced withdrawal symptoms or use cocaine to relieve or prevent withdrawal symptoms.
- Ingesting large amounts or over longer periods than intended.
- Persistently tries to reduce the use of cocaine without success.
- Spending significant time acquiring cocaine, using cocaine or recovering from the effects of cocaine.
- Reducing or eliminating social or occupational activities due to cocaine use.
- Continually using cocaine despite physical or psychological problems caused by cocaine use.

Treatment

Chronic:

- Cognitive behavioral therapy: The goal is for the patient to change behavior and develop alternative coping mechanisms than self-medicating with amphetamine.
- Narcotics Anonymous (NA): Narcotics Anonymous is a 12-step program that helps the patient stay in recovery. The 12-step program is facilitated by recovering drug abuses. In addition to the 12-step program, a member of NA volunteers to sponsor the patient. The sponsor provides one-on-one support and advice 24/7. NA has meeting 24/7 in practically every area of the country. An 800 number is available to the patient and is to be called whenever the patient feels the urge to relapse.

Withdrawal:

- Cocaine withdrawal is treated symptomatically.
- Monitor vital signs
- Administer:
  - Ativan (lorazepam), Klonopin (clonazepam), and Valium (diazepam) reduce restlessness and insomnia.
  - Thiamin, B-complex vitamins to assist in glucose metabolism and nutritional deficiency.
  - Benzodiazepines: Librium (chlordiazepoxide), Ativan (lorazepam), Xanax (alprazolam), and Serax (oxazepam) to reduce the risk of seizures

- Barbiturates: phenobarbital for sedation
- Antipsychotics: Haldol (haloperidol) to prevent psychosis and hyperactivity
- Beta blockers: Inderal (propranolol) and Tenormin (atenolol) to treat hypertension.
- Magnesium sulfate to reduce central nervous system irritability

Nursing Diagnoses

- Risk for altered nutrition less than body requirements related to decreasing food intake while intoxicated
- Risk for self-injury related to aggressive behavior
- Ineffective individual coping related to the use of cocaine to cope with life's challenges

NURSING INTERVENTION

- Patient is not withdrawing
  - Develop a therapeutic rapport with the patient
  - Be emphatic to the patient.
  - Help the patient rationalize that cocaine can be physiologically and psychologically addicting.
  - Tell the patient that the patient will be in recovery for the rest of the patient's life.
  - Discuss options for NA, inpatient rehabs, outpatient rehabs, partial hospital programs and treatment options.
  - Acknowledge that the patient has tried and failed at treatment options.
  - Tell the patient the goal is to extend the length of time between relapses.
  - Ask the patient how long is the urge to use cannabis (ie, 20 minutes, 60 minutes, 2 hours). Devise a plan that the patient can enact when the patient has the urge to use cannabis (ie, call a sponsor and friends who are in recovery).
- Patient is withdrawing
  - Focus on the physiological aspect of withdrawal.
  - Monitor the patient's vital signs.
  - Place the patient in a quiet environment
  - Monitor the patient for safety. The patient may be confused and agitated.
  - Monitor and treat symptoms of withdrawal.
  - Monitor for long-term physiological effects of cocaine on the cardiorespiratory system.

6. Hallucinogen Abuse Disorder

What Went Wrong

Hallucinogen abuse disorder occurs when the patient uses a hallucinogen to cause distortion of reality. A hallucinogen may produce a feeling of detachment from the patient's body or produce visual and special distortions. Patients may report being able to see sound and hear color. Most hallucinogens are ingested although some can be administered be injected intravenously or intramuscularly. There is no known medical use for most hallucinogen although psilocybin is used for religious rites in Mexico and peyote is used by some Native Americans. Dextromethorphan is also used for cough suppression. Common hallucinogens are as follows:

Dextromethorphan (DXM). Dextromethorphan is an ingredient in over-the-counter cough medication and produces a detachment effect in high doses that can last upward of 6 hours. Street names for dextromethorphan include red devils, dex, vitamin D, orange crush, robo, and triple C's.

Methylenedioxy-methamphetamine (MDMA, Ecstasy): Ecstasy is a synthetic hallucinogen that also has the effects of a stimulant. Ecstasy takes an effect almost immediately and lasts upward for 6 hours. Street names for Ecstasy include Club drug, Adam, bean, XTC, X, New Yorkers, Love drug, and clarity.

Lysergic acid diethylamide (LSD): LSD is a synthetic hallucinogen distributed in the form of microdots or gelatin squares. The effects of LSD are almost immediate and may last upward for 12 hours. Street names for LSD include acid, microdot, sunshine, pink robots, boomers, and superman.

Ketamine: Ketamine causes the patient to feel detached from himself or herself, and it is used at rave parties. Ketamine is called the date rape drug because it is odorless and tasteless and can be slipped into a drink without the knowledge of the person who ingests the drink. The effects of Ketamine can last upward of 12 hours. Street names for ketamine include K, special K, bump, vitamin K, super acid, ket, and psychedelic heroin.

Mescaline: Mescaline is a natural hallucinogen found in the peyote and San Pedro specifies of cactus and alters visual hallucinations and distorted perception of space that can last upward for 12 hours. Street names for mescaline include cactus, mescal, peyote, buttons, mesc, and mezc.

Phencyclidine (PCP): Phencyclidine is a synthetic hallucinogen that causes a feeling of detachment for up to 12 hours. Street names for phencyclidine include angel dust, Peter Pan, magic, black wack, crystal join, and zoom.

Psilocybin: Psilocybin is a natural hallucinogen found in the Psilocybe Mexicana mushroom. Psilocybin causes the feeling of detachment from the body. Street names for psilocybin include Mexican mushrooms, mushrooms, silly putty, magic mushroom, and shrooms.

Hallucinogens are chemicals that disrupt serotonin neurotransmitter resulting in disruption of behavioral control, muscle control, sensory perception, regulatory control, and sexual behavior.

Prognosis

The long-term effects of hallucinogens are unpredictable. Some patients experience increase anxiety and paranoia. Others have flashbacks of effects hallucinogens weeks and years after the patient stops taking hallucinogens. There is a risk of long-term psychoses.

Hallmark Signs and Symptoms

Dextromethorphan use:

- Paranoia
- Sensation of floating
- Distorted perception of time
- Audio and visual hallucinations

Ecstasy use:

- Euphoria
- Mental clarity
- Increase sexuality
- Increase alertness
- Confusion
- Dilated pupils
- Fever
- Sweating
- Distractibility
- Dehydration

Ketamine use:

- Feeling of detachment from the body
- Hypertension

- Amnesia
- Depression
- Delirium
- Impaired learning ability

LSD and mescaline use:

- Mystical experience
- Distorted perception
- Grandiose
- Hallucinations
- Sweating
- Increase salivation
- Fever
- Chills
- Tachycardia
- Arrhythmias
- Hypertension
- Muscle aches
- Loss of appetite

Phencyclidine use:

- Depersonalization
- Hallucinations
- Euphoria
- Aggressive behavior
- Numbness
- Unsteady gait
- Bloodshot eyes
- Bizarre violence

Psilocybin use:

- Visual hallucinations
- Euphoria
- Fever
- Hypertension

- Mood swings
- Seeing sound
- Hearing color
- Personality changes

Hallucinogen withdrawal:

- Diarrhea
- Hyperthermia
- Depression
- Flashbacks
- Hypertension
- Tachycardia
- Aggressive behavior
- Muscle spasms
- Psychosis
- Seizures

Common Test Results

- Urine toxicology: Positive for specific hallucinogen.
- The initial step is to rule out physiological and other mental disorders causing the symptoms before reaching a psychiatric diagnosis. The psychiatric diagnosis of cocaine abuse disorder requires the following:
  - A patient must exhibit a maladaptive pattern that has had significant impairment indicated by at least three of the following over the previous 1 month:
    - Require an increasing amount of cocaine to reach the desired effect or a decrease in the desired effect when using the same amount of hallucinogen.
    - Experienced withdrawal symptoms or use cocaine to relieve or prevent withdrawal symptoms.
    - Ingesting large amounts or over longer periods than intended.
    - Persistently tries to reduce the use of hallucinogen without success.
    - Spending significant time acquiring hallucinogen, using cocaine or recovering from the effects of hallucinogen.

- Reducing or eliminating social or occupational activities due to hallucinogen use.
- Continually using hallucinogen despite physical or psychological problems caused by cocaine use.

Treatment

Chronic:

- Cognitive behavioral therapy: The goal is for the patient to change behavior and develop alternative coping mechanisms than self-medicating with hallucinogen.
- Narcotics Anonymous (NA): Narcotics Anonymous is a 12-step program that helps the patient stay in recovery. The 12-step program is facilitated by recovering drug abuses. In addition to the 12-step program, a member of NA volunteers to sponsor the patient. The sponsor provides one-on-one support and advice 24/7. NA has meeting 24/7 in practically every area of the country. An 800 number is available to the patient and is to be called whenever the patient feels the urge to relapse.

Withdrawal:

- Hallucinogen withdrawal is treated symptomatically.
- Monitor vital signs
- Administer:
  - Ativan (lorazepam), Klonopin (clonazepam), and Valium (diazepam) reduce restlessness and insomnia.
  - Benzodiazepines: Librium (chlordiazepoxide), Ativan (lorazepam), Xanax (alprazolam), and Serax (oxazepam) to reduce the risk of seizures
  - Barbiturates: phenobarbital for sedation
  - Antipsychotics: Haldol (haloperidol) to prevent psychosis and hyperactivity
  - Beta blockers: Inderal (propranolol) and Tenormin (atenolol) to treat hypertension.
  - Magnesium sulfate to reduce central nervous system irritability

Nursing Diagnoses

- Risk for self-injury related to aggressive behavior

- Risk for confusion related to the effects of hallucinogens
- Ineffective individual coping related to the use of hallucinogens to cope with life's challenges

NURSING INTERVENTION

- Patient is not withdrawing
  - Develop a therapeutic rapport with the patient
  - Be emphatic to the patient.
  - Help the patient rationalize that the patient's addiction is the root cause of the patient's problem. No one is to blame but himself or herself.
  - Explain the physiological of addiction.
  - Tell the patient that the patient will be in recovery for the rest of the patient's life.
  - Discuss options for NA, inpatient rehabs, outpatient rehabs, partial hospital programs, and treatment options.
  - Acknowledge that the patient has tried and failed at treatment options.
  - Tell the patient the goal is to extend the length of time between relapses.
  - Ask the patient how long is the urge to use hallucinogens (ie, 20 minutes, 60 minutes, 2 hours). Devise a plan that the patient can enact when the patient has the urge to use hallucinogens (ie, call a sponsor and friends who are in recovery).
- Patient is withdrawing
  - Focus on the physiological aspect of withdrawal.
  - Monitor the patient's vital signs. The patient may have tachycardia, hypertension, and increased temperature.
  - Place the patient in a quiet environment.
  - Place the patient on seizure precaution.
  - Be alert for signs of seizures.
  - Monitor the patient for safety. The patient may be confused and agitated.
  - Monitor and treat symptoms of withdrawal.

7. Inhalant Abuse Disorder

What Went Wrong

Inhalant abuse disorder occurs when a patient inhales chemical vapors that create an altered mental state creating a euphoric feeling commonly referred to as a buzz. The vapor is released into a bag in a process called bagging or huffing. The patient inhales vapors from the bag through the patient's nose or mouth. Some patients soak a rag with the chemical and either place the rag into the bag or inhale vapors directly from the rag. The euphoric effect lasts briefly causing the patient to increase uses of the inhalant to seek the high.

There are many types of inhalants used by patients who are diagnosed with inhalant abuse disorder. Inhalants are categorized as aerosol, gases, nitrites, and volatile solvents. Commonly used inhalants are

Aerosols: paint, cooking sprays, hair sprays, and spray paint.

Gases: nitrous oxide, butane lighters, chloroform, and propane.

Nitrites: cyclohexyl nitrite, room deodorizers, butyl nitrite, and amyl nitrite

Volatile solvents: nail polish, glue, correction fluid, paints thinner, nail polish remover, and felt-tip markers.

Commonly used street names for inhalants are head cleaner, bopper, poor man's pot, gluey, climax, rush, and hippie crack.

Researchers believe that inhalants use the same mechanism as the central nervous system depressant to produce a sedated and anesthetic effect. Inhalants activate the dopamine system that produces the rewarding effect when chemicals in the inhalant interact with neurotransmitters. Other researchers believe chemicals in the inhalant increase the potentiation of the GABA neurotransmitter to reduce inhibitions. Inhalants produce signs and symptoms similar to alcohol intoxication.

Prognosis

The patient is likely to continue to use inhalants in an effort to achieve the initial euphoric feeling. Continue use interferes with the patient's activities of daily living including the capability of hold a job and responding to family demands. Furthermore, decrease appetite may leave the patient malnourished leading to medical disorders. The patient is exposed to sudden sniffing death where repeated inhalations build up in the patient's body displacing oxygen resulting in asphyxiation. The patient may also experience suffocation if the patient places the vapor-filled plastic bag over his head. Since inhalant has a sedative effect, the patient may experience a coma or choking. The patient is also at risk for seizures. Continue use can also have a neurotoxic effect impeding the patient's vision, hearing, and cognitive ability.

Hallmark Signs and Symptoms

Under the influence:

- Stains on body or clothes
- Odor of inhalant on breath or clothes

- Disoriented
- Slurred speech
- Irritable
- Depressed
- Uncoordinated movements
- Inattentiveness
- Nausea
- Decrease appetite
- Lightheadedness
- Drowsiness
- Belligerence
- Impaired functioning
- Confusion
- Muscle weakness
- Euphoria
- Increase heart rate
- Flush

Overdose:

- Delirium
- Coma
- Seizures

Inhalant withdrawal:

- Insomnia
- Aggression
- Muscle pains
- Sweating
- Headaches
- Psychosis
- Hallucinations
- Irritability
- Tremors

Common Test Results

- Blood test: The blood test reveals the level of the active ingredient in the inhalant, if the laboratory tested for specific active ingredients.
- The initial step is to rule out physiological and other mental disorders causing the symptoms before reaching a psychiatric diagnosis. The psychiatric diagnosis of inhalant abuse disorder requires the following:
- A patient must exhibit a maladaptive pattern that has had significant impairment indicated by at least three of the following over the previous 1 month:
  - Require an increasing amount of inhalant to reach the desired effect or a decrease in the desired effect when using the same amount of inhalant.
  - Experienced withdrawal symptoms or use inhalant to relieve or prevent withdrawal symptoms.
  - Ingesting large amounts or over longer periods than intended.
  - Persistently tries to reduce the use of inhalant without success.
  - Spending significant time acquiring alcohol, using alcohol, or recovering from the effects of inhalant.
  - Reducing or eliminating social or occupational activities due to inhalant use.
  - Continually using inhalant despite physical or psychological problems caused by inhalant use.

Treatment

- Chronic:
  - Cognitive behavioral therapy: The goal is for the patient to change behavior and develop alternative coping mechanisms than self-medicating with inhalants.
  - Narcotics Anonymous (NA): Narcotics Anonymous is a 12-step program that helps the patient stay in recovery. The 12-step program is facilitated by recovering drug abuses. In addition to the 12-step program, a member of NA volunteers to sponsor the patient. The sponsor provides one-on-one support and advice 24/7. NA has meeting 24/7 in practically every area of the country. An 800 number is available to the patient and is to be called whenever the patient feels the urge to relapse.

- Withdrawal:
  - Administer:
    - Thiamin, B-complex vitamins to assist in glucose metabolism and nutritional deficiency.
    - Benzodiazepines: Librium (chlordiazepoxide), Ativan (lorazepam), Xanax (alprazolam), and Serax (oxazepam) to reduce the risk of seizures
    - Barbiturates: Phenobarbital for sedation
    - Anticonvulsants: Neurontin (gabapentin), Tegretol (carbamazepine), and Trileptal (oxcarbazepine) to prevent psychosis and hyperactivity
    - Antipsychotics: Haldol (haloperidol) to prevent psychosis and hyperactivity
    - Lasix (furosemide) for over hydration
    - Magnesium sulfate to reduce central nervous system irritability

Nursing Diagnoses

- Risk for altered nutrition less than body requirements related to decreasing food intake while intoxicated
- Risk for impaired social interaction related to intoxication
- Risk for self-injury related to aggressive behavior

NURSING INTERVENTION

- Patient is not withdrawing
  - Develop a therapeutic rapport with the patient
  - Be emphatic to the patient.
  - Acknowledge that the patient's addiction to inhalants resulted in a breakdown in the patient's health, welfare, family, and support structure.
  - Help the patient rationalize that the patient's addiction is the root cause of the patient's problem. No one is to blame but himself or herself.
  - Explain the physiological of addiction.
  - Tell the patient that the patient will be in recovery for the rest of the patient's life.
  - Discuss options for NA, inpatient rehabs, outpatient rehabs, partial hospital programs, and treatment options.
  - Acknowledge that the patient has tried and failed at treatment options.

- Tell the patient the goal is to extend the length of time between relapses.
- Ask the patient how long is the urge to drink (ie, 20 minutes, 60 minutes, 2 hours). Devise a plan that the patient can enact when the patient has the urge to drink (ie, call a sponsor and friends who are in recovery).
- Patient is withdrawing
  - Focus on the physiological aspect of withdrawal.
  - Monitor the patient's vital signs
  - Place the patient in a quiet environment
  - Place the patient on seizure precaution.
  - Monitor the patient for safety. The patient may have an unsteady gait and be confused.
  - Monitor the patient's blood pressure. The patient may be hypotensive related to medication and be unable walk without assistance.
  - Place the patient on constant observation if the patient is violent. Some patient exhibit aggression when intoxicated and during withdrawal.

8. Nicotine-Dependent Disorder

What Went Wrong

Nicotine-dependent disorder occurs when the patient requires nicotine to perform activities of daily living. Nicotine is found in tobacco. The patient inhales nicotine when smoking a cigarette, pipe, or cigar. Nicotine can also enter the body by sniffing snuff and chewing tobacco. Each cigarette contains a minimum of 10 mg of nicotine and delivers 2 mg of nicotine to the bloodstream.

Nicotine is a sedative and stimulant. Long draws of a cigarette produce a sedative effect while short draws produce a stimulating effect. The effect is realized within 15 seconds and lasts upward for 50 minutes for many smokers afterward the patient experience withdrawal effects.

A patient diagnosed with nicotine-dependent disorder has both a psychological and physical dependence on nicotine. Psychological dependency occurs when the patient associates activities with smoking such as getting up from bed, eating, and drinking alcohol. These situations trigger the desire to smoke. Physical dependency occurs when the decrease level of nicotine in the bloodstream causes withdrawal symptoms requiring the patient to increase the nicotine level in the bloodstream in order to feel normal. That is, make the withdrawal symptoms go away.

Nicotine is absorbed in the lungs and in the mucosal tissues of the mouth and it travels through the bloodstream to the brain where nicotine increases dopamine levels stimulating the reward centers of the brain resulting in the feeling of pleasure. Nicotine also causes increase production of endorphins and the adrenocorticotropic hormone that causes the adrenal glands to release epinephrine into the bloodstream. Arginine vasopressin levels also increase in the bloodstream. The patient experiences hypertension, increase glucose levels, fast pulse, and increase respiration commonly called an epinephrine rush.

Prognosis

Nicotine and smoking is associated with cancer of the lung, mouth pancreas, esophagus, bladder, stomach, kidney, ureter, and cervix. There is also an increase in cardiovascular disease among patients diagnosed with nicotine-dependent disorder.

Hallmark Signs and Symptoms

Under the influence:

- Normal behavior

Withdrawal:

- Irritability
- Increased appetite
- Restlessness
- Unable to concentrate
- Craving
- Seeks sweets
- Anxiety
- Coughing

Common Test Results

- Urine toxicology test: Nicotine is detected in the patient's urine.
- The initial step is to rule out physiological and other mental disorders causing the symptoms before reaching a psychiatric diagnosis. The psychiatric diagnosis of alcohol dependency disorder requires the following:
  - A patient must exhibit a maladaptive pattern that has had significant impairment indicated by at least three of the following over the previous 1 month:

- Require an increased amount of inhalant to reach the desired effect or a decrease in the desired effect when using the same amount of nicotine.
- Experienced withdrawal symptoms or use nicotine to relieve or prevent withdrawal symptoms.
- Ingesting large amounts or over longer periods than intended.
- Persistently tries to reduce the use of nicotine without success.
- Spending significant time acquiring nicotine, using alcohol or recovering from the effects of nicotine.
- Reducing or eliminating social or occupational activities due to nicotine use.
- Continually using nicotine despite physical or psychological problems caused by inhalant use.

Treatment

- Chronic:
  - Cognitive behavioral therapy: The goal is for the patient to change behavior and develop alternative coping mechanisms than self-medicating with nicotine.
  - Smoking cessation therapy: Smoking cessation therapy is a combination of individual and group therapy that helps the patient develop alternatives to smoking when experiencing psychological and physiological withdrawal symptoms.
  - Administer:
    - Nicotine antagonist: Inversine (mecamylamine), Vivitrol (naltrexone), and Revia (naltrexone) that block nicotine receptors.
    - Silver acetate gum results in foul taste when the patient smokes.
    - Antidepressant: Zyban (bupropion)
    - Chantix (varenicline)
- Withdrawal:
  - Administer:
    - Nicotine transdermal patch gradually lowering the dose of nicotine.
    - Nicotine gum
    - Benzodiazepines: Ativan (lorazepam) and Xanax (alprazolam) to reduce irritability

Nursing Diagnoses

- Risk for impaired gas exchange related to smoking
- Risk for chronic low self-esteem related to social aversion to second-hand smoke
- Impaired comfort related to nicotine withdrawal

NURSING INTERVENTION

- Patient is not withdrawing
  - Develop a therapeutic rapport with the patient
  - Be emphatic to the patient.
  - Explain the physiological of addiction.
  - Tell the patient that the patient will be in recovery for the rest of the patient's life.
  - Discuss treatment options.
  - Acknowledge that the patient has tried and failed at treatment options.
  - Tell the patient the goal is to extend the length of time between relapses.
  - Ask the patient how long is the urge to drink (ie, 20 minutes, 60 minutes, 2 hours). Devise a plan that the patient can enact when the patient has the urge to smoke (ie, call a sponsor and friends who are in recovery).
- Patient is withdrawing
  - Focus on the physiological aspect of withdrawal.
  - Monitor the patient's vital signs
  - Place the patient in a quiet environment
  - The patient may become severely agitated exhibit aggression during withdrawal.

9. Opioid-Dependent Disorder

What Went Wrong

Opioid-dependent disorder occurs when a patient becomes psychologically and physiologically dependent on opioids. Opioids are narcotic analgesics that bind to the opioid receptors in the central nervous system, peripheral nervous system, and the gastrointestinal tract that result in the decrease perception of pain. Some opioids such as codeine are also used for suppressive coughing and stop diarrhea.

Opioids can be taken orally, transdermal or injected intramuscular or intravenous. Patients diagnosed with opioid-dependent disorder may also snort opioids. The initial sense of euphoria called a rush occurs immediately when the opioid reaches the bloodstream. The fastest route is with intravenous injection. The effect may last up to 6 hours depending on the dose.

Commonly prescribed opioids are: morphine, Demerol (meperidine), Dilaudid (hydromorphone), Alfenta (alfentanil), fentanyl, Ultiva (remifentanil), Sufenta (sufentanil), Suboxone (buprenorphine and naloxone), codeine, Vicodin (hydrocodone), Lorcet (hydrocodone bitartrate acetaminophen), Dolophine (methadone), OxyContin (oxycodone and acetaminophen), Oxycodan (oxycodone and aspirin), Vicoprofen (hydrocodone bitartrate ibuprofen), Subutex (buprenorphine), and Roxicodone (oxycodone hydrochloride).

All prescribed opioids are available illegally on the streets. In addition, heroin (diamorphine) called smack, scat, horse, and H on the street is sold as a relatively inexpensive opioid. However, the quality of heroin is questionable.

Narcan (naloxone) is an opioid antagonist and is used to immediately reverse the effect of opioids and therefore it is used in emergencies when the patient is overly medicated with opioids. Suboxone (buprenorphine and naloxone) is an opioid that is administered for opioid withdrawal. Suboxone contains naloxone and therefore should not be administered until the patient shows the first signs of opioid withdrawal. If Suboxone will place the patient in immediate withdrawal if given before the patient shows signs of withdrawal.

The terms opiate and opioid are used to describe opioid dependent. An opiate is a natural narcotic analgesic that comes from opium poppy. An opioid is not natural and is a synthetic narcotic analgesic. Many times opiate and opioid are used synonymously.

There may be confusion between Subutex and Suboxone. Both are opioids used to treat opioid dependence. Both Subutex and Suboxone contain buprenorphine hydrochloride. However, Suboxone also contains naloxone, which is an opioid antagonist used to prevent misuse of Suboxone.

Endorphins are neurotransmitters that inhibit neurons from transmitting impulses. Levels of endorphins increase during times when the patient may experience pain such as during childbirth and exercising. Morphine is the active ingredient of opioids and it has a structure similar to endorphins. Both endorphins and morphine adhere to endorphin receptors in the body producing a euphoric feeling of the analgesic effect commonly known as a high. Opioids like endorphins make the person feel good. The body regulates the amount of endorphins produced lowering the amount during less painful situations such as watching television. The desire to feel good encourages the patient to self-medicate with opioids even during less painful situations resulting in dependency. As morphine is metabolized and excreted from the body, the patient experiences an uncomfortable feeling of opioid withdrawal that is relieved by self-medicating with opioids.

Opioid withdrawal is very uncomfortable as the body is adjusting to the absence of opioids; however, the patient is not in any life-threatening danger. Opioid withdrawal symptoms resolve within 10 days.

Prognosis

Use of opioids several times a day for weeks or more may lead to physical dependency and produce withdrawal symptoms if the same level of opioids is not maintained in the bloodstream. Some patients use heroin as a recreational drug. Other patients follow a common progression in the use of heroin. The progress begins with an injury that leads to chronic pain. The patient is prescribed opioids and gradually abuses opioids by taking increased doses without the practitioner's approval. The practitioner may prescribe a 30-day supply and not return prior to 30 days. The patient may exhaust the 30-day supply in a few days and then seek other practitioners who will prescribe opioids unbeknown to the original practitioner. This process is referred to as doctor shopping. The patient may exhaust available prescribers and then turn to street dealers to provide opioids. Prescription opioids are costly. The patient then results in snorting and then using intravenous heroin, which is less costly and produces a similar effect; however, the quality of heroin is unknown. The patient is at risk for overdosing. If the patient shares IV needles, then the patient is at risk for hepatitis, HIV, and infection.

Hallmark Signs and Symptoms

Under the influence:

- Pinpoint pupils
- Uncontrollable eye movement
- Euphoria
- Clammy skin
- Constipation
- Impaired judgment
- Drowsiness
- Sweating
- Slow breathing
- Slurred speech
- Decrease appetite

Withdrawal:

- Muscle aches
- Sweating
- Agitation
- Dilated pupils
- Insomnia
- Chills
- Anxiety
- Anorexia
- Nausea
- Goose-bumps
- Vomiting
- Running nose
- Abdominal cramping
- Diarrhea
- Body pain

Overdose:

- Decrease level of consciousness
- Slow breathing
- Bluish coloring on lips and nail beds
- Muscle spasms
- Seizures
- Unable to be aroused

Common Test Results

- Urine toxicology: Positive for opioids.
- Blood test: Positive for opioids.
- The initial step is to rule out physiological and other mental disorders causing the symptoms before reaching a psychiatric diagnosis. The psychiatric diagnosis of opioid dependency disorder requires the following:
  - A patient must exhibit a maladaptive pattern that has had significant impairment indicated by at least three of the following over the previous 1 month:

- Require an increasing amount of opioid to reach the desired effect or a decrease in the desired effect when using the same amount of opioid.
- Experienced withdrawal symptoms or use opioid to relieve or prevent withdrawal symptoms.
- Ingesting large amounts or over longer periods than intended.
- Persistently tries to reduce the use of opioid without success.
- Spending significant time acquiring opioid, using alcohol or recovering from the effects of opioid.
- Reducing or eliminating social or occupational activities due to opioid use.
- Continually using opioid despite physical or psychological problems caused by alcohol use.

Treatment

- Chronic:
  - Group therapy: The goal of group therapy is to focus on underlying psychiatric problems that may be present.
  - Cognitive behavioral therapy: The goal is for the patient to change behavior and develop alternative coping mechanisms than self-medicating with opioids.
  - Narcotics Anonymous (AA): Narcotics Anonymous is a 12-step program that helps the patient stay in recovery. The 12-step program is facilitated by recovering drugs users. In addition to the 12-step program, a member of NA volunteers to sponsor the patient. The sponsor provides one-on-one support and advice 24/7. NA has meeting 24/7 in practically every area of the country. An 800 number is available to the patient and is to be called whenever the patient feels the urge to relapse.
- Administer:
  - For cravings:
    - Vivitrol (naltrexone) and Revia (naltrexone IM)
    - Suboxone (buprenorphine and naloxone) for maintenance
    - Withdrawal:
- Administer:
  - Suboxone (buprenorphine and naloxone)
  - Benzodiazepines: Ativan (lorazepam) and Xanax (alprazolam) for agitation

- Catapres (clonidine) for hypertension
  - Baclofen for muscle relaxation
- Overdose:
  - Administer: Narcan (naloxone)

Nursing Diagnoses

- Risk for ineffective relationship related to addictive behavior
- Ineffective coping skills related to self-medicating with opioids
- Risk for injury related to use of opioids.

NURSING INTERVENTION

- Patient is not withdrawing.
  - Develop a therapeutic rapport with the patient.
  - Be emphatic to the patient.
  - Acknowledge that the patient's addiction to opioid resulted in a breakdown in the patient's health, welfare, family, and support structure.
  - Help the patient rationalize that the patient's addiction is the root cause of the patient's problem. No one is to blame but himself or herself.
  - Explain the physiological of addiction.
  - Tell the patient that the patient will be in recovery for the rest of the patient's life.
  - Discuss options for NA, inpatient rehabs, outpatient rehabs, partial hospital programs, and treatment options.
  - Acknowledge that the patient has tried and failed at treatment options.
  - Tell the patient the goal is to extend the length of time between relapses.
  - Ask the patient how long is the urge to use (ie, 20 minutes, 60 minutes, 2 hours). Devise a plan that the patient can enact when the patient has the urge to drink (ie, call a sponsor and friends who are in recovery).
- Patient is withdrawing
  - Focus on the physiological aspect of withdrawal.
  - Develop a therapeutic rapport.
  - Assess how much opioids the patient has taken.
  - Monitor the patient's vital signs.
  - Monitor the patient's signs of opioid withdrawal.
  - Place the patient in a quiet environment.
  - Place the patient on constant observation if the patient is violent. Some patient exhibit aggression when during withdrawal.

REVIEW QUESTIONS

1. A patient who completed detoxing from heroin tells you that his or her family members who are not substance abusers do not understand how it feels to go through withdrawal. He or she asks you for advice. Which of the following is the best response?

   A. Tell your family members to attend Alcoholics Anonymous.

   B. Ask your family members if they ever had the flu. Tell them that withdrawal is like having the worst flu they ever had.

   C. Tell your family member that going through withdrawal is like going on a diet.

   D. Tell your family member to try heroin once.

2. A patient in heroin withdrawal comes to the nurse's station demanding a narcotic saying he or she is going to die from the withdrawal. The patient received detox medication 30 minutes ago. What is the best response?

   A. Call a rapid response before the patient has a seizure.

   B. Tell the patient he or she is not going to die from opioid withdrawal and that you will see if he or she has any PRN medications available.

   C. Tell the patient to speak with the practitioner in the morning.

   D. Tell the patient that you will call the practitioner now to see if the practitioner will order a narcotic.

3. A patient who has completed detox is ready to start recovery. He or she asks for advice. Which of the following is the best advice to give the patient?

   A. Focus on 1 day at a time. Identify your triggers and learn ways to avoid them.

   B. The goal of recovery is to lengthen periods between relapses.

   C. You will be in recovery all your life.

   D. Ask the practitioner to recommend you to a rehab program.

4. A patient is brought into the ER. The patient's BAL is 0.48 and the patient is unconscious. What is the first thing you do?

   A. Place the patient in a quiet area and wait until the patient begins to sober before continuing your assessment.

   B. Call the ED practitioner immediately.

   C. Administer Narcan to the patient.

   D. Send the patient to ICU immediately.

5. A patient is admitted to the ER and presents as very talkative, highly alert, a pupil dilated, has a relatively high temperature and is sweating. He or she tells

you he or she never needs to sleep any more. What would you suspect is causing the patient's condition?

A. The patient is under the influence of heroin.

B. The patient is under the influence of amphetamines.

C. The patient is under the influence of oxycodone.

D. The patient is under the influence of Oxycodan.

6. **A new medical resident assessed a patient who is starting withdrawal from benzodiazepine. The resident writes orders for Ativan. What is your best response?**

A. Ask the attending physician to review the orders.

B. Administer the medication as prescribed.

C. Ask the resident to clarify the orders.

D. Point out to the resident that the patient is dependent on benzodiazepine.

7. **A student nurse arrives on the unit and asks you what the rationale for treatment of withdrawal is. What is the best response?**

A. To protect the patient while the body removes the drug from the patient's bloodstream.

B. To protect the patient from relapsing during withdrawal.

C. To treat the patient's psychological dependency on the substance.

D. To treat the symptoms of withdrawal while the body removes the substance from the patient's bloodstream.

8. **During a family meeting, the patient's father called his son a bum because of his drugs use and running afoul of the law. What is the best response?**

A. Anyone can become physiologically and psychologically dependent on drugs, which can result in drug-seeking behaviors that can lead to health, financial, family, and legal problems.

B. Your son realizes his problem and is trying to change.

C. Have you thought about going to family therapy?

D. Have you heard about Nar-Anon or Al-Anon?

9. **A 43-year-old man came to the ED reporting that for short periods of time he feels detached from his body and sometimes he feels like he is floating. The patient states he had not taken any drugs and his drug toxicology test results are negative. What is your best response?**

A. Does this condition interfere with activities of daily living?

B. Did you ever take hallucinogenic at any time in your life?

C. Let me ask our psychiatrist to assess you.

D. Do you have any other symptoms?

10. Your neighbor tells you about her preteen son. It seems that he has an ongoing head cold. His sinus is congested; he is not eating regularly and is losing weight. Your neighbor reports that his head cold is so bad that he has to wear sun glasses even in the hour. She asks him to remove the glasses but he becomes agitated. You noticed her son is around the neighborhood during school hours when the rest of the family is working. What is your best response?

A. You better take your son to your doctor immediately. He might have more than a head cold.

B. Do you notice any money missing from your house?

C. Is your son going to school?

D. Your son's condition and behavior does not seem normal. Why do not you ask your practitioner to assess your son.

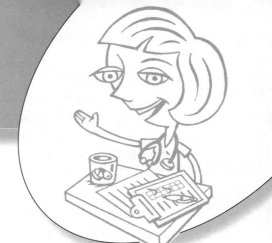

Chapter **18**

Common Laboratory and Diagnostic Tests

Abdominal Ultrasound

This is a noninvasive test and is usually painless. A transducer is guided over the abdomen, which produces sound waves that bounce off internal structures and produce a picture of internal organs and structures.

Before the test: The patient will need to be NPO (nothing by mouth).

After the test: No special care is needed.

Abdominal X-rays

These are plain x-rays, usually flat plate and upright, of the abdomen, to look for obstruction, foreign bodies, gas patterns, tumors, and other abnormalities. This test is often done to assess the major organs and structures within the abdomen. An abdominal x-ray done to specifically view the kidney, ureters, and bladder is called a KUB. Bismuth-containing medications (which are over-the-counter [OTC] products) may interfere with the test for several days after ingestion.

Before and after the test: No special care is needed.

Adrenocorticotropic Hormone Stimulation Test

This test measures the level of cortisol in a patient's blood after injection of synthetic adrenocorticotropic hormone stimulation test (ACTH). It is used to diagnose Cushing's syndrome, Cushing's disease, primary adrenal insufficiency, and ACTH insufficiency.

Before and after the test: Explain to the patient that this is often a nonfasting blood test, but high intake of carbohydrates should be avoided up to 12 hours prior to the test. A blood sample is taken before the injection of synthetic ACTH and again an hour after the injection.

Aldosterone Test

This test measures the level of the hormone aldosterone in the blood. It may be part of the workup for hypertension and is also used in diagnosing aldosteronism, adrenal adenoma, hyperplasia, nephrotic syndrome, Addison's disease, diabetes mellitus, and acute alcohol intake.

Before the test: Explain to the patient that this is a non-fasting blood test.

Allergy Skin Testing

An allergy skin test is used to confirm whether such symptoms as sneezing, wheezing, and skin rashes are caused by allergies. The test is performed by exposing an area of the skin to the extract of an allergen and then evaluating the skin's reaction. A wheal and/or erythema indicate confirmation of the allergy. An intradermal test, where the allergen is injected just under the skin, or a patch test, where an allergen patch is placed on the skin, may also be used.

Before the test: Instruct the patient to withhold antihistamines, steroids, and leukotriene modulator medications which would interfere with the results of the test. Explain to the patient what to expect.

Arterial Blood Gas

Arterial blood gas (ABG) determines the patient's ventilation, tissue oxygenation, and acid-base status. Three to five milliliters of blood is sampled from an artery in a heparinized syringe. If the sample cannot be analyzed immediately, it should be placed on ice. Usually the radial, brachial, or femoral arteries are used.

The normal ranges for results are

- pH 7.35 to 7.45
  - Increased level of pH shows alkalosis.
  - Decreased level of pH shows acidosis.
- PaO_2 80 to 100 mmHg
  - Increased level of PaO_2 shows elevated levels of oxygen, which may occur with hyperventilation.
  - Decreased level of PaO_2 shows low levels of oxygen which may be seen with respiratory difficulties.
- $PaCO_2$ 35 to 45 mmHg
  - Increased level of $PaCO_2$ indicates elevated levels of carbon dioxide, which may be seen in respiratory disorders where CO_2 is retained.
  - Decreased level of $PaCO_2$ indicates low levels of carbon dioxide, which may be seen in hyperventilation where the patient "blows off" CO_2.
- HCO_3 22 to 26 mEq/L
  - Increased level of HCO_3 indicates elevated bicarbonate, which may be seen in metabolic alkalosis (due to excess antacid use, hypokalemia, or excess gastrointestinal [GI] fluid loss).
  - Decreased level of HCO_3 indicates low levels of bicarbonate, which may be seen in metabolic acidosis (due to ketoacidosis, renal failure, diarrhea, salicylate overdose).

Before the test: Provide the laboratory with information on whether or not the patient is receiving supplemental oxygen or mechanical ventilation as well as the amount of oxygen received or the setting of the ventilator. Oxygen supplementation at the time of testing will be reported with the results. Note the patient's temperature. Alteration in temperature may alter the results of the test. Explain to the patient that arterial sticks may be more uncomfortable than venipuncture for routine laboratory work performed by the phlebotomists.

After the test: Apply mechanical pressure to puncture site for 5 minutes. Apply pressure dressing to puncture site for 30 minutes once bleeding has stopped. Monitor the puncture site for bleeding.

Arthrogram

An x-ray of a joint area is taken after the injection of a contrast medium has been injected into the joint space to enhance its visibility. In a double-contrast study, a solution is injected, followed by air. This may be done to better assess the possibility of bone chips or torn ligaments within the joint space.

Before the test: Determine if the patient has a history of allergy to contrast.

Arthroscopy

Fiberoptic scope is used to visually examine the joint, performed under some type of anesthesia (local, epidural, conscious sedation, or general). This is done to perform surgery concurrently, diagnose injuries to joint spaces, and assess response to prior treatments.

After the test: Regularly check the neurovascular status of the extremity—color, pulses, sensation, motion, and temperature. Teach patient to monitor for signs of infection—redness, swelling, fever, and increased pain.

Beta Subunit of Human Chorionic Gonadotropin

Beta subunit of human chorionic gonadotropin (beta hCG) test, better known as pregnancy testing, is used to detect early pregnancy and to diagnose or to monitor trophoblastic disease and other beta hCG secreting tumors. Using a chemiluminescent or fluorometric immunoassay, the test measures the level of beta hCG in a blood or urine sample. A detectable level of hormone will be present in the blood prior to in the urine.

Biopsy

Biopsy is removal of tissue (soft tissue, connective tissue, vascular tissue, or bone) from the body for examination to determine if cellular changes have occurred. It is one of the principal tools used in diagnosing cancer. The sample may be taken through closed (needle) biopsy or open (incisional) biopsy. *Core* or *incisional* biopsy involves removal of only a sample of tissue. When an entire lump or suspicious area of the skin or underlying tissue is removed, the procedure used is an *excisional biopsy*. *Needle aspiration biopsy* involves the removal of tissue or fluid with a needle. It is done to determine the presence of infection, cancer, muscular atrophy or inflammation, or the presence of mitochondrial disorders.

After the test: Always monitor the patient for bleeding following a biopsy.

Blood Urea Nitrogen

Urea nitrogen appears in the blood as protein breaks down. The test is typically done to evaluate kidney function. Low level of blood urea nitrogen (BUN) means fluid overload, low muscle mass, with low protein, and low carbohydrate diet; high level means renal disease, dehydration, acute MI, ketoacidosis, and excess protein intake. Use of certain medications, especially diuretics and certain antibiotics, may elevate the BUN level. Normal range is 8 to 25 mg/dL.

Bone Marrow Biopsy

Bone marrow biopsy is a biopsy or removal of bone marrow by needle aspiration for evaluation of blood cell formation. Local anesthetic is used at the site: posterior iliac crest, sternum, and ribs. Skin is cleansed per protocol for a sterile procedure. Specimen is removed from within bone, properly labeled, and delivered to laboratory.

Before the test: Informed consent is typically obtained.

Bone Scan

This is a peripheral intravenous injection of bone-seeking radiopharmaceutical followed by 2 to 3 hours delayed imaging. The patient must lie still for the duration of the scanning, about 30 to 60 minutes. It is done to diagnose osteomyelitis, bone tumors, metastatic disease, fractures, and unexplained skeletal pain.

After the test: Encourage fluids after the injection to flush the radiopharmaceutical. Monitor for reaction to the radiopharmaceutical: rash, itching, hives, and so on.

Bronchoscopy

Bronchoscopy is used to view the bronchial tree and to remove foreign obstructions, obtain tissues for biopsy or for suctioning fluid. The patient is anesthetized, and a bronchoscope is inserted into the patient's mouth and down the trachea and bronchial tree. The bronchoscope contains a tiny video camera and probes that the physician manipulates to perform the procedure.

Before the test: The patient must sign an informed consent for an invasive procedure. The patient is NPO for 8 hours except in an emergency. Withholding food and fluids reduces the chance of vomiting when the bronchoscope is passed down the throat. Patients are monitored during the procedure.

After the test: The patient remains NPO until the gag reflex returns to avoid aspiration. Check for return of gag reflex. Monitor respirations for rate, effort, use of accessory muscles, and breath sounds. Monitor heart rate and respiratory status for changes. Monitor sputum for blood due to irritation within bronchi.

Calcium Level

This test measures the level of calcium (serum) in the blood. It is used to evaluate parathyroid and renal function. Also, the level rises in certain malignancies. Excessive intake of calcium (calcium-based antacids, milk) may elevate blood levels. Vitamin D supplementation, lithium, or thiazide diuretics may also elevate levels. Low levels of calcium may mean decreased albumin levels, hyperphosphatemia, hypoparathyroidism, vitamin D deficiency, and acute pancreatitis; high level means cancer, hyperparathyroidism, hyperthyroidism, prolonged immobilization, and Paget's disease. Normal range is 8.5 to 10.5 mg/dL.

Before the test: Explain to the patient that this is a non-fasting blood test.

Cancer Antigen 125

This test measures the amount of the protein, cancer antigen 125 (CA 125), in the blood. It is performed to monitor existing endometrial and ovarian cancers. This is not a screening test. The level may also be elevated in the first trimester of pregnancy, endometriosis, pelvic inflammatory disease, benign ovarian cysts, pancreatic cancer, or fibroids.

Cardiac Catheterization

Cardiac catheterization (angiography) is an invasive procedure used to examine the coronary arteries and intracardiac structures, as well as to measure cardiac output, intracardiac pressures, and oxygenation. A radiopaque dye, which makes structures visible on x-rays, is injected through a catheter into the femoral artery in the patient's left leg or in the antecubital fossa, which is the crease of the arm; it then flows to the coronary arteries. The flow of the radiopaque dye is viewed and recorded using a fluoroscope, enabling the physician to determine obstructions to the flow and the structures of the heart.

Before the test: Blood work to assess creatinine and BUN is typically checked. These are tests to determine kidney function. Determine if the patient is allergic to seafood or iodine. If so, notify the physician immediately because the patient might be also allergic to the radiopaque dye. Ensure that written consent is obtained from the patient. Risks and benefits of the test need to be explained to the patient before commencing the test. The procedure, risks, and benefits should be explained to the patient by the healthcare provider ordering or performing the test. The patient should be NPO for 4 to 6 hours before the test to reduce the risk of aspiration. Record baseline vital signs to determine a baseline to assess for changes.

After the test: Assess for bleeding at the injection site since a major artery has been accessed. If there is bleeding, apply pressure until bleeding stops. Keep the patient on bed rest for 8 hours, so as not to dislodge a clot from the artery used for the catheter. Keep pressure on injection site for 8 hours to ensure clotting at the site. If femoral artery is used, keep left leg straight for 8 hours to minimize risk of dislodging clot. If antecubital fossa is used, keep arm straight for 3 hours to minimize risk of dislodging clot. Monitor vital signs to assess for changes. Increase fluid intake to assist the kidneys in excreting the dye.

Cardiac Enzymes

Creatine kinase (CK) and CK isoenzymes are enzymes released if there is damage to the heart muscle, cardiac troponin levels (troponin is a protein in cardiac and skeletal muscles), myoglobin (an early indication of a myocardial infarction), lactate dehydrogenase (LDH), and LDH isoenzymes. These enzymes are released when cardiac tissue is damaged and are tested in a series of blood tests if damage is suspected.

Cerebral Angiography

Contrast is injected to visualize the cerebral circulation, carotid, and vertebral arteries. This test is done to identify aneurysms, arteriovenous malformations, traumatic injuries, strictures, occlusions, and tumors. The head is immobilized during the test. A wire is inserted via the femoral arterial site and passed to the carotid or vertebral vessel under fluoroscopic guidance. Contrast dye is injected so that three-dimensional images can be obtained.

After the test: You need to monitor vital signs and perform neurologic checks and neurovascular checks of the extremity (capillary refill, peripheral pulses, skin color, and temperature). Check for bleeding at the site.

Chest X-ray

Chest x-rays are done to detect size and position of the heart and structural abnormalities of the lungs. An x-ray machine directs x-rays through the chest and onto film positioned behind the patient's back. As x-rays are directed to the patient, some are absorbed by the body and others pass through to the x-ray film. Areas of the body that absorb x-rays appear light on the x-ray film. Dark areas on the film represent x-rays that passed through the body.

Before the test: Explain to the patient that they will be asked to hold his or her breath while the x-ray is taken. Instruct the patient to remove all jewelry, zippers, hooks, and any metal on the part of the body being x-rayed.

Chloride

In laboratory analysis of a blood sample, low level of chloride (Cl) means vomiting, nasogastric suctioning, chronic respiratory acidosis, metabolic alkalosis, Addison's disease, SIADH, and excess water intake. High level means dehydration, diarrhea, metabolic acidosis, hyperparathyroidism, Cushing's syndrome, and renal tubular acidosis. Normal range is 99 to 108 mmol/L.

Coagulation Studies

(*Prothrombin time* [PT], *internationalized normalized ratio* [INR], *partial thromboplastin time* [PTT], *bleeding time, platelet count*).

These are bleeding time tests to indicate the patient's clotting ability. Most interfere at some point in the clotting cascade. INR is used to monitor the effectiveness of warfarin. PT is used to help screen patients taking warfarin. Since PT is made in the liver, this test is also useful to monitor liver function. An abnormality in the PTT indicates defects in the patient's coagulation status and with blood factors and is used to monitor heparin therapy. Bleeding time quantifies the amount of time needed to stop bleeding from a small break made in the skin. Platelet count quantifies the amount of circulating platelets. Abnormalities of shape may also be noted.

Colonoscopy

This test is used to diagnose obstruction, bleeding, change in bowel habits, and colon cancer, among other conditions. An informed consent is obtained before the patient is given any type of anesthesia. A colonoscope is passed through the rectum to visualize the anus, sigmoid, descending colon, splenic flexure, transverse colon, hepatic flexure, ascending colon, and the ileocecal valve. The colon may be insufflated to aid in visualization of the structures. Biopsies are obtained as indicated. The scope is withdrawn and anesthesia is reversed. The patient may experience abdominal distention. Risks include perforation of the large intestine. The test is commonly performed as an outpatient procedure.

Before the test: A thorough colon preparation is necessary to ensure complete emptying of the bowel prior to the procedure. The patient is NPO for several hours prior to the test due to the use of an anesthetic agent.

After the test: Assess the abdomen for bowel sounds and tenderness. Monitor vital signs. Assess the patient for side effects of anesthesia.

Complete Blood Count

- *WBC*: white blood cell count.
- *RBC*: red blood cell count.
- *Hemoglobin*: oxygen carrying capability of the blood.
- *Hematocrit*: the percentage of concentration of red blood cells within whole blood.
- *MCV*: mean corpuscular volume.
- *MCH*: mean corpuscular hemoglobin.
- *MCHC*: mean corpuscular hemoglobin concentration.
- *RDW*: red cell distribution width which tells how close in size the red cells are to each other.
- *Platelet count*: necessary for normal clotting.
- *Reticulocyte count*: elevated levels show that (immature) red blood cells are being released from the bone marrow without sufficient time to mature.
- *Neutrophils*: white blood cells, the first to respond to bacterial infection.
- *Lymphocytes*: white blood cells (comprises B cells and T cells).
- *Monocytes*: white blood cells, elevated in chronic infection and autoimmune disorders.
- *Eosinophils*: white blood cells, elevated in allergies and some infections (parasitic).

Computed Tomography Scan

Computed tomography (CT) test uses x-rays to produce cross-sectional images of the body in two-dimensional slices. Split-second computer processing creates these images as a series of very thin x-ray beams that pass through the body. A dye (contrast medium) may be injected into a vein. In some instances, a non-contrast study may be done prior to a contrast-enhanced study. The enhanced (or clearer) images produced with the dye make it easier to distinguish a tumor from normal tissue. A CT scan uses more radiation than the conventional x-rays, but the benefits of the test outweigh the risks.

Before the test: Ask the patient about any history of allergy to contrast dye or shellfish. The patient may need to be NPO, depending on the area that needs to be imaged.

After the test: No special care is needed.

Computed Tomography Angiography

CT angiography creates a three-dimensional reconstruction of the vasculature within the area imaged.

Cortisol Test

This test measures the level of the hormone cortisol in the blood. It is performed to diagnose Addison's disease, nephritic syndrome, Cushing's syndrome, acute illness, trauma, septic shock, starvation, chronic renal failure, and pregnancy.

Before the test: Explain to the patient that this is a nonfasting blood test.

Culture and Sensitivity Tests

The culture test checks for the presence of bacteria in the urine. The sensitivity test determines what antibiotics can be used to eliminate the bacteria. The laboratory divides the urine specimen in half; one part is cultured to determine which bacteria grow. A preliminary report should be available in 24 hours. The second half is used to determine to which antibiotics the organism(s) are sensitive.

Before the test: Explain to the patient that the specimen must be obtained before an antibiotic can be started or the results will be altered.

Cystoscopy

This test examines the bladder walls to check for tumors and growths. It is also used as a therapeutic tool to remove small tumors, stones, and foreign bodies and to dilate the urethra and ureters. A cystoscope is inserted into the urethra to the bladder, which allows structures to be actually visualized, that is, the urethra, bladder, ureters, and prostate.

Before the test: Explain to the patient that this test may be performed under general, light, or local anesthesia. It will be uncomfortable if the patient is awake. Obtain informed consent.

After the test: Advise the patient to increase fluids to flush out bacteria that may have been introduced with the cystoscope. Bladder muscle spasms may result. The patient should expect some pink urine following the test. Frank, red blood warrants a call to the physician. Observe for signs of a urinary tract infection (UTI)—chills, fever, frequent, uncomfortable voiding, and pelvic discomfort.

Digital Subtraction Angiography

Digital subtraction angiography (DSA) enables the physician to view arterial blood supply to the heart using an injection of radiopaque contrast material. The patient is injected with an intravascular contrast material containing iodine. Images of bone and soft tissue are viewed from fluoroscopy through the use of a computer, enabling the physician to view the cardiovascular system.

Before the test: A written consent from the patient may be needed once risks and benefits have been explained.

After the test: Determine if there is bleeding at the injection site. Encourage the patient to drink plenty of fluid to aid the kidneys in excreting the dye. Monitor the patient's vital signs to assess for changes.

Echocardiograph

An ultrasound of the heart provides a noninvasive examination of intracardiac structures and blood flow. Sound waves are directed to and deflected by the heart, causing an echo that is detected by the echocardiograph, which is interpreted by a physician.

Before the test: Describe the procedure to the patient. The patient needs to lie still during the testing to allow for clear imaging.

Electrocardiograph

The electrocardiograph (EKG, ECG) is a graphic representation of the electrical activity of the heart in a noninvasive procedure. An electrical signal is generated each time the chambers of the heart contract. Small pads containing electrodes are temporarily placed on the surface of the skin to detect the hearts electrical signal.

For a 12-lead EKG, each electrode is connected with wires to an electrocardiograph, which draws up to 12 different graphical representations of the electrical signal in designated, labeled areas on specially designed paper. There are 12 electrodes used in a typical EKG: bipolar limb leads I, II, and III; augmented limb leads AVR, AVL, and AVF; and precordial chest leads V1 through V6. In another use, the electrodes are attached to three to five leads and a continuous rhythm strip is seen on a monitor screen (either at the bedside or in a remote location). The test may also be completed as a 24-hour (or longer) test to evaluate the patient's rhythm during everyday activities. Typically a technician will perform the electrocardiograph and a healthcare provider (physician, advanced practice nurse, or physician assistant) will interpret the results of the test.

During the test: The patient must lie still for several minutes if the electrocardiograph is done during a physical or assessment. The patient can move about normally if the electrocardiograph of the patient is ambulatory or if the patient is an inpatient during monitoring. The electrodes should not get wet.

Electroencephalogram

Electroencephalogram (EEG) test records the electrical activity from the cerebral hemispheres of the brain and creates a graphic recording. It determines general brain activity as well as the site of origin of seizure activity. It is also used to diagnose sleep disorders and determine brain death.

Electromyography

Multiple small needle-type electrodes are inserted into muscle areas to test muscle potential. The patient may be asked to move the area to allow for measurement during minimal and maximal contraction of the muscle. The amount of muscle and nerve activity is recorded graphically. Electromyography (EMG) test is done to detect neuromuscular, peripheral nerve disorders, or lower motor neuron disorders, and may be done in conjunction with nerve conduction studies.

Before the test: Explain to the patient that there may be some discomfort during the testing. Certain medications may need to be stopped prior to testing: muscle relaxants, stimulants, caffeine.

After the test: The patient may complain of pain or anxiety.

Enzyme-Linked Immunosorbent Assay

Enzyme-linked immunosorbent assay (ELISA) determines if the patient's blood contains certain antigens or antibodies. A variety of different disease states can be diagnosed using ELISA. Depending on the disease being tested, the test may be a direct or indirect ELISA. The test is used to detect antibodies to human immunodeficiency virus (HIV), West Nile virus, and also to detect food allergens. In certain diseases, such as HIV, an additional test is performed for confirmation. A Western blot test is routinely used for confirmation.

Endoscopic Retrograde Cholangiopancreatography

In endoscopic retrograde cholangiopancreatography (ERCP) a thin, flexible tube (endoscope) is passed through the pharynx, the stomach, and into the upper part of the small intestine. Air is used to inflate the intestinal tract to enable the openings of the pancreatic and bile ducts to be seen. A dye is injected into the ducts through a catheter via the endoscope. X-rays are taken of the ducts. The patient may report abdominal distention from the insufflation, and a sore throat.

Before the test: The patient is NPO.

After the test: Monitor vital signs. Assess for return of gag reflex. The patient remains NPO until gag reflex returns.

Erythrocyte Sedimentation Rate

In laboratory analysis of a blood sample, low level of erythrocyte sedimentation rate (ESR) means anti-inflammatories (steroids, aspirin), blood sample not processed in timely manner (allowed to sit); high level means inflammation, hormonal effect (pregnancy, menses, oral contraceptives). Normal range is 0 to 30 mm/h.

Fecal Occult Blood Test

A stool sample is tested to determine if blood is being passed in stool, even though it cannot be seen. A chemical reagent is applied to the sample. If blood is present, a color change occurs.

Before the test: Explain to the patient to avoid red meat, beets, turnips, horseradish, aspirin, nonsteroidal anti-inflammatory drugs (NSAIDs), vitamin C, and iron for 48 hours prior to test period as they may interfere with the test result.

Fine-Needle Biopsy/Aspiration

A small needle is passed through the skin into the area to be biopsied, retrieving a small amount of fluid or tissue to be analyzed. Depending on the organ or tissue to be studied, the procedure may be done in an outpatient or inpatient setting. The test is done to look for the presence of abnormal cells.

Before the test: An informed consent is necessary, as local anesthesia will be utilized.

After the test: A dressing will be applied to the site. Monitor the site for inflammation, drainage, bleeding, increased pain, fever, or any increase in swelling. An OTC analgesic or Rx from the practitioner may be necessary.

Follicle-Stimulating Hormone Test

Follicle-stimulating hormone (FSH) test measures the level of FSH in the blood. It is done to aid in the diagnosis of hypogonadism, precocious puberty, menstrual disorders, and the inability to conceive.

Before the test: Explain to the patient that this is a non-fasting blood test.

Fructosamine Test

This test determines the average blood glucose level over the past 2 to 3 weeks. It is typically used when there have been recent changes in diabetes management to see if the change is having the desired effect. It may also be ordered when there is a physiologic change in the required insulin for the diabetic patient, such as in pregnancy or with an acute systemic illness.

Before the test: Explain to the patient that this is a non-fasting blood test.

Gastroscopy

This test is used to diagnose peptic, gastric, or duodenal ulcers and to obtain biopsies and specimens for *Helicobacter pylori* bacteria. An informed consent is obtained prior to any anesthesia. An endoscope is passed through the mouth to allow visualization of the pharynx, esophagus, lower esophageal sphincter, stomach, pyloric sphincter, and duodenum. Biopsies can be obtained at this time. Bleeding, ulcers, lesions, and polyps can be visually assessed. The back of the throat will be anesthetized to allow passage of the endoscope.

Before the test: The patient will be NPO.

After the test: Monitor vital signs. Assess for return of gag reflex. The patient remains NPO until the gag reflex returns.

Glucose Tolerance Test

A 75 to 100 g carbohydrate drink is to be swallowed by the fasting patient. Blood work and urine specimens are obtained at 30 minutes, and then hourly for 3 to 4 hours. The test is done to evaluate those with elevated blood sugars, those with risk factors for diabetes, and pregnant women to ascertain their risk for gestational diabetes.

Before the test: Explain to the patient the need for a 12-hour fast prior to the test and water only throughout the test.

Glycosylated Hemoglobin Test

Glycosylated hemoglobin A_{1C} ($HgbA_{1C}$) test measures the amount of sugar that is attached to the hemoglobin in RBCs. Because RBCs live in the bloodstream for 100 to 120 days, the $HgbA_{1C}$ test shows the average blood sugar level for the past several months. The test is done to evaluate the effectiveness of long-term diabetes management. The patient does not need to be fasting for this test. A normal result is below 6 (or equal to 120 mg/dL average blood glucose).

Before the test: Explain to the patient that the test is not affected by recent food intake, medication, or exercise.

Gram Stain

Gram stain or Gram's method is a way of differentiating bacterial species into two large groups, gram positive and gram negative based on properties of their cell walls. A stain is added to a culture on a slide which will show blue for gram-positive cells or red for gram-negative cells. This is the first step in determining the identity of a particular bacterial sample and can be used to allow empiric antibiotics to be started, before the final culture is ready.

Growth Hormone Test

A growth hormone (GH) (somatotropin) test measures the level of GH in the blood and is part of the diagnostic workup for identifying the cause of abnormal GH production. It is performed to diagnose diminished or excessive growth, immature puberty, and pituitary abnormalities. Testing usually involves either a GH stimulation test or a GH suppression test to track GH levels over time.

Before the test: Explain to the patient that stress, exercise, and low blood sugar may increase the level of GH. Instruct the patient to fast for 10 to 12 hours.

Helicobacter Pylori

This is a gram-negative bacterium that can be detected by a serum test, discovered by gastric biopsy and ELISA for anti-*H pylori* immunoglobulin G. A carbon isotope urea breath test can reveal the presence of *H pylori* (which has a false-negative rate of 5% to 15%).

Hematocrit

In laboratory analysis of a blood sample, hematocrit level will be decreased in anemia, chronic disease, hemolytic reaction, adrenal insufficiency, leukemia, and lymphoma. Normal range is 34.3% to 44.4%.

Hemodynamic Monitoring

Hemodynamic monitoring measures cardiac output and intracardiac pressure. A balloon-tipped catheter is inserted into the pulmonary artery, usually through the femoral artery. It is able to measure pressures in the heart's various chambers and vessels.

Before the test: Obtain written consent from the patient to ensure he or she understands risks and benefits.

After the test: Determine if there is bleeding at the injection site. Look for signs of infection at the injection site (redness, warmth, swelling, or increasing discomfort). Examine for complications: air embolus, arrhythmia, and clots. Assess for decrease in respiratory effort, increase in respiratory rate, dyspnea.

Hemoglobin

In laboratory analysis of blood sample, hemoglobin level will be decreased in anemia, cancer, hemolytic reaction, liver disease, kidney disease, hyperthyroidism, systemic lupus erythematosus (SLE); increased in chronic obstructive pulmonary disease, hemoconcentration, polycythemia, burns. Normal range is 11.5 to 15.2 g/dL.

Hepatitis Panel

Tests for acute viral hepatitis include:

- Hepatitis B surface antigen (HBsAg)
- Hepatitis A virus antibody (anti-HAV)
- Hepatitis B core antibody immunoglobulin M (IgM anti-HBc)
- Hepatitis C virus antibody (anti-HCV)

Tests for chronic hepatitis include:

- Hepatitis B surface antigen (HBsAg)
- Hepatitis C virus antibody (anti-HCV)
- Hepatitis D virus antibody (anti-HDV)
- HAV is confirmed by detecting an IgM antibody to HAV (IgM anti-HAV).
- HBV is confirmed by detecting HBsAg and IgM anti-HBC (when hepatitis B early antigen (HBeAg) is detected, patient is highly infectious).

- HCV is confirmed by detecting ELISA-2 and RIBA-2.
- HDV is confirmed by detecting anti-HDV and serologic markers for HBV.
- HEV—only research-based tests are available at this time.

Herpes Simplex Virus Culture

Herpes simplex virus (HSV) culture test is performed by taking a fluid sample from the lesions within 3 days of appearance. The virus, if present, can be detected in this fluid sample in a few days. Blood testing can also be performed to identify antibodies for the particular type of herpes virus.

Hysterosalpingogram

Hysterosalpingogram (HSG) is an x-ray test that examines the inside of the uterus and fallopian tubes and the surrounding area. It is used to identify abnormalities, reasons for infertility, tubal pregnancy or infections in the uterus and tubes. A contrast dye is inserted through the vagina into the cervix and x-ray pictures are taken as the dye flows through the uterus and fallopian tubes.

Before the test: Explain to patient NPO for 6 to 8 hours before the procedure and that it is normal to experience some cramping during and after the test. Obtain informed consent.

After the test: Monitor the patient after the test for any allergic reaction to the dye. Monitor for excessive vaginal bleeding.

Hysteroscopy

This test directly examines the lining of the uterus to determine the cause of abnormal bleeding and infertility. A thin viewing tube called a hysteroscope is moved through the cervix into the uterus via the vagina. A light and a camera are hooked to the hysteroscope so that the lining of the uterus can be viewed on a video screen.

Before the test: Explain to patient that she must be NPO for 6 to 8 hours before the procedure. Obtain informed consent.

After the test: Monitor for excessive vaginal bleeding.

Immunologic Blood Studies

These tests are used to identify immunologic factors in the blood:

- *ANA*: The antinuclear antibodies test is a screening test for the detection of antibodies to nuclear antigens. Close to 100% of patients with SLE will show positive evidence.

- *ESR*: The erythrocyte sedimentation rate is useful in differentiating between inflammatory and neoplastic disease. Serial values are helpful to track disease severity.
- *SS-A* and *SS-B*: SS-A antibodies can be detected in about 30% of SLE patients. SS-B antibodies have a high specificity for the sicca complex, caused by diminished secretion from glands.
- *Rheumatoid factor*: Rheumatoid factor is an IgM antibody that is associated with rheumatoid arthritis. Blood is drawn from a vein and a study is conducted to determine if the blood contains this immunoglobulin antibody. Fifty percent of the patients with rheumatoid arthritis have this antibody.
- *Scleroderma autoantibodies*: The scleroderma antibody is found in venous blood of patients who have scleroderma. The autoantibodies are positive in about 25% to 40% of scleroderma patients.

A small amount of blood is removed from the patient and is examined for immunoglobulins, and their antibodies, antinuclear antibodies, rheumatoid factor, and lupus erythematosus cell preparation. A positive finding indicates that the patient has the corresponding immunologic disease, or has had some exposure.

International Normalized Ratio
In laboratory analysis of a blood sample, high ratio means clotting ability is diminished; spontaneous bleeding is possible with international normalized ratio (INR) level greater than 6.0. Normal range is 0.69 to 1.37.

Iron Studies
- *Serum iron*: determines the amount of iron within the circulation.
- *TIBC*: total iron-binding capacity, levels are inverse to iron. If iron levels are low, the TIBC is elevated (showing that there are increased sites available to bind with iron) and if iron levels are high, the TIBC will be low.
- *Transferrin saturation*: the amount of serum iron divided by the TIBC $\times$ 100.
- *Ferritin*: shows the amount of iron stores within the body.
- *Vitamin B_{12} levels*: measures the amount of vitamin B_{12} (used to evaluate macrocytic anemia).
- *Folate*: measures the amount of folate (used to evaluate macrocytic anemia).

Kidney, Ureter, Bladder X-ray Study

The kidney, ureter, bladder (KUB) study is an abdominal x-ray used to detect kidney stones, abdominal abscesses, paralytic ileus, or obstruction.

Before the test: Explain to the patient that this is not an invasive procedure.

Liver Biopsy

Here, a small sample of tissue is removed from the liver and examined under a microscope, allowing for a definite diagnosis. A thin cutting needle, through the skin of the abdomen, is used to obtain the sample. Needle biopsies are relatively simple procedures requiring only local anesthesia. Risks include bruising, bleeding, and infection.

Before the test: Informed consent will be needed.

After the test: Monitor vital signs for drop in blood pressure as well as an increase in pulse or respiration. Check the site for bruising or bleeding. Check skin for pallor or sweating.

Liver Function Tests

These comprise several tests, obtained through a venipuncture, which show hepatic function. These generally include alanine aminotransferase (ALT), alkaline phosphatase (ALP), aspartate aminotransferase (AST), bilirubin, gamma-glutamyl transpeptidase (GGPT), LDH, PT, and PTT.

- *Alanine transaminase (ALT)*: An enzyme found mainly in liver cells, ALT helps the body to metabolize protein. When the liver is damaged, ALT is released in the bloodstream.

- *Aspartate transaminase (AST)*: The enzyme AST plays a role in the metabolism of alanine, an amino acid. An increase in AST levels may indicate liver damage or disease.

- *Alkaline phosphatase (ALP)*: ALP is an enzyme found in high concentrations in the liver and bile ducts, as well as some other tissues. Higher-than-normal levels of ALP may indicate liver damage or disease.

- *Albumin and total protein*: Levels of albumin—a protein made by the liver—and total protein show how well the liver is making proteins that the body needs to fight infections and perform other functions. Lower-than-normal levels may indicate liver damage or disease.

- *Bilirubin*: Bilirubin is a red-yellow pigment that results from the breakdown of RBCs. Normally, bilirubin passes through the liver and is excreted in stool. Elevated levels of bilirubin (jaundice) may indicate liver damage or disease.

- *Gamma-glutamyl transferase (GGT)*: This test measures the amount of the enzyme GGT in the blood. Higher-than-normal levels may indicate liver or bile duct injury.
- *Lactate dehydrogenase*: LDH is an enzyme found in many body tissues, including the liver. Elevated levels of LDH may indicate liver damage.
- *Prothrombin time (PT)*: This test measures the clotting time of plasma. Increased PT may indicate liver damage.

Lumbar Puncture

A spinal needle is inserted into subarachnoid space at a level of L3–L4 or L4–L5 with patient lying on side with knees drawn up to chest. This test is performed under local anesthesia. It is done to obtain pressure readings, obtain cerebrospinal fluid for analysis, inject contrast medium or air for diagnostic tests, inject medications, or reduce increased intracranial pressure.

After the test: The patient must lie flat for several hours to reduce the risk of spinal headache due to leakage of spinal fluid. Encourage oral fluid intake.

Luteinizing Hormone Test

This test measures the amount of luteinizing hormone (LH) in a sample of blood or urine. It is to evaluate reasons for infertility, menstrual problems, precocious puberty, and delayed puberty.

Before the test: Explain to the patient that this is a non-fasting test. The patient may be asked to stop taking certain medications, including birth control pills, for up to 4 weeks before the test.

Lymphangiography

This test produces a radiographic image of the lymphatic system to determine if there are any abnormalities, such as edema of the legs, Hodgkin's disease, lymphoma, lymphadenopathy, and lymphatic metastasis. The results are useful in the staging of lymphoma and Hodgkin's disease and to determine the efficacy of treatment. A radiopaque dye is injected via a catheter into the lymphatic system and then the patient is x-rayed. The dye remains for some time after the test so that repeat testing can be done without further injection of dye.

Before the test: Consent is needed for the test. Ask the patient about any allergies, especially to other radiologic dyes. Check renal function tests prior to the injection of the dye, as the kidneys process the dye.

During the test: Monitor the patient for allergic reaction.

After the test: Encourage fluids to enhance renal clearance.

Magnesium

In laboratory analysis of a blood sample, low level of magnesium means hemodialysis, blood transfusion, hypoparathyroidism, malabsorption, chronic disease, and chronic pancreatitis; high level means renal failure, diabetic acidosis, Addison's disease, hypothyroidism, and antacid use.

Magnetic Resonance Imaging

Use of a superconducting magnet and radio frequency signals causes hydrogen nuclei to send out an individual signal. As the radio waves bounce off the tissues in the body, different signals are sent based on the density of the tissues. The computer will create detailed images based on the information it receives. Contrast may be injected intravenously. The magnetic resonance imaging (MRI) diagnoses problems within joints, soft tissue (tendons, ligaments), spine, intervertebral discs, and spinal cord. It is able to detect differences in tissue integrity. Gadolinium may be used to enhance the clarity of the images.

Before the test: Ask the patient about possible metallic objects (surgical clips, implants), pacemakers or implanted infusion pumps (may cause dysfunction of devices), or pregnancy. Ask the patient about history of claustrophobia: closed machines are somewhat restrictive, while open machines are less claustrophobic. Tests typically last between 15 and 60 minutes, sometimes longer. Warn the patient that loud banging noises are typical. Headphones and/or ear plugs are typically used during the test. The patient may need to be NPO, depending on the area that needs to be imaged.

Mantoux Intradermal Skin Test

This determines if the patient has antibodies to the *Mycobacterium tuberculosis* bacteria, which indicates that the patient has been exposed to the bacteria. An injection of tuberculin is given intradermally. The test is positive if an indurated area appears at the injection site after 48 to 72 hours. A positive test indicates the presence of antibodies. Further testing is used to confirm that the patient has TB. Following a positive Mantoux intradermal skin test (PPD), the patient will typically be sent for a chest x-ray and may have a sputum culture for *Mycobacterium* done.

Before the test: Explain to the patient why the test is being done, and that a positive result means that the patient has been exposed to TB.

During the test: The injection needs to be given intradermally on the forearm. If it is given at the wrong depth, the reading will not be accurate and there may be irritation or damage to the tissue.

After the test: Patients need to return in 48 to 72 hours to have the injection area evaluated for induration. A positive test result means that the patient has been exposed to the disease. There may be slight redness at the injection site later on the day of injection. This does not mean that the test is positive or that the patient has TB.

Myelography

This is an injection of contrast medium into the subarachnoid space of the spine to allow for better visualization of the vertebral column, intervertebral discs, and spinal nerves. This is done when the patient is not a candidate for MRI or CT scan.

After the test: The patient typically is sitting to keep the contrast medium low in the spinal column, away from the brain.

Mammogram

A radiologic study of the breast tissue in which the breasts are positioned and compressed within a special device to allow optimal imaging. At least two images are taken of each breast. This test is used to detect growths within the breast tissue, as part of recommended screening for breast cancer.

Before the test: Explain to patient that she must avoid using lotions, powders, and deodorants the day of the tests.

Nuclear Cardiology

These noninvasive tests determine myocardial perfusion and contractility of the heart, ischemia, infarction, wall motion, and ejection fraction. Radioisotopes (thallium, sestamibi, tetrofosmin) are injected through the IV. A scanning device monitors the uptake of the radioisotope by the heart muscle. Myocardial perfusion study is the most commonly used of these tests.

Before the test: A written consent from the patient may be necessary to ensure he or she understands the risks of the test.

After the test: Monitor for any bleeding or reaction at the injection site.

Papanicolaou Smear Test

Papanicolaou (Pap) smear test is a screening test for cervical cancer. During the test the doctor takes a sample of cells from the cervix and sends the sample to a laboratory which then checks the sample for changes in the cervical cells.

Parathyroid Hormone Test

Parathyroid hormone (PTH) test measures the level of PTH in the blood. It is used as a means of assessing the level of blood calcium, since PTH is one of the major factors affecting calcium metabolism. The test is performed to evaluate parathyroid function and to check for abnormal calcium levels.

Before the test: Explain to the patient to have nothing to eat or drink from midnight until after the test the next morning. Some prescription drugs affect the PTH test and the patient may be asked to stop taking them prior to the test.

Partial Thromboplastin Time

In laboratory analysis of a blood sample, low level of PPT in early Disseminated intravascular coagulation (DIC) and in extensive cancer; high level means blood is thin due to clotting disorder or medication such as heparin. Normal range is 25.8 to 34.6 seconds.

Positron Emission Tomography

Positron emission tomography (PET) tells about the function of the brain involving glucose and oxygen metabolism. The test is done to detect areas of altered metabolism such as dementia, epilepsy, neoplasm, or degenerative disorders. The patient is given a tagged isotope on deoxyglucose. There will be increased glucose uptake by areas with increased metabolic activity.

Phosphorus

In laboratory analysis of a blood sample, low level of phosphorus means hyperparathyroidism, elevated insulin level, diabetic coma, vomiting, renal tubular acidosis; high level means renal insufficiency, hypothyroidism, hypocalcemia, excess intake of alkali, Addison's disease, and healing fractures.

Platelet Count

In laboratory analysis of a blood sample, low level of platelet count means diminished clotting ability, very low counts mean spontaneous bleeding may occur; high count means increased clotting ability, potential for platelet clumping. Normal range is 132 to 413 × 103/mm^3.

Potassium

In laboratory analysis of a blood sample, low level of potassium means GI loss, renal loss, diuretic use, eating disorders, wound drainage, respiratory alkalosis, licorice intake; high level means dehydration, renal failure, metabolic acidosis, diabetic ketoacidosis, sickle cell anemia, and interstitial nephritis. Normal range is 3.4 to 5.2 mmol/L.

Potassium Hydroxide Preparation

Potassium hydroxide preparation (KOH) test is done to provide a rapid, differential diagnosis of fungal infections of the hair, skin, or nail. A solution of KOH mixed with a blue-black dye is added to a slide containing cells from the infected tissues, and the slide is viewed under a microscope.

Prolactin Test

This test measures the level of prolactin in the blood. The test is done to determine the cause of galactorrhea (inappropriate lactation), to diagnose infertility and erectile dysfunction, and to assess for pituitary adenomas.

Before the test: Explain to the patient that this is a non-fasting blood test.

Prostate-Specific Antigen Test

Prostate-specific antigen (PSA) test measures the level of PSA in the blood. The level will be elevated in patients with benign prostatic hypertrophy (BPH) or prostate cancer. Elevated PSA levels alone do not give doctors enough information to distinguish between benign prostate conditions and cancer; however, the doctor will take the test results into account when deciding whether to order additional screening for prostate cancer. The test is also used to monitor treatment and to test for recurrences of prostate cancer.

Before the test: Explain to the patient that rectal and prostate exams, ejaculation, UTI, and prostatitis will all elevate a PSA level.

Prothrombin Time

In laboratory analysis of a blood sample, high PT means blood less likely to clot; increases with anticoagulants (Coumadin), deficiency in vitamin K, factors II, V, VII, X, liver disease, DIC. Normal range is 9.9 to 13.1 seconds.

Pulmonary Angiography

This provides a view of the pulmonary circulatory system so that the healthcare provider can determine the condition of blood flow to the lungs. Radiopaque dye is inserted into the patient's veins after a catheter has been passed through the heart into the pulmonary artery fluoroscopically. The image is viewed on a screen as the dye flows through the pulmonary circulatory system.

Before the test: Verify that the patient is not allergic to contrast dye, iodine, or shellfish. If the patient is, then either another diagnostic study may be ordered, or the patient may be premedicated for this test if no other test is deemed appropriate. Diphenhydramine and prednisone may be given prior to the test to lessen or prevent an allergic reaction while closely monitoring the patient. The patient must sign an informed consent based on institutional policy. The patient may experience a flushed feeling when the dye is injected intravenously.

During the test: Monitor patient for tolerance of procedure and possible reaction to dye.

After the test: Monitor the insertion site for bleeding. Monitor patient's vital signs, color, and respiratory effort.

Pulmonary Function Test

Pulmonary function test (PFT) assesses the lungs' ability to move air, monitors change from normal function, and helps differentiate obstructive from restrictive disease. The patient takes a deep breath. The spirometer is inserted into the patient's mouth and the patient breathes outward quickly at full force until all air is expelled. A deep breath is then taken in through the mouthpiece and this process is repeated three separate times. A computer then calculates the lungs' volume and vital capacity by measuring the amount of air moving in and out. The force of the air flow is measured. The duration of time of exhalation is measured.

Before the test: The patient should not smoke prior to the test. Smoking may have an effect on the outcome of the test. Instruct the patient to take a deep breath and then exhale completely into the spirometer, followed by deep inhalation.

After the test: Administration of bronchodilators after the initial testing may be done, followed by repetition of the test if indicated. This will show the effect of bronchodilators on pulmonary function. Albuterol or levalbuterol is typically used.

Pulse Oximetry

This determines the abbreviated arterial oxygen saturation of the blood. The full arterial oxygen saturation is determined by the ABG test. An infrared light passes through the patient's nail bed or skin. The amount of infrared light passing through determines the amount of arterial oxygen saturation of the blood.

Before the test: Clamp the sensor on the patient's finger over the nail bed, toe, ear lobe, or bridge of the nose. Make sure that the site is clean. Nail polish or artificial nails may interfere with the reading.

Radioallergosorbent Test

Radioallergosorbent test (RAST) is a blood test used to screen for an allergy to a specific substance or substances. It measures the amount of IgE antibody that reacts specifically with the suspected allergen.

Red Blood Cell Count

This test measures the amount of red blood cells (RBCs). It may be decreased in anemia, bleeding, SLE, chronic infection, Addison's disease, Hodgkin's disease, leukemia, multiple myeloma; increased in polycythemia; relative increase in dehydration, severe burn, and shock. Normal range is 3.71 to 5.25 × 106/mm^3.

Rhesus Factor

Rhesus (Rh) factor is a serum test used to check the presence of a protein, Rh D antigen, on the surface of the RBCs. It is used to assess for blood compatibility between mother and fetus.

Before the test: Explain to the patient that this is a non-fasting test.

Semen Analysis

This test evaluates the male aspect of a couple's inability to conceive.

Before the test: Explain to the patient that he must abstain from sex for 2 days before a specimen is collected, which is then microscopically evaluated for volume, sperm motility, and count. The specimen must be delivered to the laboratory within an hour of collection.

Single-Photon Emission Computed Tomography

Single-photon emission computed tomography (SPECT) involves an intravenous injection of a radiopharmaceutical to enhance the image. It is done to detect cerebral blood flow, stroke, dementia, amnesia, neoplasm, head trauma, seizures, persistent vegetative state, brain death, and psychiatric disorders. This test is not for pregnant women.

Skin Biopsy

A skin biopsy is usually done to diagnose an abnormal area of the skin, such as a growth or mole for cancer. It is also used to diagnose a bacterial or fungal skin infection or other abnormal skin condition. A sample of tissue is taken for analysis by a pathologist to determine if cellular changes have occurred. There are several types of biopsy which are as follows:

- *Punch biopsy*: where a small cylindrical fragment of tissue is removed from the affected area, by a sharp cookie-cutter-like tool (punch).
- *Shave biopsy*: where a superficial piece of skin is removed from the affected area with a sharp, sterile blade.
- *Excisional biopsy*: where a larger area of skin is removed, allowing for analysis of deeper skin structures or removal of the entire lesion. A local anesthetic is typically used.

After the test: Monitor the area for healing.

Sodium

In laboratory analysis of a blood sample, low level of sodium (Na) means diarrhea, vomiting, edema, excess water intake, diuretic use, nasogastric suction, Addison's disease, hypothyroidism; high level means dehydration, bronchitis, Cushing's disease, diabetes insipidus, and insufficient water intake. Normal range is 136 to 146 mmol/L.

Sputum Culture and Sensitivity

Sputum is collected from the patient in a sterile container and sent to the laboratory where the sample is placed in Petri dishes and incubated to grow the bacteria. Samples of the bacteria are stained and examined under a microscope to identify the bacteria. The samples are checked periodically but are usually given 72 hours to complete the testing process. Once identified, bacteria are exposed to known antibiotics to determine which antibiotic kills the bacteria.

Explain the proper manner to obtain a sputum sample. Use a sterile specimen container to determine that the bacteria that grow in the laboratory have come from the patient and not from contamination. Collect sputum only and not saliva—there are bacteria naturally found in the mouth, so saliva samples will grow bacteria in the laboratory even though it is not causing any infection.

Syphilis Testing

Rapid plasma regain (RPR), venereal disease research laboratory (VDRL), fluorescent treponema antibody test (FTA-ABS), and treponema pallidum particle agglutination (TP-PA) are blood tests used to diagnose syphilis.

Triiodothyronine Test

Triiodothyronine (T3) test measures the level of T3 in the blood in order to determine whether the thyroid is functioning properly. It is used primarily to help diagnose hyperthyroidism and is usually ordered following an abnormal thyroid-stimulating hormone (TSH) or T4 test.

Before the test: Explain to the patient that this is a non-fasting blood test.

Thoracentesis

Thoracentesis is removal of fluid from the pleural sac to drain fluid or identify the contents of the fluid. The patient either sits at the edge of the bed leaning forward (with arms folded on a bedside table for support) or lies on the unaffected side with the head of the bed slightly elevated. The affected site is anesthetized. A needle is inserted into the plural sac and fluid is drained using a syringe.

Before the test: The patient must sign an informed consent for an invasive procedure.

During the test: Monitor the patient for tolerance during the procedure. Monitor respiratory status for rate, effort, skin color, use of accessory muscles, and breath sounds.

After the test: Position the patient on the affected side for an hour following the procedure. This applies direct pressure to the puncture site, reducing the chance of bleeding. Monitor the injection site for leakage; reinforce dressing if drainage noted. Monitor respiratory status for changes.

Thyroxine Total Test

Thyroxine total (T4) test measures the amount of T4 in the blood and is ordered to evaluate the thyroid function and to help diagnose hyperthyroidism and hypothyroidism.

Before the test: Explain to the patient that this is a non-fasting blood test.

Thyroid-Stimulating Hormone Test

Thyroid-stimulating hormone blood test measures the level of TSH in the blood and it is used to check thyroid gland problems. It may be done at the same time as tests to measure T3 and T4.

Before the test: Explain to the patient that this is a non-fasting blood test.

Thyroid Scintiscan

A radioactive substance is orally given to the patient, who returns at a designated time for a thyroid scan (Thyroid Scintiscan). The test is done to assess nodules as either hot (functioning) which often indicates a goiter or a benign mass or cold (nonfunctioning) which may indicate a cancer, thyroiditis, or other disease process.

Before the test: Find out whether the patient has any allergies to iodine or shellfish. Speak to the practitioner about withholding thyroid medications before the test. It is a noninvasive test.

24-Hour Urine Collection

This is a diagnostic test that involves collecting a patient's urine for 24 hours. It is typically used to measure volume and various other factors of kidney function as well as to determine the daily elimination of such substances as proteins, electrolytes, etc.

Before the test: Explain to the patient that the test is started in the morning. Discard the first-voided specimen, and then save subsequent specimens, ending with the first-voided specimen the following day. The urine collection jug should be kept on ice or under refrigeration.

Ultrasound

Sound waves are used to generate an image. This is done to determine the presence and location of mass, fluid, or surgical hardware.

Urinalysis

Urinalysis is the physical, chemical, and microscopic examination of urine. It involves a number of tests to evaluate the urine specimen for appearance, color, clarity, pH, specific gravity, and the presence of bacteria, blood, casts, glucose, ketones, leukocytes, proteins, RBCs, and WBCs. The tests are used to confirm symptoms of a UTI, to check diabetics for excess glucose levels, and to monitor the kidney function of renal patients.

Before the test: Explain to the patient that many drugs affect a urine specimen. Some samples, as when ascertaining the presence of an infection, may need to be "clean catch" or "midstream clean" collection. The perineum or urethral opening should be cleansed, and the voiding stream started. Without stopping the stream, position the sterile container into the flow of urine. When the container is more than half full, withdraw from the flow of urine. Allow the patient to finish emptying the bladder. Tightly cap and send to the laboratory immediately.

Urinary Catecholamines

This test, a 24-hour urine test, measures the amount of the hormones epinephrine, norepinephrine, and dopamine in the body. The test is done to assess for pheochromocytoma (tumor of the adrenal gland) as the cause of elevated blood pressure.

Before the test: Instruct the patient to collect urine in a special container for a 24-hour period. Explain to the patient that the test is started in the morning. Discard the first-voided specimen, and then save subsequent specimens, ending with the first-voided specimen the following day. A preservative has been added to the container and it must be refrigerated.

Urine Flow Studies

Urine flow studies, also known as uroflowmetry, measure the strength and volume per second of urine flow from the bladder when a patient urinates into a test machine. They help identify an obstruction or abnormality of the urinary tract and assist in evaluating how well or poorly a patient is urinating.

Before the test: Explain to the patient not to urinate for a few hours before the test and to drink enough fluids to develop an urge to urinate. It is not an invasive test. They will need to void into a flowmeter.

Urine Toxicology Screening

This test detects the presence of drugs in the urine. Urine screening is preferred to blood screening because urine samples contain the substance for several days after its use, whereas blood levels diminish after several hours. Hair and nail samples may also be required for certain tests. The test is done to detect commonly used drugs, such as alcohol, anabolic steroids, amphetamines, barbiturates, benzodiazepines, cannabinoids, cocaine, methamphetamines, opiates, phencyclidine, and propoxyphene.

Before the test: Obtain informed consent if the specimen is needed for medical/legal purposes. Urine specimen collection must be monitored to ensure that the specimen has not been altered in any way. Be aware of which prescription medications the patient is taking as some may alter the test results.

Vasopressin Challenge Test

This test is performed to assess the ability of the kidneys to concentrate urine and to help determine which type of diabetes insipidus is present. Vasopressin is injected subcutaneously. Serum and urine samples are collected at 1 to 2-hour intervals after the injection, and the osmolality of these samples is measured in the laboratory.

Before the test: Explain to the patient that fluids are restricted the evening before the test and the patient must be NPO after midnight. Any extra fluid or food intake invalidates the test.

Venogram

This x-ray test takes pictures of the blood flow through the veins. It is used to identify and locate blood clots and to determine the condition of the valves in the veins. An iodine dye is injected into the vein, making the vein visible in a fluoroscope; this allows the physician to visualize the flow of venous blood.

Before the test: Assess latest chemistry to check on BUN, creatinine, and creatinine clearance. Determine if the patient is allergic to seafood or iodine. If so, notify the physician immediately because the patient might be also allergic to the dye. Obtain written consent from the patient to assure adequate knowledge of risks and benefits. Explain the procedure to the patient and its possible effects. The patient may experience effects from the dye, such as flushing of the face, nausea, urge to urinate or chest pain.

After the test: Check for bleeding at the injection site to assess for hemorrhage. If bleeding, apply pressure until bleeding stops. Monitor for infection at the injection site. Look for redness, warmth, and oozing of purulent matter. Increase fluid intake to assist the kidneys in excreting the dye.

Ventilation-Perfusion Scan

Ventilation-perfusion scan (V/Q scan) test enables visualization of the flow of blood in the lungs to determine if lung tissue is adequately perfused. The patient inhales radioactive gas mixed with oxygen for the ventilation phase. Radioisotopes are intravenously injected into the patient's veins using an IV access for the perfusion phase.

Before the test: Explain the procedure to the patient. The patient must lie still for the testing, holding his or her breath as directed.

Voiding Cystogram

This test involves taking an x-ray image of the bladder and urethra during urination. A radiopaque contrast material is instilled into the bladder via a Foley catheter. After x-rays are taken, the catheter is removed. The patient voids while more x-rays are obtained. This test is performed to look for defects of the urinary system, for tumors of the bladder, ureters, and urethra, or for reflux of urine from the bladder to the ureters.

Before and after the test: Explain to the patient that the presence of the catheter will feel like the urge to urinate. Obtain informed consent. Check for allergies to contrast material. Advise the patient to increase oral fluids before and after test to aid the kidneys in removal of contrast material.

Western Blot Tests

This test looks for the presence of viral proteins in the patient's blood to confirm disease. It may be used to confirm presence of HIV infection, Lyme disease, and herpes among others.

White Blood Cell Count

This test measures the amount of WBCs in the current circulation. WBCs are responsible for fighting infection in the body. There are five subtypes of WBCs: neutrophils, basophils, eosinophils, lymphocytes, and monocytes. WBCs are often tested to determine infection, inflammation, allergic response, and parasitic infection. The result may be decreased in viral infection, bone marrow depression or disorder, heavy metal intoxication, irradiation, hypersplenism; increased in bacterial infection. Normal range is 3.8 to $10.8 \times 10^3/mm^3$.

X-ray

Body part to be imaged needs to be positioned properly to see underlying bone structure, identify fractures, and detect foreign bodies. The patient may need to lie, sit, or stand, depending on the body part to be imaged. Typically, two different views are taken of the same body part to allow better diagnostics. Fractures, misalignment, calcifications, or dislocation may be identified.

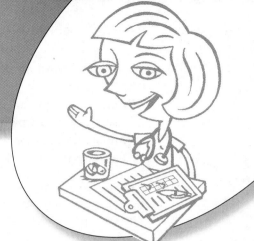

Final Exam Questions

1. **Joan is apprehensive about undergoing bronchoscopy. You respond by saying:**
   A. The thought of this procedure seems to be disturbing you. You will be sleeping during this procedure. I will ask your physician to visit you again and answer any questions that you might have regarding the procedure.
   B. Your physician has performed this procedure frequently.
   C. I had it performed 3 years ago and I was fine.
   D. You would not feel a thing. You will be fine.

2. **A patient with sickle cell anemia will be given supplemental oxygen and which of the following?**
   A. IV fluids to adequately hydrate.
   B. Narcotic pain management when pain is severe.
   C. Transfusion of red blood cells to correct anemia.
   D. All of the above.

3. **Joan asks you why she is being administered so many arterial blood gas tests. You respond by saying:**
   A. This test determines if your liver and kidneys are functioning properly.
   B. This test determines if you have sufficient WBC to fight infection.
   C. This test determines if you are hyperglycemic, which is a side effect of your medication.
   D. This test determines how well your tissues are oxygenated.

4. **Tim presents with an acute episode of gout. You expect the physician to prescribe:**

    A. Nonsteroidal anti-inflammatory medications and colchicine.

    B. Allopurinol and aspirin.

    C. Antibiotics and acetaminophen.

    D. Bisphosphonates and calcium.

5. **Following treatment with fluoxetine, a selective serotonin reuptake inhibitor for depression, Mary hardly sleeps, is hyperactive, easily distracted, and appears elated. You would expect her physician to:**

    A. Continue the selective serotonin reuptake inhibitor.

    B. Start a mood stabilizer.

    C. Switch to a tricyclic antidepressant.

    D. Add a monoamine oxidase inhibitor.

6. **Mandy is a 17-year-old adolescent girl. On physical examination you note partial erosion of her tooth enamel and callus formation on the posterior aspect of the knuckles of her hand. This is indicative of:**

    A. A connective tissue disorder; she should be referred to dermatology.

    B. Self-induced vomiting; she likely has bulimia nervosa.

    C. Self-mutilation; this correlates with anxiety.

    D. A genetic disorder; her siblings should also be tested.

7. **Denise is recovering from an open cholecystectomy. You know that because of the location of the surgery, she has an increased chance of postoperative:**

    A. Myocardial infarction.

    B. Respiratory complications.

8. **Steve, who is diagnosed with pneumonia following recent intrathoracic surgery, will likely be prescribed:**

    A. Cephalosporin, such as cefazolin.

    B. Penicillin, such as amoxicillin.

    C. Fluoroquinolone, such as levofloxacin.

    D. Tetracycline, such as doxycycline.

9. **Bob reports chest pains when performing strenuous work. The pain goes away when he sits. What is he likely to be experiencing?**

    A. Indigestion.

    B. Stable angina.

    C. Unstable angina.

    D. Prinzmetal's angina.

10. **Anne returned from carpal tunnel surgery. Her hand and arm must remain elevated above the heart after the surgery. She asks you why. You respond by saying:**

    A. To reduce lymphatic drainage.

    B. To restrict hand movements.

    C. To decrease possibility of nosocomial infection.

    D. To reduce postoperative swelling.

11. **What is the priority intervention for a patient admitted to your unit diagnosed with advanced amyotrophic lateral sclerosis (ALS)?**

    A. Develop a method of communication.

    B. Provide six small meals high in protein and assist with feeding.

    C. Do not involve the patient in decisions about his healthcare because he is not in the mental state to respond.

    D. Provide six normal meals high in protein and assist with feeding.

12. **Signs of clotting and bleeding concurrently indicate:**

    A. Hemophilia.

    B. Multiple myeloma.

    C. Disseminated intravascular coagulation.

    D. Polycythemia vera.

13. **A patient is diagnosed with Bell's palsy and has signs of unilateral facial paralysis and is unable to close his right eye. What eye care is required?**

    A. The patient will need to instill artificial teardrops and use an eye patch.

    B. None, since the symptoms will disappear in a few weeks.

    C. Increase fluid intake to prevent dryness of the eye.

    D. Wear sunglasses.

14. **A 55-year-old smoker who is normally in good health reports having had a bad cough for the past 3 weeks. He does not have crackles, rhonchi, or discolored blood-tinged sputum. What would you expect his physician to rule out?**

    A. Asthma.

    B. Pneumonia.

    C. The flu.

    D. Lung cancer.

15. **Patients returning from the operating room (OR) should be monitored for atelectasis. Why is this important?**

    A. Immobility, anesthesia, and lack of deep breathing place the patient at risk for collapsed lung.

    B. All postoperative patients are at risk for infection.

C. Postoperative patients might have received too much oxygen during surgery.

D. Postoperative patients do not receive enough oxygen during surgery.

16. **Chronic hepatitis C may be treated with:**

    A. Sulfasalazine.

    B. Interferon and ribavirin.

    C. Metronidazole or ciprofloxacin.

    D. Acetaminophen.

17. **An inflammatory bowel disorder in which the patient develops abdominal pain, bloody diarrhea, tenesmus (feeling of incomplete defecation), and weight loss is:**

    A. Crohn's disease.

    B. Diverticulitis.

    C. Ulcerative colitis.

    D. Appendicitis.

18. **Mary, who is diagnosed with osteomyelitis, may not heal properly unless she has:**

    A. Debridement and drainage of the area.

    B. Immobilization of the area.

    C. Ice packs alternating with moist heat, applied externally.

    D. Internal fixation device inserted.

19. **Your postoperative patient develops a cellulitis in her leg. Your nursing treatments would include:**

    A. Keeping both her legs elevated as much as possible.

    B. Encouraging ambulation as much as possible to help with the blood flow.

    C. Application of ice four times a day for an hour each to reduce inflammation.

    D. Application of moisturizing lotion three times daily to keep the skin moist.

20. **Donna is a healthy, 46-year-old woman scheduled for elective surgery next week. You would include in her preoperative preparation:**

    A. A pulmonary function test and chest x-ray.

    B. A complete blood count (CBC), chemistry panel, and pregnancy test.

    C. Urine culture, thyroid panel, and cortisol level.

    D. Glucose tolerance test, ankle-brachial index, and electrocardiogram (EKG).

21. **Felicia's family is concerned because Felicia states that she is hearing voices. This is a sign of:**

    A. Bipolar disorder.

    B. Schizophrenia.

C. Panic disorder.

D. Bulimia nervosa.

22. **Gregory has gastrointestinal bleeding and is experiencing hematochezia. You recognize this as:**

A. Vomiting of bright red or maroon blood.

B. Passage of black, tarry stool.

C. Passage of red or maroon-colored stool.

D. Coffee ground emesis.

23. **Bob is diagnosed with idiopathic thrombocytopenic purpura (ITP). You realize that he has an increased risk of bleeding and you must monitor:**

A. WBC and bleeding time.

B. Prothrombin time (PT) and partial thromboplastin time (PTT).

C. Platelet count and RBC.

D. Iron and ferritin levels.

24. **The patient asks you what the clip on his finger is for. The best response is:**

A. This is a cardiac monitor that alerts us to any arrhythmia that you might experience during the night.

B. This measures your temperature.

C. This is pulse oximetry and is used to give us an idea of how much oxygen is in your blood.

D. This tells us the number of red blood cells you have. These cells provide oxygen throughout your body.

25. **For your patient with a CD4 count, less than 200, the most important nursing assessment would include:**

A. Bowel movements.

B. Urinary output.

C. Fever.

D. Blood pressure.

26. **Upon hearing that he has acute pericarditis, the patient asks how he could have contracted the disease. The best response is:**

A. The upper respiratory viral infection that you experienced a couple of weeks ago could have led to acute pericarditis.

B. It is a genetic condition that you received from your father.

C. It is a genetic condition that you received from your mother.

D. It is the weakening of the left side of your heart.

27. **While you are talking with the patient, she becomes confused and begins slurring her words. What would you expect the physician to do?**

    A. Assess if the patient had an ischemic or hemorrhagic cerebral vasospasm (CVS).
    B. Administer thrombolytic agent (TPA) since this is within 3 hours of the cerebrovascular accident (CVA).
    C. Tell the patient to go home, get rest, and to call the physician in the morning if the symptoms continue.
    D. Admit the patient and place her on bed rest.

28. **A father asks you how to prevent another asthmatic attack in his son. You respond by:**

    A. Saying asthmatic attacks cannot be prevented.
    B. Asking his son's physician to change his medication.
    C. Instructing him to move his family immediately to a dry climate.
    D. Helping him identify triggers that cause asthmatic attacks and showing him how to avoid them.

29. **Your patient's physician told him that he has hemophilia. You are asked to teach the signs and symptoms of this disease. You respond by saying:**

    A. Clot formation, especially in the veins of the lower extremities.
    B. Low blood counts and fatigue due to lack of adequate red blood cell production.
    C. High blood counts and clot formation under the nails.
    D. Excessive bleeding after minor trauma.

30. **Priority treatment of a fracture is:**

    A. Surgical reduction of the fracture.
    B. Immobilization of the area.
    C. Insertion of an internal fixation device.
    D. Reduction of the fracture.

31. **Anne asks how she developed iron deficiency anemia. You respond by saying:**

    A. Insomnia.
    B. An increase in iron intake.
    C. Heavy menses or an inadequate intake of iron.
    D. Low salt intake.

32. **Treatment of the patient with appendicitis includes:**

    A. Transfusion to replace blood loss.
    B. Bowel preparation for cleansing.
    C. Surgical removal of appendix.
    D. Medications to lower pH within stomach.

33. **When assessing a skin lesion, you look for A—asymmetry, B—irregular borders, C—variegated colors, D—diameter, and E—**

    A. Edema.
    B. Erythema.
    C. Elevation.
    D. Ever-changing.

34. **To clean a wound, it is best to use:**

    A. Hydrogen peroxide to bubble away the debris.
    B. Tap water.
    C. Saline.
    D. It is best not to disturb a healing wound.

35. **Mary is diagnosed with a brain tumor and is unable to speak. Where is the tumor probably located?**

    A. Occipital lobe.
    B. Cerebellum.
    C. Frontal lobe.
    D. Parietal lobe.

36. **Mary, who is scheduled for a thoracentesis, asks why there is so much fluid in the pleural space. You respond by saying:**

    A. Your body is unable to remove fluid, resulting in a buildup of fluid in the pleural space around your lungs.
    B. An error occurred and you were administered too much IV medication.
    C. This is the result of oxygen therapy.
    D. This is a normal side effect of bumetanide, which is medication ordered by your physician.

37. **Tom is diagnosed with congestive heart failure and asks why fluid accumulates in his lungs. You respond by saying:**

    A. Because of the excessive volume of IV fluid that is being administered.
    B. The right side of your heart is weakened and is losing the capability to pump blood to your lungs.
    C. You stand too long at work.
    D. The left side of your heart is weakened and is losing the capability to pump blood to your lungs.

38. **You are caring for a patient who has had a transurethral resection of the prostate for benign prostatic hypertrophy. There is continuous bladder irrigation setup. You would notify the physician if you noted:**

    A. Any signs of hematuria.
    B. A change from clear red output to thicker, bright red output.

C. A decrease in the amount of blood in the urine.

D. The development of uremic pruritis.

39. **A nurse criticizes the attending physician and suggests that a different physician should care for the patient. What is your best response?**

    A. Call the nurse away from the patient and remind him that the patient can still hear even if unconscious.

    B. Report the nurse to the attending physician.

    C. Ask the nurse why he has such feelings.

    D. Simply nod your head in agreement.

40. **Roger presents with blurred and double vision, muscle weakness, and intolerance of temperature changes. In order to rule out multiple sclerosis, the physician will likely order:**

    A. CBC showing a very low WBC count.

    B. Endocrine function study showing a low growth hormone and high T3 and T4.

    C. CT scan showing plaque formation.

    D. Fasting glucose test showing a result over 300 mg/dL.

41. **Tom arrives in the Emergency Room (ER) and is unable to move his legs as a result of an automobile accident that occurred 30 minutes ago. You respond by saying:**

    A. Swelling due to the initial trauma prevents you from moving your legs.

    B. There are good rehabilitation centers that will help restore sensation to your legs.

    C. Swelling due to the initial trauma may make the injury seem more severe than it actually is. A more accurate assessment will be made once the swelling goes down.

    D. You should have been wearing your seatbelt.

42. **Tom reports abdominal pain that started over the periumbilical area and moved to the right lower quadrant area. Tom probably has:**

    A. Crohn's disease.

    B. Cholecystitis.

    C. Appendicitis.

    D. Diverticulitis.

43. **On assessment of the abdomen in a patient with peritonitis, you would expect to find:**

    A. A soft abdomen with bowel sounds every 2 to 3 seconds.

    B. Rebound tenderness and guarding (protecting).

    C. Hyperactive, high-pitched bowel sounds and a firm abdomen.

    D. Ascites and increased vascular pattern on the skin.

44. **Which member of the surgical team does not scrub in the OR?**

    A. The surgeon.
    B. The circulating nurse.
    C. The scrub nurse or surgical tech.
    D. The holding area nurse.

45. **Josie is the mother of a healthy 19-year-old having surgery tomorrow. After the surgeon discusses the surgery, risks, and benefits with the patient and her mother, the mother wants to sign the consent form. The most appropriate response to this would be:**

    A. Of course she can sign the consent form; after all, the patient is her daughter.
    B. While you appreciate the concern for her daughter, the patient is a consenting adult and legally has to sign her own consent form.
    C. No consent form must be signed.
    D. Why do not both the patient and her mother sign the form?

46. **Alex is a 78-year-old married man with sudden onset of confusion and disorientation; he is exhibiting combative behavior. He has no previous psychiatric history. A psychiatric consultation has been called. You suspect Alex has:**

    A. Delirium.
    B. Psychosis.
    C. Depression.
    D. Panic disorder.

47. **Tom has Guillain-Barré syndrome and asks what causes his burning, prickling feeling. You respond by saying:**

    A. You are lying too long on the affected side.
    B. This is in response to your medication.
    C. The myelin cover of the nerve endings is absent.
    D. This is secondary to dysphagia.

48. **A confirmatory laboratory test for HIV includes:**

    A. Western blot.
    B. Low WBC.
    C. Comprehensive metabolic panel.
    D. Enzyme-linked immunosorbent assay (ELISA).

49. **Bob, who has Huntington's disease, tells you that he sees the same symptoms of the disease in his 13-year-old son. You respond by saying:**

    A. Your son probably has the early symptoms of the disease.
    B. Symptoms usually appear between the ages of 30 and 50; however, you may want to ask your physician about genetic testing that can detect if your son has the gene that is associated with Huntington's disease.

C. Symptoms usually appear before the age of 30; you may want to ask your physician about genetic testing.

D. Huntington's disease is genetically transmitted.

50. **The patient experiences sudden pain in his right calf while sitting at home. He is diagnosed with deep vein thrombosis (DVT). The first intervention is to:**

A. Apply ice packs to the affected area every 4 to 6 hours.

B. Increase dietary intake of foods rich in vitamin K.

C. Monitor platelet counts daily.

D. Use intermittent warm soaks of the affected area.

51. **The best treatment for mononucleosis is:**

A. Antibiotics.

B. Physical therapy.

C. Nonsteroidal anti-inflammatory drugs (NSAIDs).

D. Rest and fluids.

52. **Joan is a data-entry specialist who types most of the day. She has an increased risk for:**

A. Osteomyelitis.

B. Osteoporosis.

C. Fracture of the overused area.

D. Carpal tunnel syndrome.

53. **Tom reports a history of carpal tunnel syndrome. What else would you expect to find in his history?**

A. Crepitus (grating feeling on palpation over joint during range of motion) due to loss of articular cartilage and bony overgrowth in joint.

B. Excessive forward curvature of the thoracic spine (kyphosis) due to pathologic vertebral fractures and collapsing of the anterior portion of the vertebral bodies in the thoracic area.

C. Pain and numbness or tingling sensation in the hand over the palmar surface of the thumb, index, and middle fingers, and lateral aspect of the ring finger, that is worse at night.

D. Acute onset of excruciating pain in joint due to accumulation of uric acid within the joint.

54. **Tom is diagnosed with an aortic aneurysm. He asks why this did not show up on his annual physical examination. You respond by saying:**

A. It did show and your physician did not want to alarm you.

B. You probably do not remember that your physician told you about your condition.

    C. Aortic aneurysms are asymptomatic.

    D. Aortic aneurysms are always symptomatic.

55. **Sam is diagnosed with having a myocardial infarction after experiencing chest pain and pain radiating to his arms, jaw, and back. He asks what a myocardial infarction is. You respond by saying:**

    A. You had a heart attack.

    B. Your aortic valve was malformed at birth, causing a disruption in blood flow.

    C. All patients who are as overweight as you will have a heart attack

    D. One or more arteries that supply blood to your heart are blocked, thereby preventing blood from flowing to your cardiac muscles.

56. **Patients with a paralytic ileus typically have:**

    A. Intravenous fluid replacement and a nasogastric tube connected to suction.

    B. Surgical correction of the problem.

    C. Endoscopic injection of botulinum toxin or esophageal dilation.

    D. Endoscopy to allow biopsy followed with broad-spectrum antibiotics.

57. **Sue is having a minor procedure performed. Which type of anesthesia is most likely to be used?**

    A. General.

    B. Epidural.

    C. Regional.

    D. Conscious sedation.

58. **Three days after surgery, Mark notices that the wound site is more painful now than it was the day before. When you inspect the surgical site you are looking for redness or inflammation. Other indicators of infection would include:**

    A. Elevated RBC and elevated respiratory rate.

    B. Elevated WBC and elevated temperature.

    C. Elevated erythrocyte sedimentation rate and decreased pulse.

    D. Decreased platelets and decreased blood pressure.

59. **Sixty-five-year-old Dominic is being transferred into the postanesthesia care unit (PACU) from the OR. Once there, initial assessment will focus on:**

    A. Airway, breathing, circulation, and wound site.

    B. Intake, output, and intravenous access.

    C. Abdominal sounds, oxygen level, and level of consciousness.

    D. Pulse oximetry, pupil responses, and deep tendon reflexes.

60. Joan has osteoporosis. She has an increased risk for:

   A. Infection in the bone.
   B. Peripheral blood clot formation.
   C. Fracture formation.
   D. Painful joint inflammation.

61. When assessing a patient for anaphylaxis, you would be alert for:

   A. Chest pain and indigestion.
   B. Hives and dyspnea.
   C. Hypertension and blurred vision.
   D. Headache and photophobia.

62. Your patient is often fatigued as a result of having anemia. She asks you why she is fatigued. You respond by saying:

   A. Destruction (hemolysis) of the red blood cells.
   B. Paleness (pallor) of the skin.
   C. Lack of nutritional intake of essential nutrients, such as iron or B_{12}.
   D. Decreased oxygen-carrying capability of the blood.

63. When assessing the patient, you notice that there is contraction of his facial muscle after tapping the facial nerve anterior to his ear. This is a sign of:

   A. Hyponatremia.
   B. Hypokalemia.
   C. Hypomagnesemia.
   D. Hypocalcemia.

64. Tom presents with sudden difficulty breathing, tachypnea, tachycardia, and localized chest pain. The physician suspects a pulmonary embolism and would order what test?

   A. EKG.
   B. Helical CT scan.
   C. ECC.
   D. Vital capacity.

65. Your patient is experiencing exacerbations of systemic lupus erythematosus. What would you expect the physician to prescribe?

   A. Antiemetics.
   B. Corticosteroids.
   C. Antineoplastics.
   D. Antibiotics.

66. **Joan is diagnosed with a gastric ulcer. What symptoms would she exhibit?**
    A. Epigastric pain worse before meals, pain on awakening, and melena.
    B. Decreased bowel sounds, rigid abdomen, rebound tenderness, and fever.
    C. Boring epigastric pain radiating to back and left shoulder, bluish-gray discoloration of periumbilical area, and ascites.
    D. Epigastric pain that is worse after eating and weight loss.

67. **A patient with a history of pulmonary embolism asks how to lower the risk of experiencing another pulmonary embolism. You respond by saying:**
    A. Take vitamin K with heparin.
    B. Avoid confined spaces.
    C. Avoid sitting and standing for too long and do not cross your legs.
    D. Jog 5 miles each day.

68. **Build-up of bile salts may cause the systemic symptom of:**
    A. Hypotension.
    B. Pruritis (itching).
    C. Ecchymosis (bruising).
    D. Urticaria (hives).

69. **Paralytic ileus may occur as a postoperative complication. Which of the following patients would cause you the greatest concern about the development of paralytic ileus?**
    A. Kim, a 27-year-old postlaparoscopic appendectomy.
    B. Joyce, a 39-year-old post–open right hemicolectomy.
    C. Nancy, a 56-year-old postmediastinoscopy.
    D. John, a 47-year-old post–total joint replacement.

70. **Steps to prevent a pressure ulcer may include:**
    A. Not disturbing the patient.
    B. Changing the position of a bedbound patient every 4 hours.
    C. Vigorously rubbing the skin with alcohol.
    D. Avoiding pressure on the heels of a bedbound patient.

71. **Patient teaching for risk reduction of skin cancer should include:**
    A. Having suspicious moles checked by a dermatologist.
    B. Daily sun exposure every 1/2 hour.
    C. Daily sun exposure of 1 hour to build tolerance.
    D. Applying moisturizer.
    E. DVT.
    F. Wound infection.

72. **Sue is diagnosed with congestive heart failure. What medication would you expect to administer to strengthen myocardial contractility?**

    A. Nitroprusside.
    B. Digoxin.
    C. Nitroglycerine ointment.
    D. Furosemide.

73. **Following a bone marrow transplant, the patient has an increased risk for:**

    A. Bleeding.
    B. Infection.
    C. Clot formation.
    D. Nausea and vomiting.

74. **Which of the following would have the highest priority in septic shock?**

    A. Monitoring temperature.
    B. Monitoring pupillary reaction.
    C. Monitoring airway, breathing, circulation (ABC).
    D. Monitoring ANA and RF levels.

75. **The primary mode of treatment for ankylosing spondylitis is:**

    A. Relaxed posture for comfort.
    B. Physical therapy.
    C. Strict bedrest.
    D. Respiratory therapy.

76. **Bob presents with emphysema. He has difficulty breathing and has a barrel chest. He asks why increasing oxygen therapy does not relieve his difficulty breathing. You respond by saying:**

    A. You must lie on your right side for oxygen therapy to work properly.
    B. Your barrel chest has decreased, causing your lungs to overly expand.
    C. You must take deeper breaths when receiving oxygen therapy.
    D. Your difficulty in breathing is due to air trapped in your lungs, reducing the lungs' ability to exchange oxygen and carbon dioxide. Increasing oxygen does not resolve the trapped air.

77. **The patient asks when she should take bisphosphonate medications for treatment of osteoporosis. You tell her:**

    A. On a full stomach.
    B. Just before getting into bed.
    C. First thing in the morning on an empty stomach with a full glass of water, 30 to 60 minutes before eating, and without lying down.
    D. With an acidic liquid such as orange juice.

78. **Anne asks how a chest x-ray would help the physician examine her heart. You respond by saying:**

    A. A chest x-ray is used to rule out that a fractured rib caused your pain.
    B. The chest x-ray is an error. I will cancel the order.
    C. A chest x-ray is used to detect the size and position of the heart.
    D. All patients who are admitted must have a chest x-ray.

79. **Mary is diagnosed with gastroesophageal reflux disease. You need to teach Mary to:**

    A. Avoid coffee, tea, and other caffeine-containing beverages.
    B. Take histamine 2 blockers, such as ranitidine, as directed.
    C. Avoid acidic foods such as citrus or tomato.
    D. All of the above.

80. **Joan is diagnosed with a ruptured aneurysm. She wonders why this was not picked up in her annual physical. You respond by saying:**

    A. The physician must have misread the x-ray.
    B. The aneurysm must have developed since the physical.
    C. Aneurysms are often asymptomatic.
    D. Do not be too concerned because this happens all the time.

81. **A patient with a second-degree burn has a greater risk for:**

    A. Constipation.
    B. Infection.
    C. Hypotension.
    D. Hyperglycemia.

82. **You are caring for a patient with an infected wound. You would expect:**

    A. To prepare for sutures to close the wound.
    B. To use steri strips to hold the edges together.
    C. To leave the wound open.
    D. To cover the wound with a loose, fluffy dressing.

83. **Appropriate treatment for a patient with cellulitis includes:**

    A. Petrolatum and vitamin A and D ointment.
    B. Antibiotics, such as cephalexin, and over-the-counter analgesics.
    C. Weight-bearing exercises and diuretics, such as furosemide.
    D. Wet to dry dressings and steroids.

84. Karen is suspected of having a hormone imbalance. What would you expect to monitor?

A. Electrolyte levels.

B. Thyroid studies, follicle-stimulating hormone (FSH), and luteinizing hormone (LH).

C. Caloric intake.

D. All of the above.

85. You have been caring for a patient with osteomyelitis. In preparing the patient for discharge, you include teaching about:

A. The importance of multiple-week treatment with antibiotics.

B. The side effects and interactions of the medications.

C. Symptoms that necessitate a call to the physician, nurse practitioner, or physician assistant.

D. All of the above.

86. Mary asks how the pulmonary function test ordered by her physician is performed. You respond by saying:

A. You breathe into a spirometer to measure your lung capacity.

B. You breathe through a mouthpiece into a spirometer until all air in your lungs is expelled; then you take a deep breath through the mouthpiece. This is done three times and a computer calculates the capacity of your lungs.

C. A computer is used to measure your volume and vital capacity.

D. A tube is inserted into your lungs while you are asleep to expand your lungs to their full capacity.

87. Mary tells you that she has an undiagnosed case of hypothyroidism. What symptoms would you expect her to present?

A. Polydipsia and polyphagia.

B. Fatigue and cold intolerance.

C. Weight loss and hyperglycemia.

D. Tachycardia and diarrhea.

88. It is important to teach a patient who is receiving immunosuppressive therapy for a bone marrow transplant to:

A. Avoid other people with signs of infection.

B. Report signs of infection, such as sore throat or fever.

C. Take the medications as directed.

D. All of the above.

89. The first priority to care for the patient with a new fracture includes assessing:

    A. Respiratory rate and effort, as well as pulse.
    B. The fracture site for bleeding.
    C. For signs of infection at the wound site of an open fracture.
    D. For circulation and sensation distal to the fracture site.

90. Mary has been dieting and exercising daily. Her weight is well below the recommended minimum for her height. Assessment for Mary would include looking for:

    A. Ecchymosis and extraocular movements.
    B. Temporal wasting and irregular heart rhythm.
    C. Peripheral edema and rales.
    D. Periorbital edema and chorea.

91. Patients with pernicious anemia are treated with:

    A. Oral iron.
    B. Oral folic acid.
    C. Parenteral vitamin B_{12}.
    D. Oral prednisone.

92. Mary presents difficulty breathing, fatigue, orthopnea, and palpitation, and is diagnosed as having aortic insufficiency. After undergoing aortic valve repair, what medication would you expect her physician to prescribe?

    A. Ativan.
    B. Haldol.
    C. Heparin.
    D. Thorazine.

93. A patient with a history of asthma is scheduled for an appendectomy. Because of her asthma, you would include as part of the preoperative teaching the need to perform postoperatively:

    A. Coughing and deep breathing exercises.
    B. Leg exercises.
    C. Wound dressing changes.
    D. All of these.

94. When staging a pressure ulcer, you correctly recognize a stage II ulcer as:

    A. Redness, with no break in the skin.
    B. Shallow ulcer with red base.
    C. Dermis involvement with eschar.
    D. Bone visible with no drainage.

95. **Sue has a mild dermatitis rash and asks for advice. You respond by saying:**
    A. Wash the area with an antiseptic soap frequently to keep the area clean.
    B. Use an antifungal ointment.
    C. Use talcum powder to soothe the inflamed skin.
    D. Use a mild steroidal cream.

96. **What cell ingests invading or foreign cells?**
    A. Macrophage.
    B. T cell.
    C. B cell.
    D. Erythrocyte.

97. **Patients with rheumatoid arthritis typically have pain:**
    A. With activity.
    B. Only upon awakening.
    C. Late in the evening.
    D. All day without remission.

98. **Instructions for a patient at risk for testicular cancer include:**
    A. Restrict potassium, phosphate, sodium, protein in diet.
    B. Self-catheterization of ileal reservoir.
    C. Testicular self-exam.
    D. Change in color of urine is to be expected.

99. **The joints most commonly involved with rheumatoid arthritis include the:**
    A. Spine, from the sacrum to the cervical spine.
    B. Symmetrical involvement of major joints.
    C. Small joints of hands and feet.
    D. Slightly movable joints of the axial skeleton.

100. **John presents with bronchitis. He thinks that he might have chronic bronchitis and asks you to explain the difference between them. You respond by saying:**
    A. Acute bronchitis lasts for 3 consecutive months and is reversible.
    B. Acute bronchitis lasts 7 to 10 days.
    C. Chronic bronchitis lasts 3 consecutive months in 2 consecutive years. This results in a blockage of the airways which cannot be reversed. Acute bronchitis is caused by a viral or bacterial infection and lasts about 10 days. Blockage of the airways is reversible in acute bronchitis.
    D. I will ask your physician to explain the differences during his rounds.

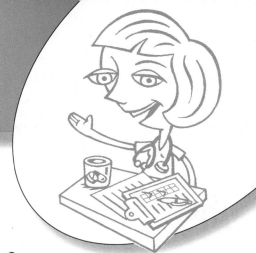

Answers to Review Questions and Final Exam Questions

Chapter 1
1. b
2. a
3. d
4. b
5. b
6. a
7. a
8. d
9. a
10. b

Chapter 2
1. c
2. c
3. b
4. a

5. b
6. c
7. a
8. b
9. a
10. c

Chapter 3
1. c
2. b
3. d
4. c
5. d
6. a
7. c
8. a
9. c
10. b

Chapter 4
1. b
2. c
3. a
4. a
5. a
6. b
7. c
8. a
9. d
10. c

Chapter 5
1. c
2. a
3. a
4. d

5. b
6. a
7. b
8. b
9. a
10. c

Chapter 6

1. b
2. a
3. a
4. d
5. d
6. b
7. a
8. c
9. d
10. a

Chapter 7

1. c
2. a
3. b
4. b
5. d
6. a
7. b
8. a
9. d
10. c

Chapter 8

1. c
2. a
3. a
4. d
5. d
6. b
7. d

8. a
9. a
10. a

Chapter 9

1. d
2. c
3. d
4. b
5. b
6. a
7. a
8. c
9. c
10. a

Chapter 10

1. d
2. a
3. b
4. b
5. b
6. c
7. d
8. d
9. a
10. c

Chapter 11

1. b
2. d
3. c
4. a
5. b
6. b
7. c
8. c
9. a
10. d

Chapter 12

1. d
2. b
3. c
4. a
5. c
6. d
7. b
8. b
9. b
10. d

Chapter 13

1. b
2. a
3. c
4. d
5. d
6. a
7. b
8. b
9. b
10. c

Chapter 14

1. c
2. b
3. a
4. d
5. b
6. c
7. a
8. a
9. d
10. a

Chapter 15

1. c
2. c

3. c
4. a
5. b
6. d
7. a
8. a
9. d
10. a

Chapter 16

1. b
2. d

3. c
4. a
5. d
6. a
7. b
8. b
9. b
10. c

Chapter 17

1. b
2. b

3. a
4. b
5. b
6. b
7. d
8. d
9. b
10. d

Final Exam

1. a	35. c	69. b
2. d	36. a	70. d
3. d	37. d	71. a
4. a	38. b	72. b
5. b	39. b	73. b
6. b	40. c	74. c
7. b	41. c	75. b
8. c	42. c	76. d
9. b	43. b	77. c
10. d	44. d	78. c
11. a	45. b	79. d
12. c	46. a	80. c
13. a	47. c	81. b
14. d	48. a	82. c
15. a	49. b	83. b
16. b	50. d	84. d
17. a	51. d	85. d
18. a	52. d	86. b
19. a	53. c	87. b
20. b	54. c	88. d
21. b	55. d	89. a
22. c	56. a	90. b
23. c	57. d	91. c
24. c	58. b	92. c
25. c	59. a	93. a
26. a	60. c	94. b
27. a	61. b	95. d
28. d	62. d	96. a
29. d	63. d	97. a
30. b	64. b	98. d
31. c	65. b	99. c
32. c	66. d	100. c
33. d	67. c	
34. c	68. b	

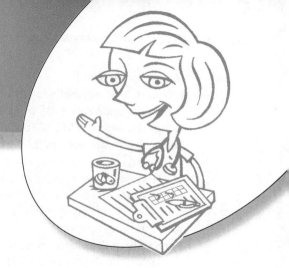

Glossary

Chapter 1

ABG: A test that measures the arterial blood gas.

ANA complement: Antinuclear antibody test that measures the amount of autoimmune antibodies.

Antecubital fossa: Triangular cavity of the elbow joint.

AST/ALT: Enzymes released by liver tissue when the liver is damaged. Their levels are used as a measure of liver function.

BNP: A test that measures the presence and severity of heart failure.

Bradycardia: A heart rate lower than 60 beats per minute.

Cardiac troponin levels: A troponin test checks for elevated levels of those proteins which are released when there is damage to the heart or skeletal muscle.

Cardiomyopathy: A disease of the heart muscle.

Complete Blood Count (CBC): A test used to determine the general health of the patient.

CK isoenzymes: Enzymes released if there is damage to the heart muscle.

CK-MB: An enzyme released by damaged cardiac tissue 2 to 6 hours following an infarction.

Creatine kinase (CK): Enzyme released if there is damage to the heart muscle.

Creatinine: A waste product from protein metabolism and muscle that is removed by the kidneys in urine. Creatinine is tested to determine kidney function.

CXR: Chest x-ray.

DVT: Deep vein thrombosis.

Endocarditis antibiotic prophylaxis: Antibiotic given to prevent a bacterial infection.

Erythrocyte sedimentation rate (ESR): See sed rate.

Fowler's position: A position where the client is semi-sitting with knees flexed.

Guaiac: A test to locate hidden (occult) blood in stool.

HTN: Hypertension.

Hypoxia: Decreased oxygen to tissues.

IM: Intramuscular.

International normalized ratio (INR): A medical blood test used to determine the coagulation capability of a patient's blood.

Ischemia: Reduced blood flow due to an obstructed vessel.

Lactate dehydrogenase (LDH): Enzymes released when there is tissue damage in the heart, liver, kidney, skeletal muscle, or lungs.

LDH isoenzymes: A test to check the level of lactate dehydrogenase in the blood.

Myoglobin: A protein in the heart and skeletal muscles. A rising level of myoglobin is an early indication of a myocardial infarction.

NPO: Nothing by mouth.

Partial thromboplastin time (PTT): A medical blood test used to measure the coagulation capability of a patient's blood.

Percutaneous coronary intervention (PCI): Commonly referred to as angioplasty where the diameter of a narrow blood vessel is increased.

Prothrombin time (PT): A medical blood test used to determine the coagulant capability of the patient's blood.

PT/PTT/INR: Tests that help detect and diagnose bleeding disorders. Also it used to determine the effectiveness of anticoagulants.

RA: Rheumatoid arthritis.

Radiopaque dye: Makes structures visible on x-rays.

Sed rate: The rate at which red blood cells settle in a test tube. A high rate indicates inflammation.

Troponins: Proteins in cardiac and skeletal muscles.

Chapter 2

Alpha$_1$-antitrypsin deficiency: A lack of a liver protein that leads to emphysema and liver disease.

Beta$_2$-agonist: A bronchodilator that relaxes muscles around the airway thereby opening the airway during an asthma attack or in COPD.

Cardiac glycoside: Medication that improves cardiac output and reduces distention of the heart.

Caseous granulomas: Destructive tissue that enters the bronchus causing tuberculous bronchopneumonia.

Chronic obstructive pulmonary disease (COPD): A lung disease where excess mucus in the airways interferes with gas exchange in the lungs resulting in frequent coughing.

Computed tomography (CT) scan: A three-dimensional image of the body structure created from a series of cross-sectional images of the patient.

D-dimer: A blood test to diagnose conditions that cause hypercoagulability, a tendency to produce inappropriate blood clots.

Eosinophils: White blood cells that respond to allergic diseases, parasitic infections, and other disorders.

Exudate: Fluid from the circulatory system that enters into areas of inflammation.

FEV$_1$: A measurement of the volume of air exhaled in the first second.

Ghon's complex: Infection caused by *Mycobacterium tuberculosis* that usually results in primary tuberculosis.

Granulomatous: Inflamed granulation tissue associated with ulcerated infections.

Helical CT scan: Computed tomography scan produced by a scanner with a continuously rotating gantry. This innovation enabled a very quick scan time.

Histamine: A substance that is released from mast cells that causes itching, sneezing, and nasal congestion related to an allergic reaction.

Incentive spirometer: A device that improves the functioning of lungs by exercising breathing muscles. It is used to prevent development of pneumonia following surgery.

Indurated area: A raised thick or hardening area.

Induration: The process of becoming extremely firm or hard.

Leukotrienes: A substance, released by mast cells during an allergic reaction, constricts the bronchial passages in an asthma attack.

Mast cells: These are cells that make and release histamine during an allergic reaction.

Mediastinum: The middle section of the chest cavity.

Pulmonary function test (PFT): A test that measures how well the lungs take in and exhale air and how efficiently they transfer oxygen into the blood.

Postural drainage: The patient is positioned with the head lower than the chest allowing gravity to clear secretions from the lungs.

Prostaglandins: A hormone-like substance that dilates and constricts blood vessels as well as contracts and relaxes smooth muscles during an immune response.

Serous fluid: Pale yellow and transparent body fluid.

Chapter 3

Bamboo spine: Spinal fusion gives a bamboo-like appearance on an x-ray.

Buccal mucosa: Inner lining of the cheeks and lips.

CMV: Herpes virus found in healthy individuals without causing symptoms.

Coagulopathies: A defect in the body's blood-clotting mechanism.

IgM antibody: The first immunoglobulin antibody made in response to an infection.

Lymphadenopathy: Disease of the lymph nodes.

NSAID: A medication that is anti-inflammatory and pain killer such as ibuprofen.

ROM: Range of motion.

Sicca complex: Dryness of mucous membranes in the absence of connective tissue disease.

Synovial: A cavity filled with synovial fluid.

Chapter 4

Ataxia: Loss of muscle coordination.

Bilirubin: A substance, part of bile, is formed when red blood cells (RBCs) are broken down.

DDAVP: Medication that mimics the action of an antidiuretic hormone.

Demyelination: The loss or breakdown of myelin, which is the protective coating on nerve cells.

Erythropoiesis: Formation of RBCs.

Mean corpuscular hemoglobin (MCH): The amount of oxygen-carrying hemoglobin inside RBCs.

Mean corpuscular volume (MCV): The average size of RBCs.

Myeloid: Relating to bone marrow.

Parenteral: Any type of injectable medication.

Parietal cells: Stomach cells that produce hydrochloric acid.

Petechiae: Small red, purple, or brown spots on the skin or mucosa.

Proprioception: Subconscious awareness of position, posture, movement, and changes in equilibrium.

Red cell distribution width (RDW): A calculation of various sizes of RBCs.

Reagent: Substance used to produce a chemical reaction.

Reticulocytes: Immature RBCs without a nucleus that are normally found in the circulation.

Romberg test: A neurologic test to detect poor balance.

Shilling test: Determines vitamin B_{12} deficiency.

Chapter 5

ADL: Activities of daily living.

Afferent: Nerve signals that travel from the peripheral nervous system to the central nervous system.

Aphasia: Unable to speak, write, and/or understand due to brain damage.

Arachnoid mater: The middle portion of the meninges that encloses the brain and spinal cord.

Bi-level positive airway pressure (BiPAP): Device used to provide oxygen to a person who has sleep apnea.

Continuous positive airway pressure (CPAP): Device used to provide oxygen to a person who has sleep apnea.

Diabetes insipidus: A condition characterized by excessive thirst and increased urination.

Efferent: Nerve signals that travel from the central nervous system to the peripheral nervous system.

Lumen: The hollow area of a tube.

NG: Nasal gastric.

Nystagmus: Rapid involuntary eye movement.

Petechial: Small purple spot caused by a hemorrhage.

Pia mater: The inner portion of the meninges that encloses the brain and spinal cord.

Postictal stage: The final stage of an epileptic seizure in which the patient gradually recovers. It is also known as ictal.

Stenosis: Abnormal narrowing of a passage.

Vagal: Related to the vagus nerve.

Chapter 6

C-reactive protein (CRP): Increases during the inflammatory process and is part of an early defense system against infections.

Haversian canals: Tubes around the channels in the region of a bone called compact bone.

Uricosuric agent: Medication that increases the excretion of uric acid.

Chapter 7

A & D ointment: All purposes skin protection ointment.

ALT: Serum glutamic-pyruvic transaminase is an enzyme that is elevated in liver disease.

AST: Serum glutamic-oxaloacetic transaminase is an enzyme that is elevated in liver disease.

Cast: A cylindrically shaped aggregation of some particulate in the urine. There are several different types, such as hyaline casts, red blood casts, etc.

Colostomy: An opening into the colon usually from outside the body.

Encephalopathy: A degenerative brain disease.

Fecalith: Hard mass of fecal matter.

Fistulas: Abnormal connection between vessels or organs that normally do not connect.

Glomerulonephritis: Inflammation of the kidney.

HAV: Hepatitis A.

HBeAg: A test that measures hepatitis B antigen.

HBsAg: A test that measures hepatitis B surface antigen.

HBV: Hepatitis B.

HCV: Hepatitis C.

HDV: Hepatitis D.

Hepatocellular: Liver cells.

IgM: A class of immunoglobulin involved in fighting blood infections.

IgG: A class of immunoglobulin that is the most common serum antibody. It is passed from mother to fetus.

Manometry: Measures pressure of the rectum and anus muscles.

Polyarteritis nodosa: Inflammation of the arteries caused by an autoimmune disease.

Polycast: Presence of many casts in the urine.

RIBA-2: Recombinant immunoblot assay.

Septicemia: Blood poisoning.

Chapter 8

Dysmetabolic syndrome: Abnormalities in serum insulin/glucose levels.
Ectopic: Tissue growing in an unusual location.

Chapter 9

Cryptorchism: Absence of one or both testes from the scrotum.
Hematuria: Blood in urine.
Hydronephrosis: Enlarged kidney resulting from urine accumulation in the upper urinary tract caused by a blockage of the urinary tract.
Median sulcus: Shallow midline groove.
Stoma: A surgical opening in the abdominal wall.

Chapter 10

Atopic: Predisposition to allergies.
Radioallergosorbent test (RAST): A test used to measure allergic reactions in the blood.

Chapter 11

Ketones: By-product of fat metabolism.
mEq/L: Milliequivalents per liter.
mOsm/L: Osmolarity per liter.
Paresthesia: Numbness, prickly sensation or tingling of the skin.
Rhabdomyolysis: Degeneration of skeletal muscle.
SLE: Systemic lupus erythematosus.

Chapter 12

Caries: Tooth decay.
Ecchymosis: Bruise.
Hypoxia: Oxygen reduction.
NMDA: Receptors in the brain.

Chapter 13

Asepsis: Without infection.
Atelectasis: Collapse of part or the entire lung.
Chemoreceptor trigger zone: This is the part of the brain responsible for nausea.

Cholecystectomy: Surgical removal of the gallbladder.

Laparoscopic: A surgical procedure performed through small incisions in the abdominal wall using a camera transmitting images to a video monitor.

Paralytic ileus: Movement loss in the small intestine.

Stridor: High-pitched respiratory sound usually occurring in inspiration.

Chapter 14

Adnexal: An appendage of an organ.

Beta hCG: A fragment of the human chorionic gonadotropin (hCG) complex used to determine pregnancy.

Brain hormone (BH): Hormone that causes stimulation of growth.

CA-125: A cancer marker for ovarian cancer.

Dyspareunia: Painful intercourse.

Dysplasia: Noncancerous abnormal cells.

I&O: Intake and output of fluids.

Laparoscopically: A surgical procedure, using a camera transmitting images to a video monitor, performed through small incisions in the abdominal wall.

Myomectomy: A surgical procedure to remove fibroids from the uterus.

MMR: Measles, mumps, and rubella vaccine.

Nulliparity: Never pregnant.

Peritonitis: Inflammation of the peritoneum.

RhoGAM: Rh immunoglobulin prevents an Rh-negative mother's antibodies from attacking the fetus's Rh-positive cells.

Rapid plasma reagin test (RPR): A new test to diagnose syphilis.

Salpingitis: Inflammation of the fallopian tubes.

Venereal disease reference laboratory (VDRL): Older test to diagnose syphilis.

Chapter 15

Adjuvant modalities: Additional methods of treatments given in addition to the primary treatment.

Epistaxis: Nosebleed.

Chapter 16

Bradykinesia: A lack of spontaneous movement or movement that is slow.

Dysphagia: Inability to swallow or difficulty in swallowing.

Dyspnea: Difficult or labored breathing.

Immune senescence: Gradual loss of immune function often associated with aging.

Myelofibrosis: Disorder where bone marrow is replaced by fibrous, scar tissue, disrupting normal production of blood cells.

Myelopathy: Spinal cord dysfunction.
Normal decline: A process by which the capacity for cell division, growth, and function is reduced over time.
Polypharmacy: Use of multiple medications by a patient.
Pharmacodynamics: Effects of drugs on the body and their mechanism of action.
Pharmacokinetics: Movement of drugs within the body.
Polycythemia vera: An abnormal increase in blood cells, primarily RBCs.
Thrombocythemia: The overproduction of platelets in the blood.

Chapter 17

Abuse: Overindulgence in or dependence on an addictive substance, especially alcohol or drugs.
Addiction: A primary, chronic disease of brain reward, motivation, memory and related circuitry characterized by inability to consistently abstain, impairment in behavioral control, craving, diminished recognition of significant problems with one's behaviors and interpersonal relationships, and a dysfunctional emotional response.
Blood alcohol level: The concentration of alcohol detected in a blood sample.
Cravings: A powerful desire for a substance.
Delirium tremens (DT): A psychotic condition typical of withdrawal in chronic alcoholics, involving tremors, hallucinations, anxiety, and disorientation.
Dependency: The state of needing a certain drug in order to function normally.
Detoxification: The process of reducing a substance level in the body.
Hallucinogen: A drug that causes hallucinations.
Narcotics Anonymous (NA): A nonprofit fellowship or society of men and women for whom drugs had become a major problem and who seek to abstaining from drugs.
Neural transmission: A chemical released from a neuron that stimulates another neuron.
Physical dependency: A physical condition caused by chronic use of a tolerance forming drug, in which abrupt or gradual drug withdrawal causes unpleasant physical symptoms.
Psychological dependency: A form of dependence that involves emotional-motivational withdrawal symptoms upon cessation of drug use.
Recovery: A commitment to being totally abstinent from the substance.
Substance dependency: An adaptive state that develops from repeated drug administration, and which results in withdrawal upon cessation of drug use.
Tolerance: A reduced reaction to a drug following its repeated use.
Triggers: Any form of stimuli that initiate the desire to engage in addictive behavior.
Withdrawal: The group of symptoms that occur upon the abrupt discontinuation or decrease in intake of drugs.

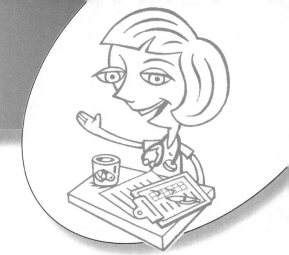

Index